Medical Coding Evaluation and Management

Medical Coding Evaluation and Management

Kate Gabriel-Jones
CPC, CGSC

Larry Bohn
Ph.D., OSCS(SW) USN Ret.

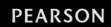

Boston   Columbus   Indianapolis   New York   San Francisco   Upper Saddle River
Amsterdam   Cape Town   Dubai   London   Madrid   Milan   Munich   Paris   Montreal   Toronto
Delhi   Mexico City   São Paulo   Sydney   Hong Kong   Seoul   Singapore   Taipei   Tokyo

Editor in Chief: Marlene Pratt
Executive Acquisition Editor: Joan Gill
Editorial Project Manager: Bronwen Glowacki
Editorial Assistant: Stephanie Kiel
Director of Marketing: David Gessell
Production Project Manager: Debbie Ryan
Cover Designer: Suzanne Behnke
Art Director: Jayne Conte

Interior Designer: Christopher Weigand
Cover Image: Shutterstock
Full-Service Project Management: Mohinder Singh/ Aptara®, Inc.
Composition: Aptara®, Inc.
Printer/Binder: Courier/Kendallville
Cover Printer: Lehigh-Phoenix Color/Hagerstown
Text Font: Plantin Std Regular 9/11

Credits and acknowledgments borrowed from other sources and reproduced, with permission, in this textbook appear on the appropriate page within text.

Microsoft® and Windows® are registered trademarks of the Microsoft Corporation in the U.S.A. and other countries. Screen shots and icons reprinted with permission from the Microsoft Corporation. This book is not sponsored or endorsed by or affiliated with the Microsoft Corporation.

Many of the designations by manufacturers and sellers to distinguish their products are claimed as trademarks. Where those designations appear in this book, and the publisher was aware of a trademark claim, the designations have been printed in initial caps or all caps.

Library of Congress Cataloging-in-Publication Data

Gabriel-Jones, Kate.
   Medical coding evaluation and management / Kate Gabriel-Jones, Larry Bohn.
      pages cm
   ISBN-13: 978-0-13-288156-2
   ISBN-10: 0-13-288156-X
   1. Nosology—Code numbers.   2. Medicine—Nomenclature—Code numbers.   I. Bohn, Larry.   II. Title.
   RB115.G33 2014
   616.001'2—dc23
                                                                                        2012036299

10 9 8 7 6 5 4 3 2 1

PEARSON

ISBN-10:   0-13-288156-X
ISBN-13: 978-0-13-288156-2

DEDICATION

KATE GABRIEL-JONES

This text is dedicated to . . .

- my wonderful husband of 21 years, Seth, and our beautiful teenage daughter, Rhiannon, who have both encouraged me during the process of writing this text
- the many physicians and clinicians who work tirelessly, providing care and comfort for patients every day
- every professional medical coder and every nonclinical healthcare staff member who provides professional support for the physicians and clinicians
- every patient who shares his or her own story of health with a physician or clinician

LARRY BOHN

This text is dedicated to my beautiful wife of 32 years, Margaret, and my children—Nathan, Joshua, Katie, Zack, Stephen, and Andrew.

BRIEF CONTENTS

CONTENTS

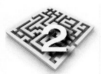

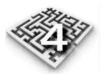

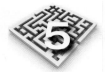

Overall History Level 52

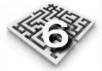

Physical Examination—1995 Documentation Guidelines 61

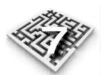

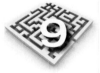

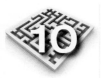

Medical Decision Making: Amount and/or Complexity of Data to Be Reviewed   131

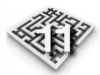

Medical Decision Making: Risk of Complication, Comorbidity, or Mortality   143

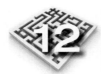
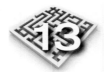

SECTION II UNDERSTANDING EVALUATION AND MANAGEMENT CODING

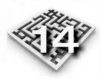

Categories Requiring Content of Service 183

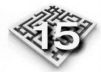

Categories Requiring More Than Content of Service 204

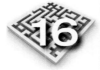

Prolonged Services, Newborn Care, and Critical Care   221

Evaluation and Management Modifiers   238

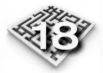

Evaluation and Management: Resources and Summary 250

The foundation of this text is two documents and a manual that have been the source of nearly all rules, requirements, and standards for evaluation and management coding: "1995 Documentation Guidelines for Evaluation and Management Services," "1997 Documentation Guidelines for Evaluation and Management Services," and the *Current Procedural Terminology* (CPT) manual published by the AMA.

Although written in 1995 and 1997, the Documentation Guidelines provide extensive direction for the performing physician's documentation of the evaluation and management service visit. On the whole, the 1995 and 1997 documents present redundant guidelines for almost all elements of the content of service *except* for the requirements for the physical examination. In this one regard, the two documents present extremely different guidelines and requirements. As a result, this text devotes three chapters to the physical examination. Chapter 6 introduces the physical examination performed during an evaluation and management service visit and also analyzes the more general documentation requirements identified in the 1995 Documentation Guidelines. Chapters 7 and 8 present much more detailed explorations of the rigorous documentation requirements for the physical examinations identified in the 1997 Documentation Guidelines, which demand a greater understanding of human anatomy and physiology. Chapters 7 and 8 build on the information presented in Chapter 6, while addressing the nuances inherent in the 1997 guidelines.

Although the CPT manual provides specific guidelines and requirements for each category of evaluation and management service, it utilizes the documentation requirements identified in the 1995 and 1997 Documentation Guidelines. Repeatedly, these two documents have set the standard for the physician's documentation of the evaluation and management service visit. Unfortunately, however, the content of these essential documents is rarely introduced to new coders, and without this knowledge, the requirements for documenting the content of service remain elusive and intimidating. On the other hand, medical coders with a broader understanding of the guidelines and the service components can approach the category requirements with confidence.

Given the scrutiny under which healthcare now operates, medical coders must approach their work both informed and empowered. More than ever, it is important for medical coders to be able to think critically as they read physician documentation and query the physicians, nurse practitioners, and other clinicians as needed. In a manner reminiscent of the axiom "Knowledge is power," well-informed, knowledgeable medical coders can step into evaluation and management coding with the understanding needed to code appropriately and also advocate for themselves, the physicians with whom they work, and the healthcare organizations in which they operate.

This text has been written for anyone in the medical field who is unfamiliar with the documentation guidelines for evaluation and management services, as well as the related coding. An understanding of basic anatomy is expected; however, the text is intended for new coders with little experience, as well as established coders with more experience. Some of the material has been inspired by interchanges with physicians for whom I have had the honor of providing education about the 1995 and 1997 Documentation Guidelines, whereas other parts of the material have been informed by my encounters with new coding students. Every part of this text has been designed to inform and empower anyone who deals with evaluation and management services.

The scheme of the text is intended to inspire critical thinking on the part of the reader. Evaluation and management services are medical visits between a patient and a performing physician during which therapeutic or diagnostic services are provided by the physician. These services are divided into separately identified categories, each of which represents one of the different places in which an evaluation and management service may occur. Specific guidelines for each category inform the selection of the appropriate evaluation and management service code. For many readers, this will be the first introduction to evaluation and management coding, and as with a well-designed building, the stronger the foundation, the longer the building can last. Therefore, this text builds on the strength inherent in the evaluation and management guidelines, allowing the reader to develop an understanding of service documentation before delving into the specific category guidelines. This text also presents a variety of challenging exercises requiring the reader to build on cumulative knowledge of evaluation and management services. From this evolving position of strength, the reader is empowered to not only discern the evaluation and management documentation, but also approach the specific category guidelines with strong critical-thinking skills.

THE ORGANIZATION OF THIS TEXT

Nearly half of the evaluation and management categories require documentation of the content of service by the physician who has performed the service. The content of service refers to the history, physical examination, and medical decision making performed by the physician; and each component reflects a different aspect of the performed service. These key components of the content of service are each composed of several different elements, each of which stands as an important part of the documented evaluation and management service.

The first 13 chapters of this text focus on an exploration of the key components of evaluation and management. Even though some of the components may seem similar, each one stands apart and provides a unique glimpse into the documented performance of the evaluation and management service. Understanding the differences among these elements offers important skills for the reader and encourages critical thinking in reading the documentation of an evaluation and management service visit.

Given the importance of distinguishing among these elements in medical documentation, the first 12 chapters use excerpts of evaluation and management documentation to encourage discernment and understanding of each element. These chapters provide the building blocks for evaluation and management documentation. With this strong foundation of the content of service, the related service categories become less intimidating, the guidelines become more understandable, and the coder becomes more confident. For greater comprehension and easy review, all of the content of service elements are presented in a compiled worksheet in Appendix D, whereas Appendix C shows how these elements function together in the E/M medical documentation.

To minimize confusion, one evaluation and management scenario is repeated throughout the first 13 chapters: the documentation of service for a patient named Johnny, who has an irritating cough. Although the basic premise of the clinical scenario remains the same, the content of the service provided changes throughout the 13 chapters to provide challenging hands-on experience with each element of the content of service. Every presentation of the clinical scenario in the examples and exercises requires careful consideration and thought on the reader's part. This approach provides greater educational opportunities without the distraction of extensive clinical variation and supports continuity throughout these 13 chapters.

With this strong understanding of the content of service, the reader can then explore the evaluation and management categories. Chapters 14 through 18 employ a variety of coding exercises that challenge the reader, build on the reader's developing knowledge, and require careful critical thinking in reviewing the evaluation and management categories. The categories of evaluation and management service that require the key components are explored, even as the different requirements of other categories are examined.

FEATURES OF THIS TEXT

Chapter Objectives Each chapter begins with a list of specific learning objectives that state what students will achieve upon successful completion of the chapter.

Key Terms and Abbreviations Terms and their definitions appear at the beginning of each chapter, as well as in the narrative and comprehensive glossary.

Introduction A brief introduction at the beginning of each chapter highlights the concepts presented in the chapter.

Examples Medical documentation examples are provided to elucidate various concepts and inform the reader about important aspects of evaluation and management service coding. Throughout the chapters that specifically address the content of service, one basic clinical scenario is utilized—"Johnny's Irritating Cough." The specific content of this medical documentation changes from example to example, depending on the material being presented. When simpler concepts are introduced, "Johnny's Irritating Cough" presents less complicated documentation for the reader to review. Contrarily, when more challenging concepts are addressed, the medical documentation for "Johnny's Irritating Cough" becomes more complex. As a result, these examples become multifaceted illustrations that the reader can not only read and review, but reference during a developing career in medical coding.

Exercises Exercises in each chapter are designed to stimulate detailed critical thinking on the part of the reader. However, throughout the text, different exercises require different mental exertion, depending on the material being covered. The exercise for Chapter 1 exposes readers to medical documentation of an evaluation and management visit, especially important since the majority of readers have had little experience with medical documentation of an evaluation and management service. In Chapters 2–13, the exercises follow the developing understanding of the elements of the content of service, whereas the exercises in Chapters 14–18 challenge readers to utilize prior and new material when reviewing the categories of evaluation and management services.

Figures and Tables Tables and illustrations appear throughout the text to summarize, clarify, and reinforce key topics.

Summary   Each chapter ends with a bulleted list of summary points, which correlate to each of the chapter learning objectives presented at the beginning of the chapter.

Chapter Review   Each chapter ends with multiple-choice questions, including medical documentation exercises, to assess student understanding of the concepts presented in the chapter.

Case Study   Every chapter contains at least one case study for the reader to review at the conclusion of the chapter. Each case study is designed to challenge the reader's retention of the material, while inspiring confidence in the reader's understanding of the presented material. To this end, some of the case studies may be similar from chapter to chapter in order to reinforce the differences among related concepts, such as those in the chapters dedicated to the three distinct elements of history. Since the information presented in the chapters is cumulative, the case studies reflect and challenge the reader's developing knowledge.

Coding Challenge   At the end of Chapters 14–17, coding exercises are included to help the reader understand and identify both the specific evaluation and management category *and* the specific evaluation and management CPT code. Each question in the coding challenge requires the reader to utilize all of the textual material in order to ascertain the appropriate CPT category and code. Each coding challenge is presented in the form of a documented evaluation and management service visit, requiring the reader to utilize comprehensive knowledge of anatomy, content of service, and the clinical setting, as well as critical thinking skills, in order to identify the particular code and/or modifier that best reflects the documented evaluation and management service.

ABOUT THE AUTHORS

Larry Bohn, OSCS (SW) USN Ret., PhD, EMBA, retired as a Senior Chief Petty Officer in the United States Navy after 21 years of service and has over 30 years of experience in developing and delivering training in the academic, corporate, and government arenas. He has taught in community college, university, and seminary settings, both face-to-face and online.

Kate Gabriel-Jones, CPC, CGSC, has taught at multiple levels over the past 20 years—preschool, high school English, and online college courses. In her career as a certified professional coder and certified general surgery coder, her skill with language has helped her design and implement clinical documentation improvement programs, as well as advocate on behalf of medical coders, clinicians, and support staff for the importance of clinical documentation.

SUPPLEMENTS PACKAGE

For the Student

- *Companion Website for Medical Coding Evaluation and Management* includes the Coder's Index, a link to a trial encoder, active web links to Coder's Toolbox resources, any code updates, and activities such as Terminology Games, Fill in the Blanks, Matching and Multiple Choice questions.
- **Access your free trail of Pearson's SpeedECoder at http://sec.pearsonhigered.com.**

For the Instructor

- MyTest
- PowerPoint Lecture Notes
- Instructor's Resource Manual (download only)

ACKNOWLEDGMENTS

I, Kate, wish to thank Larry Bohn for the many hours he spent listening to me extol the nuances of evaluation and management documentation and for introducing the idea of this text to Pearson Education. Many sincere thanks go also to Elizabeth Glover for the many hours she devoted to proofreading the content of service material—you helped to keep me grounded during this process, Elizabeth! And to Sylvia S. Spragg, I cannot extend enough thanks for your support and for being the mentor I've always dreamed of. In addition, I extend humble and extensive gratitude to my development editor, Alexis Breen Ferraro, for her assiduous support and encouragement and her remarkable editorial skills, which have helped to bring this text to fruition.

REVIEWERS

The publisher and authors would like to thank the following reviewers for their valuable feedback:

Lori Bentley, RMA, CMRS
Allied Health Instructor
Remington College, TN

Kelly Berge, MSHA, CPC, CBCS
Medical Instructor
Dover College, NJ

Cindi Brassington, MS, CMA
Professor of Allied Health Quinebaug Valley
Community College, CT

Linda H. Donahue, AS, RHIT, CCS, CCS-P, CPC
Assistant Professor, Health Information Technology/Medical Coding
Delgado Community College, LA

Michelle Edwards, AA, CCP, CMRS, CPMB
Medical Billing and Coding Lead Instructor
University of Antelope Valley, CA

Missy Hamilton, MBA, RHIT
Assistant Professor, Program Director, Health Information Management
Zane State College, OH

Susan Holler, MSEd, CMRS
Allied Health Faculty
Bryant and Stratton College, NY

Deborah McGichen, BS
Medical Coding Instructor
Allstate Career, MD

Norma Mercado, MAHS, RHIA
Department Chair, Professor
Health Information Technology
Austin Community College, TX

Trasey Pfluger, MA, CMAA, CBCS, NCICS
Program Director
Health Information Technology
Fortis College, FL

Amy Semenchuk, RN, BSN
Rockford Career College
Roscoe, IL

Julia Steff, RHIA, CCS, CCS-P
Assistant Professor, Department Chair
Health Information Technology
Palm Beach State College, FL

Medical Coding Evaluation and Management

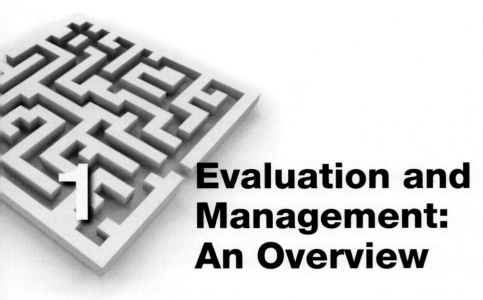

Evaluation and Management: An Overview

Learning Objectives

After completing this chapter, you should be able to do the following:

- Spell and define the key terms and abbreviations presented in this chapter
- Identify the importance and challenges of medical documentation
- Define *evaluation* and *management* in the context of healthcare
- Identify the importance of documentation guidelines for evaluation and management (E/M) visits
- List the six constituent elements that comprise the format of every E/M service

Key Terms

American Medical Association (AMA)

assisted living facility

category

Centers for Medicare and Medicaid Services (CMS)

clinician

content of service

Current Procedural Terminology (CPT)

Documentation Guidelines (DGs)

established patient

evaluation

healthcare

history

inpatient hospital

management

medical decision making

medical documentation

nature of the presenting problem

new patient

outpatient

physical examination

place of service

subcategory

type of service

Abbreviations

AMA American Medical Association

CMS Centers for Medicare and Medicaid Services

CPT *Current Procedural Terminology*

DGs Documentation Guidelines

E/M evaluation and management

INTRODUCTION

Nearly every person has some experience with a doctor's visit. This foundational experience occurs around the world, whether a child is seen by the family physician for a persistent cough, an adult is brought to an emergency department after an automobile accident, or the evening news shows a physician examining patients in a refugee camp. Regardless of the situation, a doctor's visit represents a specific kind of healthcare: a physician spends time with an individual patient in order to provide medical, professional, or other healthcare services specifically for that individual. A patient's **healthcare** is a little bit like a story; there is a beginning, middle, and end to each clinical encounter. In the beginning, the patient feels unwell and goes to the doctor. The middle of the story occurs when the doctor, with the patient's involvement and help, evaluates the patient's condition and assesses the patient's health. The end of the story occurs when the doctor identifies and treats the condition in order to bring relief and health back to the patient. Once this particular condition resolves, this specific chapter of the patient's healthcare story might end; however, the patient's entire story of health will continue on. Every evaluation and management service represents another portion of the patient's story of health and is recorded in the patient's medical documentation by the physician or other healthcare professionals who have provided the service.

WHAT IS MEDICAL DOCUMENTATION?

Many people have heard the phrase "A picture is worth a thousand words." In healthcare, words form the basis of medical documentation and prove to be more valuable than a thousand pictures.

Medical documentation is the record of healthcare that has been provided for the patient. Every healthcare facility is required to maintain that medical documentation for each patient. This record is most commonly an electronic medical record, but medical documentation can also be handwritten or typed narratives of provided care; reported results of diagnostic tests, images, or scans; or any other record of the patient's care received at that specific healthcare facility. Medical documentation does more than tell the story of provided care; it provides the foundation for the continuation of care for the patient and the coordination of care for the **clinician**, as well as peace of mind. The recording of pertinent facts, specific findings, observations, assessments, and/or recommendations proves to be the connection between clinician, patient, insurance payer, other medical healthcare agencies, and any other party involved in providing healthcare for the patient. Regardless of who reads the patient's medical documentation, this record clearly reflects the medical, professional, or other healthcare services that have been provided for the patient.

Medical documentation requirements are very simple. Whatever was done by the clinician must be properly recorded to facilitate the coordination, continuity, and communication of care for the patient. This can help to ensure not only proper payment for the clinician, but also thorough oversight for all of the clinicians involved in the patient's care. Every time a patient visits a clinician for a healthcare concern, the medical documentation provides another part of the patient's story for the patient's medical record; each part of the story provides insight into the healthcare provided for each individual patient. Wherever the patient's medical documentation travels, that story can facilitate consistent, proper healthcare.

Documentation might seem simple to accomplish: this was done, that was done, and this is what happened. However, documenting a performed activity is more difficult than it appears, and the ability to thoroughly document a performed action should be respected and admired. Consider the process of shaking someone's hand. Think about documenting every part of that process—from lifting and extending your hand, to the feel of the person's skin, and so on through every step—without using the phrase "shake hands."

healthcare the promotion and preservation of physical health and well-being through clinical assessment, diagnosis, treatment, and, if necessary, management of disease and illness

medical documentation the record of healthcare provided to the patient at the healthcare facility, which may be in the form of handwritten or typed narratives, reported diagnostic results, diagnostic images or scans, or other records

clinician a healthcare professional dedicated to the care and treatment of patients in a healthcare setting; includes a physician, nurse practitioner, registered nurse, or other trained healthcare professional who is most commonly licensed through an overarching professional organization

Documentation of Shaking Hands

While still walking toward Jane, I lifted my right hand in an upward motion, extending my fore-arm to be nearly perpendicular to my torso, with my fingertips reaching toward her. Jane, who had also raised her right hand, stepped toward me; both she and I faced one another. I slid the palm of my hand onto the palm of Jane's hand and gently closed my fingers around the back of her hand, while her fingers also closed around the back of my hand. Although her grip was firm, it did not feel too tight around my fingers. I noticed the warmth of her palm, while the tips of her fingers felt cold. The space between both palms felt slightly sweaty. In one motion, both Jane and I lifted our own right hands a few inches and proceeded to make slight pumping motions up and down, a total of four or five times. Jane and I maintained eye contact throughout, while simultaneously engaging in light, welcoming conversation. I released the pressure of my fingers when I felt Jane's fingers loosen around my hand; I allowed my right hand and arm to return to a relaxed position at my side.

Notice that the "Documentation of Shaking Hands" records every part of the act of shaking hands. With this documentation, a person could identify every specific part of this greeting. In healthcare, medical documentation requires this same kind of focus, attention, and specificity. Fortunately, clinicians receive professional training on how to document clinical encounters; however, it is also important for those charged with reading the clinical notes to understand the importance of the medical documentation, especially the documentation of evaluation and management services.

| Exercise 1.1 | Documentation Exercise |

Instructions: Document two of the following four everyday activities. Follow the previous documentation example for shaking hands, providing specific details about the activity without using the title of the exercise within the documentation.

A. Tying your shoes (avoid any version of the phrase "tie my shoes")

B. Brushing your teeth (avoid any version of the phrase "brush my teeth")

C. Brushing your hair (avoid any version of the phrase "brush my hair")

D. Tying a tie in a Windsor knot (avoid any version of the phrase "tie the tie")

Exercise used with permission from JoAnne Wolf, RHIT, CPC.

EVALUATION AND MANAGEMENT SERVICES

In healthcare, patients experience many different kinds of services including surgery, radiology, and clinical lab or pathology services, along with a variety of medicinal services such as physical therapy, psychiatry, dialysis, ophthalmological treatment, diagnostic cardiology studies, neuromuscular procedures, and more. However, the one healthcare service with which most people are familiar is the evaluation and management service—nearly every person has "gone to see the doctor."

During an evaluation and management service, a specific patient presents to a certain clinical setting for a particular medical need(s). During an evaluation and management service visit, the clinician must perform an **evaluation** of the patient's medical need(s) and create a plan of care for the **management** of that need(s). This evaluation and management service, commonly referred to as E/M, is identified by a series of codes that represent nearly every variety of E/M visit, from a routine office checkup to a complex cardiology evaluation of a chronically ill patient.

evaluation a review and/or assessment of a patient to ascertain a clinical judgment of the patient's diagnosis, current health status, and/or condition

management identification of an appropriate clinical treatment to promote the patient's health, recovery, and wellness

Examples of evaluation and management services include these:

- A 10-year-old boy visits the pediatrician with a high fever and "juicy" cough.
- A 20-year-old woman is brought to the emergency room by her roommate after the woman was struck by a car.
- A teenager visits his family doctor 2 days after a violent tackle on the football field during the last game.
- A 56-year-old woman is brought to the emergency room for chest pain and nausea; she is then admitted to the hospital for observation.
- A young father visits his physician for abdominal pain; his physician suspects appendicitis. After emergency surgery for a ruptured appendix, the young man remains in the hospital for 1 week.
- An elderly woman spends 3 days in the hospital after a hip replacement and is transferred to a nursing home for rehabilitative therapy.
- A young pregnant woman experiences early, obstructed labor and heavy blood loss. She remains in the hospital for 2 weeks and then is discharged to home, where she is seen by a home health nurse to ensure a full recovery.
- A newborn baby boy experiences respiratory distress and is transferred to the neonatal intensive care unit (NICU) in critical condition.

During an E/M service, the clinician must identify and document many different factors, each of which may constitute an important building block in that specific clinical visit. The term *evaluation* means the clinician will do the following:

- Ask the patient questions about his or her current health concern and health history to help identify the nature of the presenting problem
- Assess the current status of the patient's health at the time of the visit to determine the impact of the presenting problem on the patient's health
- Provide and/or identify some recommendation or plan of care for the patient

The term *management* means the clinician will do the following:

- Identify any conditions that may make the patient's condition worse, make the patient sicker, or potentially be fatal to the patient
- Review any medical records or diagnostic or pathology results to assist in the diagnosis and treatment
- Suggest or prescribe a plan of care to manage the patient's specific condition

Each one of these factors represents a different part of the physician's interaction with the patient, telling a different part of the patient's story. The documentation of the E/M service not only tells the story of the patient's health, but also ensures consistent care for the patient: wherever the medical documentation travels, the story of the patient's health can be told for future clinicians. Therefore, proper documentation of the E/M service becomes vital.

GUIDELINES FOR DOCUMENTATION

American Medical Association (AMA)
the largest nonprofit professional organization for physicians and medical students in the United States

Centers for Medicare and Medicaid Services (CMS) the administrative branch of the U.S. Department of Health and Human Services responsible for the oversight of Medicare and Medicaid services, including guidelines, regulation, payment for services, coverage policies, and many other aspects

Documentation Guidelines (DGs) standardized requirements for medical documentation as defined by the Centers for Medicare and Medicaid Services in 1995 and 1997

Current Procedural Terminology (CPT) the book of numeric and alphanumeric codes that identify and describe the healthcare service provided to the patient; maintained and published annually by the AMA

Without consistent guidelines for the documentation of an E/M service, discrepancies in documentation and billing existed across the medical industry. In 1995 the **American Medical Association (AMA)**, in cooperation with the **Centers for Medicare and Medicaid (CMS)**, developed a set of guidelines specifically for E/M services. Titled "1995 **Documentation Guidelines** for Evaluation and Management Services" and known as the 1995 **DGs**, these guidelines provided consistency for the documentation and billing of E/M services; they identified the structure, expectations, and requirements for the documentation of any E/M Service. The first principle of medical record documentation, that "the medical record must be complete and legible,"[1] means that anyone should be able to read the document, which brings up a host of bad jokes about the stereotypical handwriting of physicians. However, legibility can be an issue with typed documentation as well; omission of a key word can turn a sentence into a jumble of words. The "1995 Documentation Guidelines for Evaluation and Management Services" provided direction and clarity for the proper documentation of an E/M service.

The 15 pages of the DGs left some lingering questions regarding the complete documentation of a physical examination. Therefore, in 1997 CMS developed a new, more comprehensive version of the DGs, which delineated much more detailed guidelines for the documentation of a physical examination during an E/M service.

Along with the 1995 and 1997 Documentation Guidelines, the AMA maintains and publishes a compilation of medical codes known as *Current Procedural Terminology (CPT)*. Within the CPT manual, different medical procedures and services are represented by specific codes, including E/M services. Every patient is a unique individual with specific needs, which means that each E/M service is unique for each individual patient. However, to ensure consistency and clarity, there are several different guidelines for the many E/M services, each clearly listed throughout the "Evaluation and Management Service" section of the AMA's CPT manual.

THE SIX CONSTITUENT ELEMENTS THAT COMPOSE THE E/M SERVICE

In the initial guidelines for E/M services, the CPT manual clearly states the basic format for most of the E/M categories, which builds on the factors that constitute different parts of the clinical visit. According to the AMA, each of the many kinds of E/M services follows a similar format of constituent elements that form a specific, individual E/M service:

1. Place of E/M service
2. Type of E/M service
3. Unique code identified with the E/M service

---

[1]Centers for Medicare and Medicaid, "1995 Documentation Guidelines for Evaluation and Management Services," p. 1; "1997 Documentation Guidelines for Evaluation and Management Services," p. 3.

4. Amount of time typically required to perform the specific E/M service
5. Nature of presenting problem
6. Content of the service

Each of these constituent elements reflects a different part of the patient's E/M service.

Place of Service (Site of Service)

As mentioned earlier, E/M services occur in a variety of places:

- Office (also called **outpatient**), which is any location that does not require the patient to be admitted for evaluation and management
- **Assisted living facility**, which is a residential facility with self-contained living units or apartments that provides daily assessment of each resident's needs as well as on-site medical support, 24 hours a day, 7 days a week
- **Inpatient hospital**, which is any facility, other than psychiatric, that provides diagnostic, therapeutic, and rehabilitative services by or under the care or supervision of physicians. Care, which can be both surgical and nonsurgical, is provided to patients who have been admitted to the facility for a variety of conditions.

The **place of service** defines the category of the service. The **category** indicates the facility in which the E/M service occurs, and provides tremendous help in determining the appropriateness of an E/M service code and, most of all, the documentation requirements for that specific visit.

Why does the site of service make such a difference? Consider the differences between these two clinical scenarios:

1. A critically injured patient with multiorgan shut-down that requires very complex care and coordination of treatment for a high-risk condition
2. An elderly patient requiring therapeutically planned care that can be available 24 hours a day

These two scenarios are very different and deserve individual representation—and thus, different categories.

Type of Service and Unique Listed Code

The **type of service** addresses the extent of clinical experience between the patient and the clinician or facility, specifically whether the patient is an **established patient** or a **new patient**. The term *new patient* means the patient has not received any clinical or professional care from the physician, or another physician of the same specialty or subspecialty who belongs to the same group practice, within the previous 3 years. An established patient has received previous healthcare services from the physician, or another physician of the same specialty or subspecialty who belongs to the same group practice, within the previous 3 years; in other words, the patient is known to, and has received clinical care from, the clinician/facility within the last 3 years.

The difference between new patient and established patient affects the clinician's effort required to evaluate and manage the patient's care. After all, the more familiar a clinician is with a patient, the more information is available for the clinician when evaluating and managing a patient's care. The clinician who can access a patient's previous medical records has an established patient, even if the patient presents with a new problem; the patient's medical and treatment history are known to the clinician/facility. Conversely, a new patient requires a much more thorough evaluation of the patient's health history, that is, the patient's past health status.

Even as the place of service indicates the specific location, or category, in which the patient receives the E/M service, the type of service indicates the subcategory of the E/M service. **Subcategories** indicate whether the patient has received clinical care at the place of service. The subcategory provides insight into the extent of the clinical relationship between the clinician and the patient: Is there a long history between the clinician and the patient, or is this visit a first between the clinician and the patient? Many of the categories are separated into at least two subcategories, to further clarify the nature of the E/M service.

For example,

- Physician clinic office for a first-time visit
  - Category: Office/outpatient
    - Subcategory: New patient
- Patient in the hospital for 3 days
  - Category: Hospital inpatient services
    - Subcategory: Subsequent hospital care
- Patient in the hospital for observation only, first calendar day
  - Category: Hospital observation services, first day
    - Subcategory: Initial observation care

outpatient any clinical location that does not require the patient to be admitted for evaluation and management; most commonly identified as a clinical setting to which a patient presents for medical care and then leaves after the service is completed, such as a physician's clinic office

assisted living facility a residential facility with self-contained apartments, or units, that provides assessment of the resident's needs as well as healthcare support 24 hours a day, 7 days a week, in addition to other services

inpatient hospital a category of evaluation and management services that occur when the patient has been admitted to a hospital setting for the purpose of evaluation and/or treatment

place of service the facility or location where the evaluation and management service visit occurs, such as a clinic office or an emergency room

category the group of CPT codes that identify evaluation and management services performed in a similar healthcare setting or location

type of service identification of the clinical experience provided for the patient by the clinician or facility

established patient a patient who has received professional, medical, or other healthcare services from a specific physician, or from another physician of the exact same specialty and subspecialty who also belongs to the same group practice, during the 3 years prior to the evaluation and management service in question

- Emergency room visit
  - Category: Emergency department
    - Subcategory: New or established patient
- Nursing home, admission into facility
  - Category: Nursing facility services
    - Subcategory: Initial nursing facility care
      - Subsubcategory: New or established patient

Requirements exist for each of these categories and subcategories; fortunately, the E/M Service section of the CPT book lists these requirements clearly, providing the foundation and structure for E/M service codes and the E/M services represented by the codes. Understanding these requirements requires an understanding of the building blocks—the factors and components—that provide the foundation and constitute the structure of the E/M documentation requirements.

Typical Time

Reflect on the difference between an E/M service visit in a private physician's office for a patient receiving a routine physical and a 90-minute E/M service visit for a critically ill patient. Since these two E/M scenarios represent different kinds of care, the E/M service categories and subcategories have different requirements to reflect the care provided; some requirements are based on time in minutes, whereas other requirements use a "per diem" or calendar-day guideline. Other guidelines list the time as a block of time during which a specific visit typically can be performed, whereas certain E/M services do not recognize time as a requirement at all. Fortunately, the CPT book clearly defines these guidelines and requirements for the documentation of time in the E/M Service section of the AMA's CPT book.

Nature of Presenting Problem

A patient presents for healthcare evaluation and management for a specific reason. This reason may be a condition, an illness, an injury, a complaint, or some other indicator. This reason for the patient's arrival in the healthcare facility is known as the **nature of the presenting problem**. This can influence the complexity of the patient's E/M service visit.

Example: The Nasty Cough

A mother brings her 10-month-old daughter to her family physician because the child has had a cough. During the course of the visit, the physician comments that the child's weight has gone down since the last visit and asks if the baby girl has been sick in any way in the past month. The mother recalls that her daughter had a very high fever for 3 days about a week ago, but the fever had cleared up, leaving her daughter with a nasty cough that has prevented her daughter from sleeping more than an hour at a time. It turns out that the 10-month-old child has contracted pertussis, otherwise known as whooping cough, and has developed a secondary viral respiratory infection. The mother is tested for pertussis as well, is found positive, and both the mother and her daughter are treated for whooping cough.

This is a great example of how the nature of a presenting problem can differ from the reason the patient originally sought care. In this example, the little girl presented to the physician with a bad cough, even though the presenting problem was actually much more serious. Through their hard work, intelligence, knowledge, and skill, clinicians may determine the presenting problem through the course of the E/M visit.

Content of Service

The documentation of any E/M service contains several essential pieces of information. The obvious pieces of information—such as the patient's name, the date, and the name of the clinician performing the E/M visit—help ensure consistency of care through the maintenance of complete and correct medical records. However, there are three other elements often considered the building blocks for many E/M services: **history**, **physical examination**, and **medical decision making**. These three elements make up the **content of service** and tell the story of the patient's health, both before and during the E/M service; they also identify what could happen or should happen after the patient's visit. Each one of these elements tells part of the story of the E/M visit.

- History tells about the patient's health before the visit, or what has already happened.
- Physical examination tells what is happening in the patient's health at the time of the visit, as determined by the clinician.
- Medical decision making tells the complexity of the presenting problem and the risk this could pose to the patient, as well as what could happen or should happen in the patient's health in the future.

content of service the three elements that are considered the building blocks of evaluation and management services: history, physical examination, and medical decision making

Every documented E/M service adds another part of the patient's story of health; each one of these last three elements—history, physical examination, and medical decision making—provides insight and detail that helps every person involved in the healthcare of the patient. Even as each one of these elements tells a different part of the story, each element has a different set of requirements that facilitate a more complete and thorough documentation of the patient's story of health. The documented content of these specific elements correlates to the level of that specific element, which in turn determines the content of the E/M service.

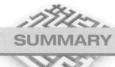

SUMMARY

- Because medical documentation tells the healthcare story of the patient, legibility and completeness are important. However, medical documentation does more than relate the clinical interaction with the patient. Medical documentation provides the foundation for the continuation of care for the patient and the coordination of care for the clinician, as well as the connection between clinician, patient, insurance payer, other medical healthcare agencies, and any other party involved in providing healthcare for the patient. E/M services represent a specific kind of healthcare service between one physician and one patient. These services may occur in a variety of facilities, or locations.

- One of the most important requirements for medical documentation can also prove to be a challenge: Any professional

or clinical services provided by the clinician must be written down and maintained in the medical documentation. Because of the importance of clear, complete medical documentation, CMS provided specific documentation guidelines for E/M services in the 1995 and 1997 "Documentation Guidelines for Evaluation and Management Services."

- Every E/M service is built on the foundation of six constituent elements: the place of service, the type of service, the specific correlating code, the typical time required for the performance of the E/M service, the nature of the presenting problem, and the content of the service.

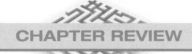

CHAPTER REVIEW

Multiple Choice

Choose the letter that best answers each question or completes each statement.

1. What does the DGs abbreviation mean in "1995 DGs" or "1997 DGs"?
   a. Deadline Goals
   b. Disease Graphing
   c. Documentation Guidelines
   d. Doctor's Guidelines

2. E/M stands for
   a. everyday medicine.
   b. enduring monotony.
   c. evaluation of medicine.
   d. evaluation and management.

3. What does the acronym CMS represent?
   a. Centers for Medical Supervisors
   b. Clinical Management Standards
   c. Centers for Medicare and Medicaid Services
   d. Center for Clinical Managing Medical Services

4. Medical documentation should be
   a. alphabetically listed because order is important, and all records should make sense.
   b. complete, thorough, and legible so that anyone can read the document and understand the story of the patient's health and disease.

   c. written in English regardless of what language the patient or the clinician happens to speak.

   d. typed and never handwritten.

5. After the 1995 DGs for E/M services was written, what changed in the 1997 DGs for E/M services?

   a. The 1997 DGs provided more detailed guidelines for the language in which the medical record documentation of the E/M service should be written.

   b. The 1997 DGs provided more detailed guidelines for how long the patient should wait for the clinician during an E/M service.

   c. The 1997 DGs provided more detailed guidelines for a physical examination during an E/M service.

   d. The 1997 DGs provided more detailed guidelines for the amount of time spent by the clinician during an E/M service.

6. Which of the following is NOT a constituent element of a specific, individual E/M service?

   a. Place of service

   b. Type of service

   c. Individually listed code

   d. Language spoken by the patient

7. What does the term "place of service" define?

   a. The location of the clinic in relation to the nearest hospital

   b. The category of service, indicating the facility in which the E/M service occurs

   c. The place where the clinician documents the E/M service

   d. The subcategory, which often suggests whether the patient is a new or established patient

8. What does the type of service define?

   a. The time of day when the E/M service begins

   b. The category of service, indicating the facility in which the E/M service occurs

   c. The presence or absence of a specifically trained clinician, such as a nurse

   d. The subcategory, which often suggests whether the patient is a new or established patient

9. The content of the service is composed of

   a. the length of time the clinician spends with the patient in counseling or conversation.

   b. history, physical examination, and medical decision making.

   c. the devices used by the clinician during the E/M visit.

   d. documentation methods, such as recorders, utilized at the time of the E/M visit.

10. What does AMA stand for?

   a. All Medical Abbreviations

   b. American Medical Association

   c. American Medical Management Alliance

   d. Asphyxiation Mitigation Assessment

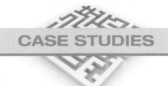

CASE STUDIES

Note: The case studies at the end of every chapter of this text are intended to help the reader utilize the information learned. To provide consistency throughout the 18 chapters of *Medical Coding Evaluation and Management*, certain aspects of the case studies may be familiar throughout the text. For instance, the patient in Case Study 1-2, Franklin, appears in several case studies, although the clinical scenario may change. The case studies help the reader identify the subtleties of evaluation and management and recognize the significant differences among the elements of an E/M service.

Case Study 1-1

Please read the following medical documentation, and then answer questions 1–10.

Edna is a 79-year-old woman who is well-known to me after many years of treatment and care. Edna presents to the clinic today because of lower leg bruising and swelling. Yesterday afternoon she tripped on an ottoman in her house. She has not reported any dizziness or shortness of breath after the fall; however, her adult daughter noticed a large bruise forming on the anterior surface of her mother's lower left leg. This morning Edna noticed that her lower left leg was swollen and the bruise was darker and warmer than the surrounding skin. Edna's adult daughter encouraged her to seek medical attention because of her antiplatelet therapy: aspirin-diprydamole twice daily. Edna suffered a stroke 3½ years ago.

Exam: Temperature, 98.2; Pulse, 60; Blood pressure, 110/81. Edna is gregarious and delightful with a cheerful attitude toward her bruising. She remembers everything about yesterday with clear recall and without slurring. Eyes are clear without signs of jaundice. Heart and lungs are clear without abnormal sounds. She does not appear uncomfortable during the abdominal examination. Edna displays a full range of motion when extending her left knee and ankle with no referring pain along upper leg or in hip. She has full sensation of toes and soles of left foot with good identification of toe pinch. Toes are warm with good circulation.

Plan: Because of Edna's antiplatelet therapy, a PT/INR test is important to identify clotting concerns. Edna has been educated about the signs and symptoms of a clot. The dangers of a deep vein thrombosis have been stressed. Edna expresses understanding. Recheck of bruising in 3 days.

1. Which of the following best describes the service in this medical documentation?

   a. Surgical procedure

   b. Radiology test

   c. Evaluation and management

   d. Medical diagnostic test

2. Which of the following best reflects the place of service of this documented service?

   a. Emergency department

   b. Nursing facility care

   c. Inpatient hospital

   d. Physician's office

3. Which of the following best reflects the type of service, or the patient type?

   a. Established patient

   b. New patient

   c. One-time visit

   d. The documentation does not reflect this.

4. Which of the following options best supports the type of service, or the patient type?

   a. This is a new patient type of service because the problem is new to the physician.

   b. This is an established patient type of service because the patient has been treated by the physician within the previous 3 years.

   c. This is neither a new nor an established patient because the physician did not specifically document the patient type.

   d. Patient type is not applicable to this scenario.

5. Which of the following best reflects the nature of the presenting problem?

   a. Yesterday afternoon, Edna tripped on an ottoman in her house.

   b. Bruise on lower left leg is swollen, bruise is darker and warmer than the surrounding skin, and patient is undergoing antiplatelet therapy.

   c. Patient's adult daughter is concerned about her mother's health.

   d. PT/INR test is ordered to identify clotting concerns, and patient has been educated about the signs and symptoms of a clot as well as the dangers of a deep vein thrombosis.

6. Which of the following best reflects the history in this documentation?

   a. Eyes are clear without signs of jaundice . . . heart and lungs are clear without abnormal sounds . . . she does not appear uncomfortable during the abdominal examination . . . she displays a full range of motion when extending her left knee and ankle with no referring pain along upper leg or in hip.

   b. Patient tripped on an ottoman in her house . . . no reported dizziness or shortness of breath after the fall . . . large bruise formed on the anterior surface of her lower left leg . . . this morning she noticed that her lower left leg was swollen and the bruise was darker and warmer than the surrounding

skin . . . patient is currently undergoing antiplatelet therapy . . . patient suffered a stroke 3½ years ago.

   c. Because of Edna's antiplatelet therapy, a PT/INR test is important to identify clotting concerns. Edna has been educated about the signs and symptoms of a clot.

   d. No history has been documented for this service.

7. Which of the following best reflects the physical examination in this documentation?

   a. 79-year-old woman who is well known to me after many years of treatment . . . patient is being treated with aspirin-diprydamole twice daily after a stroke 3½ years ago.

   b. Antiplatelet therapy warrants a PT/INR test to identify clotting concerns; patient has been educated about the signs and symptoms of a clot and the dangers of deep vein thrombosis.

   c. There is no physical examination documented for this service.

   d. Eyes are clear without signs of jaundice . . . heart and lungs are clear without abnormal sounds . . . she does not appear uncomfortable during the abdominal examination . . . she displays a full range of motion when extending her left knee and ankle with no referring pain along upper leg or in hip.

8. Which of the following best reflects the medical decision making in this documentation?

   a. Her adult daughter noticed a large bruise forming on the anterior surface of her mother's lower left leg and encouraged patient to seek medical attention because of her antiplatelet therapy.

   b. No medical decision making has been documented for this service.

   c. Patient tripped on an ottoman in her house . . . no reported dizziness or shortness of breath after the fall . . . large bruise formed on the anterior surface of her lower left leg . . . this morning she noticed that her lower left leg was swollen and the bruise was darker and warmer than the surrounding skin.

   d. Antiplatelet therapy warrants a PT/INR test to identify clotting concerns; patient has been educated about the signs and symptoms of a clot and the dangers of deep vein thrombosis.

9. In the medical documentation, what does the patient express understanding about?

   a. The bruise being hotter than the surrounding skin

   b. Her adult daughter's concern about Edna's health

   c. The signs and symptoms of a clot and dangers of a deep vein thrombosis

   d. The toe pinch test

10. Which of the following is NOT documented in the case of Edna's bruise?

   a. The circumstances surrounding the onset of the bruise

   b. The patient's physical responses to the toe test and the range of motion of her left leg

   c. The performance of the PT/INR test

   d. The medication regimen the patient is currently undergoing, specifically the aspirin-diprydamole

Case Study 1-2

Read the following E/M medical documentation. Then, in your own words, briefly describe the events reflected in the medical documentation in the lines provided.

Complaint: Franklin is well-known to me and presents for sharp left flank pain over the past 2 days, with dark-colored urine. Franklin is accompanied by his wife, Mary. Three weeks ago, Franklin was involved in a minor ATV accident. Directly after the accident, Franklin's primary complaint involved injuries to his chin and chest, both of which suffered contusions and lacerations. At the subsequent visit 1 week after the accident, both chin and chest contusions and lacerations were healing well; however, his wife reported that Franklin was holding his abdomen carefully when he rose from a sitting position, and Franklin admits today that his abdominal pain has gradually moved to his left flank and increased in intensity. Two days ago, Franklin tripped on the computer cords in his home office, and his left flank pain became extreme in severity. Pain was not relieved after Excedrin and a hot bath. This morning Franklin vomited once, and his temperature was elevated to 101.6°F. Other than Excedrin, Franklin has taken no medications.

The contusions and lacerations Franklin sustained in the ATV accident have healed appropriately. Other than his abdominal and flank pain and fever, Franklin has been in good health. He reports no loss of memory or dizziness since the accident and denies any joint, muscle, or bone pain. No shortness of breath reported, and patient denies any chest pain, heart palpitations, or tingling in arms or fingers. Bowel movements have been normal, regular, and painless. Franklin reports painful urination has caused him to postpone urination at times; however, postponing urination does not relieve his flank pain or painful urination. Other than his fever this morning and one episode of vomiting, Franklin denies chills, night sweats, or any reported fever since the ATV accident. There is no history of kidney disease, pyelonephritis, or diabetes in Franklin's past or Franklin's family. He has never had a urinary tract infection.

Physical Exam: T, 101.3; BP, 126/86; P, 78. Eyes clear without jaundice. Head is atraumatic without tenderness, nodules, or swelling. Neck soft without masses. Auscultations of lungs clear without wheezes or rub. Auscultation of heart reveals regular rate and rhythm with no abnormal sounds noted. No cervical spine tenderness. No thoracic spine tenderness and no lumbar spine tenderness; however, costovertebral tenderness noted upon palpation. Palpation of abdomen reveals guarding, tenderness with rebound. Franklin expressed nausea upon palpation and vomited immediately after abdominal exam. His face became quite flushed. Although palpation of lower abdomen caused significant pain, bladder was palpable even though Franklin provided copious urine specimen before examination. No rashes noted during abdominal exam, along groin, or on penis. Urinary meatus clear, without redness or inflammation.

Laboratory: Urinalysis notable for pH of 6. Nitrate positive and leukocyte esterase positive with a small amount of blood noted. Electrolytes notable for a BUN and creatinine of 14 and 8. White blood count is 18,000. An abdominal CT scan was reviewed with radiologist. Scan showed a normal right kidney. Left kidney scan revealed no evidence of trauma, inflammation, or infection; however, the mid-left ureter was slightly dilated with mild inflammation, consistent with an upper urinary tract infection and perhaps a recent mild obstruction. Review of KUB revealed significant stool within sigmoid and rectum.

Assessment: Franklin has an upper urinary tract infection. Due to the intensity of Franklin's upper urinary tract infection, I believe it would be prudent to begin oral Augmentin treatment at 875 mg twice a day for 7 days and increase fluid intake. Follow-up in 10 days for recheck.

_____
_____
_____
_____
_____
_____

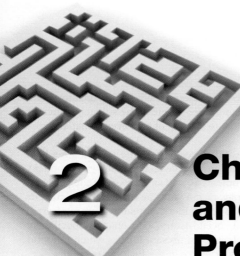

2 Chief Complaint and History of Present Illness

Learning Objectives

After completing this chapter, you should be able to do the following:

- Spell and define the key terms and abbreviations presented in this chapter
- List and define the chief complaint
- Identify the eight elements of history of present illness
- List and define the two levels of history of present illness
- Identify the history of present illness in the medical documentation

Key Terms

associated signs and symptoms
brief history of present illness
chief complaint
comorbidity
context
duration
extended history of present illness
history of present illness (HPI)
location
modifying factor
over-the-counter medication

quality
severity
sign
symptom
timing

Abbreviations

CC chief complaint
HPI history of present illness
Hx history
OTC over-the-counter medication
S/S signs and symptoms

INTRODUCTION

What does *history* mean? Does it refer to the pyramids of Egypt? the American Civil War? the story of a 35-year-old man breaking his leg at the age of 8 when he fell from a tree? Whether the subject is ancient Egyptian pharaohs or events from childhood, the word *history* refers to a series of past events that are usually described in chronological terms.

Considered the first component of the E/M service, **history (Hx)** pertains to the patient's medical background, specifically as it relates to the reason for the patient's current visit. The history component includes the patient's own personal description of the current problem, as well as a review of the patient's previous health and the circumstances of the patient's life that may, or may not, be related to the current problem. Four different elements constitute the history component: the chief complaint, history of present illness, review of systems, and the patient's past, family, and social history. This chapter specifically addresses the first two history elements: the chief complaint and history of present illness, which function in concert with one another to portray the reason for the patient's presence at the healthcare facility.

CHIEF COMPLAINT

Although certain exceptions exist, many E/M visits occur for a specific reason; the patient feels ill, sick, or unwell and presents to the healthcare facility. The **chief complaint (CC)** is the patient's personal account of the symptoms, pain, discomfort, or illness that brought the patient to seek medical care. Consider the following interview between a clinician and patient:

- **Clinician:** What brings you in today?
- **Patient:** I feel sick to my stomach, and my belly hurts a whole lot.

The sentence "I feel sick to my stomach, and my belly hurts a whole lot" begins the story of the patient's health or disease and, most importantly, is expressed to the clinician in the patient's own words. However, this does not mean that the medical documentation of the E/M visit should be in dialogue form. The previous interchange may be documented in the clinical note as

Patient presents today complaining of upset stomach and painful abdomen.

Notice that this summary encompasses the patient's "sick to my stomach" and "belly hurts a whole lot" in a more concise manner while remaining true to the patient's description. The CC could present a minor risk to the patient's health, such as a minor head cold, or a small splinter of wood embedded in the palm of the patient's hand. Contrarily, for a patient managing a more chronic condition such as type II diabetes, the CC could represent a change in health since the patient's last visit with the clinician. Most of all, the CC describes in simple terms without a lot of detail the reason the patient has presented for the current E/M visit. The history of present illness provides the necessary detail about the CC.

HISTORY OF PRESENT ILLNESS

CMS defines the **history of present illness (HPI)** as a chronological description of the development of the patient's CC. This development refers to what the patient noticed about the CC, as either of the following:

1. An acute condition, identifying the onset of the CC and the first **signs** and/or **symptoms**
2. A chronic condition, identifying any change in the CC since the last clinical visit

To include all possible clinical variations, CMS expanded the definition of *history of present illness* to the following:

The history of present illness (HPI) is a chronological description of the development of the patient's present illness from the first sign and/or symptom or from the previous encounter to the present.

Every patient is unique, and each patient experiences pain, discomfort, or disease differently; the history of present illness provides the initial insight into the nature of the CC, providing the first clues about the patient's condition. The 1995 and 1997 Documentation Guidelines have determined that the history

history in response to questions posed by the clinician, the patient's description of the current health complaint and the status and function of the patient's body, as well as past medical history, genetic medical history, and/or any social habits that may impact the patient's health

chief complaint the patient's description of the specific health issue, complaint, or disease for which the patient came to the clinician

history of present illness (HPI) any of eight standardized descriptions with which the patient may provide a visceral (embodied or instinctive), personalized description of the specific health issue, complaint, or disease for which the patient came to the clinician

sign objective evidence of an illness, condition, or pathology that can be scientifically observed and quantified

symptom a patient's subjective report of the discomfort, pain, illness, or disease currently experienced

of present illness is the only history element that must be documented by the clinician at the time of the visit. Only the performing clinician can know what questions to ask the patient. Only the performing clinician can see the patient's demeanor at the time of the visit, hear the patient's voice, and notice the intonation of the voice as the patient answers the questions about the pain or discomfort currently experienced.

THE EIGHT ELEMENTS OF HISTORY OF PRESENT ILLNESS

Descriptions can prove to be inconclusive without clear parameters. After all, 10 different people experiencing back pain may describe the pain in 10 completely different ways. Identifying the clear parameters for objective documentation of such subjective topics can make all the difference in understanding the history of the patient's present illness.

CMS lists eight different elements for the history of present illness: location, severity, timing, duration, quality, context, modifying factor, and associated signs and symptoms. Each of these elements addresses a different aspect of the patient's present illness, providing a broader understanding of the patient's current experience.

1. Location (a specific place of pain or discomfort in or on the patient's body)
2. Severity (the pain or discomfort described in degrees or on a scale of 1–10)
3. Timing (how often the condition occurs)
4. Modifying factor (anything that has helped the pain or discomfort)
5. Quality (what the pain is like, the most subjective of all eight elements)
6. Duration (how long ago this condition started—hours, days, weeks, months)
7. Context (what was happening around the time this condition began)
8. Associated signs/symptoms (anything else that hurt or that the patient noticed as distressing or painful, whether it is related or not)

All eight of the history-of-present-illness elements may not be discussed during an E/M visit and/or documented in the clinical note; only a few of the history-of-present-illness elements are needed to provide a more in-depth description of the patient's CC. Consider the following paragraph:

Patient presents with pain in **location** abdomen. Patient reports pain began **duration** ago and has gotten **severity** in the past **timing** hours. Patient reports pain as very **quality**, taking her breath away. Patient reports that just prior to onset of pain, patient **context** occurred, leaving patient breathless for about 20 minutes. Patient has taken **modifying factor** but has not felt any relief from the pain. Patient has noticed **associated sign and symptom** when urinating.

Notice that each of the eight history-of-present-illness elements provides a little bit more detail for the CC. Language matters when dealing with the HPI, specifically what words are used as well as how these words are used. Since the HPI portrays the patient's discomfort and pain in vivid detail, these elements may be considered the "empathy elements," which provide a visceral understanding of the patient's CC. Consider this clinical interview of the unfortunate patient with the abdominal pain:

- **Clinician:** What brings you in today?
- **Patient:** I feel sick to my stomach, and my belly hurts a whole lot.
- **Clinician:** Where does your belly hurt?
- **Patient:** Right here . . . just below my belly button.
- **Clinician:** On a scale of 1–10, how much does your stomach hurt?
- **Patient:** This weekend my belly hurt so much I couldn't get out of bed; an 8 or 9 out of 10.
- **Clinician:** How bad was your nausea?
- **Patient:** I never threw up, but I wished I had; maybe it might have helped.
- **Clinician:** How long has your stomach hurt?
- **Patient:** All weekend, since Friday evening.
- **Clinician:** Did anything happen last week, maybe on Thursday or Friday; were you around anyone who was sick?
- **Patient:** No, no one was sick at the office all week, and there was a potluck party at work Friday afternoon.
- **Clinician:** What kind of food was at the potluck party?
- **Patient:** Chips and this really good spinach dip.
- **Clinician:** Do you know who made the dip?

- **Patient:** No one made it; it came from the grocery store. Come to think of it, Judy went crazy over the dip, and then she went home early throwing up.
- **Clinician:** Have you vomited?
- **Patient:** No, I've felt really awful though.
- **Clinician:** Have you experienced any other stomach problems: diarrhea, cramping, sharp pains, anything like that?
- **Patient:** I did have really, really bad diarrhea on Saturday morning, but that's all. After that, I just hurt all the time.
- **Clinician:** Has anything helped you feel better this weekend?
- **Patient:** Yeah, eating saltines and drinking ginger ale helped a little.

In this example, the clinician asks questions to find out more about the CC. Through the interview, the clinician has received answers to those questions:

- Why did you seek medical attention today? (CC: abdominal pain and nausea)
- Where does it hurt? (HPI element, location: pain just below the belly button)
- How badly does it hurt? (HPI element, severity: so bad—an 8 or 9 out of 10—the patient couldn't get out of bed)
- When did it start hurting? (HPI element, duration: Friday afternoon, just before the weekend)
- What (if anything) has helped you feel better? (HPI element, modifying factor: saltines and ginger ale)
- Did any specific event occur before or surrounding the onset of symptoms? (HPI element, associated signs and symptoms: very bad diarrhea)

Each one of these HPI elements provides a little bit more information about the patient's CC.

Location

location the specific anatomic area in or on the body in which signs and symptoms have occurred

Location identifies the place in or on the body in which signs and symptoms have occurred. Considered the "where" element, location refers to a specific anatomical site that can be clearly understood. These words or short phrases point to the specific anatomical location where the patient is currently experiencing, or has experienced, the chief complaint.

> **Examples of Words and Short Phrases That Support Location**
>
> | | |
> |---|---|
> | Right side of head | Distal (far) |
> | Lower left side of abdomen | Proximal (near) |
> | Upper chest | Third digit |
> | Lower back | Left hand |
> | Posterior | Head |

In the medical documentation, the location of the CC may be found in brief, stand-alone phrases or embedded within longer sentences. Regardless of how the location is documented, this element of the HPI reflects a specific anatomical location where the patient experiences the signs and/or symptoms of the CC.

> **Medical Documentation Examples of Location**
>
> 1. Face hurts, especially on the right cheek beneath eye.
> 2. Stomach hurts, down low on the right side.
> 3. Low back hurts, down by beltline.

Severity

severity an objective measurement of the patient's experience of the sign or symptom

Severity describes in objective terms the degree or intensity of the sign, symptom, pain, or discomfort. These words or phrases objectively measure the pain or discomfort and reveal how the pain or discomfort has affected the patient's life. The HPI element of severity should be considered the "ouch" element, because these words and phrases clearly and objectively describe the significance of the patient's pain, discomfort, sign, or symptom being experienced.

> **Examples of Words and Short Phrases That Support Severity**
>
> | | |
> |---|---|
> | Getting worse | Patient fell 3 feet |
> | Improving | Increased |
> | Severe pain | Complicated |
> | Moderate pain | Progressive |
> | A 7 on a pain scale of 1–10 | |

Regardless of whether the severity of the CC is documented with words, phrases, or numeric identifiers, this element of the HPI clearly indicates how the patient experiences the sign and/or symptom.

> **Medical Documentation Examples of Severity**
>
> 1. Face hurts so much patient feels that she can't open her eyes all the way.
> 2. Stomach hurts really very badly . . . an 8 on a pain scale.
> 3. Low back pain is very severe.

Timing

Timing provides an objective indication of how the patient experiences the pain, discomfort, sign, or symptom during day-to-day activities. Findings that support the timing element often identify the occurrences of a symptom within an hour, day, week, or specific block of time, such as overnight. These words or phrases reflect the frequency of symptomatic occurrences during such periods of time, to better identify the impact of the symptom, pain, discomfort, or sign. The HPI element of timing could be considered the "how often" or the "interruption" element, because it portrays how the pain, symptom, discomfort, or sign has interrupted the patient's life.

timing a measurable, objective indication of how the pain, discomfort, sign, or symptom has affected or currently affects the patient's day-to-day life

> **Examples of Words and Short Phrases That Support Timing**
>
> | | |
> |---|---|
> | Twice | Occasionally |
> | Daily | Twice a week |
> | Constant (it never goes away) | Recurrent |
> | Intermittent | Upon rising |
> | Sporadic | While sleeping |
> | Frequent | 20 minutes after ___ |
> | Persistent | At noon |
> | Rarely | |

Documentation of the timing indicates how, if, or when the patient's sign or symptom interrupts a day, an hour, a week, or any other span of time. Therefore, this element of the HPI describes the CC within the context of the patient's life.

> **Medical Documentation Examples of Timing**
>
> 1. The pain in face is constant.
> 2. Stomach doesn't hurt all the time, but it's worst in the morning after getting up.
> 3. The pain in low back is sporadic, mostly when standing after sitting for a while.

Modifying Factor

We live in the modern age of accessible, over-the-counter pain relief, analgesics, and other pharmaceutical medications and tools that can provide relief for discomfort or pain. Sometimes when a person experiences significant discomfort or pain, grandmother's old-fashioned remedies might not seem so far-fetched. This HPI element, **modifying factor**, is considered the "tried it, and it helped" or "tried it, and it did not help" element, because it reflects the actions taken by the patient, or other clinicians, to modify or lessen the pain, sign, symptom, or discomfort.

modifying factor any treatment taken by a patient in an attempt to alleviate or change the sign or symptom; may include over-the-counter or prescription medication, a specific activity or therapy, such as ice packs or massage

Examples of Words and Short Phrases That Support Modifying Factor

- Relieved by applying an ice pack, heating pad, analgesic cream, etc.
- Not affected by ice pack, heating pad, analgesic cream, etc.
- Children's Tylenol did not lessen the fever.
- Slept all night and felt better the next morning
- Improved after taking ibuprofen
- Antacids did not (or did) help the heartburn.
- Taking an oatmeal bath helped the itching.
- Tried grandfather's Windex trick, and the swelling decreased
- Rubbed Vicks VapoRub on the soles of feet at night

Regardless of the nature of the treatment or remedy, this element of HPI reflects any measures taken by the patient in an attempt to alleviate, improve, or resolve the sign or symptom.

Medical Documentation Examples of Modifying Factor

1. Alka-Seltzer Cold helped only in the morning.
2. Stomach feels better after patient eats breakfast.
3. Ibuprofen used to help, but now it does not help back pain anymore.

Quality

Some descriptive words provide general impressions, whereas other descriptions give visceral illustrations. The **quality** element subjectively measures the pain or discomfort in a very personal way; being subjective, these words or phrases are not often measured in degrees. Considered the "ewwww" element, words or phrases that support the quality element translate the patient's experience of the pain or discomfort into personal understanding for the clinician and anyone reviewing the documentation.

quality a subjective description of the pain or discomfort that illustrates the patient's personal experience of the sign or symptom

Examples of Words and Short Phrases That Support Quality

Sharp (abdominal) pain	Green phlegm
Cramping discomfort	Runny diarrhea
Smelly urine	Dull pain
Stabbing pain	Clear sputum
Throbbing discomfort/pain	Green puslike drainage
Watery diarrhea	Productive cough with brownish green sputum
Hot, shooting pain	Hacking cough
Painful urination	Cloudy urine
Crushing pressure	
Pyritic drainage	

Of all of the elements of HPI, quality sometimes proves to be the most subjective, which can pose challenges when identifying this element. For this reason, the quality of a sign or symptom most often generates a vivid image of the sign or symptom.

> **Medical Documentation Examples of Quality**
>
> 1. Stabbing pain beneath right eye
> 2. Pain is sharp and burning in lower stomach.
> 3. Low back pain is sharp and throbbing.

Duration

Duration defines how long the patient has experienced the sign, pain, discomfort, or symptom, by identifying the starting point or the length of time the symptom, pain, or discomfort has affected the patient's life or the point of time when a complication arose during the management of a chronic condition. The HPI element duration should be considered the "how long" element, because these words/phrases give a definite sense of the length of time the patient has experienced the pain, discomfort, symptom, or sign.

duration the measurement of elapsed time since the patient began to experience the sign, pain, discomfort, or symptom, either by identifying the starting point; the length of time the symptom, pain, or discomfort has impacted the patient's life; or the point of time when a complication arose during the management of a chronic condition

> **Examples of Words and Short Phrases That Support Duration**
>
> For the past 2 days
> 2 hours
> Since yesterday
> Until today
>
> For 1 week
> Since last visit
> For most of patient's life

Duration is sometimes confused with timing, since both of these elements address the sign or symptom within the context of the patient's life. However, duration objectively expresses how long the patient has experienced this sign or symptom.

> **Medical Documentation Examples of Duration**
>
> 1. My face started hurting like this about 3 days ago.
> 2. The pain became really bad last week.
> 3. I have had low back pain for about 20 years, since I was first in the service.

Context

Often, an event bears some relevance for, or may even affect, a patient's health, and that event can provide tremendous information about the patient's current condition. The HPI element **context** includes any pertinent external events or occurrences in the narrative of the patient's story of health. The context element might be best considered the "Oh, really?" element, because context provides a fuller picture of the patient's life surrounding the pain, sign, discomfort, or symptom.

context narration of the circumstance or event that occurred prior to or coincidentally with the onset of the patient's sign, symptom, or disease; may or may not be related to the sign or symptom

> **Examples of Words and Short Phrases That Support Context**
>
> - Occurred at the same time as the car crash
> - Burned hand while taking cake from oven
> - During the snowball fight
> - While the patient (pt) was playing bingo
> - Fell off ladder while putting up Christmas lights
> - The pain was insidious (slow, stealthy, sneaky) in onset.
> - Fell from tree
> - Tripped off curb

Whereas many of the HPI elements offer subjective or objective descriptions of the patient's signs and symptoms, this element places the CC within the larger context of the patient's life.

> **Medical Documentation Examples of Context**
>
> 1. Pt had been caught in rain while camping a week days ago.
> 2. Pt's child had stomach flu last week.
> 3. Pain noticed shortly after pt played touch football with adult children on Thanksgiving.

Associated Signs and Symptoms

Everything in the body is connected; swelling in one part of the body may or may not radiate to another part of the body, which may show a possible relationship between the swelling and the pain. Sometimes when a patient feels discomfort or pain, another symptom may be overlooked. The HPI element **associated signs and symptoms (s/s)** offers the opportunity for any other discomfort, pain, sign, or symptom to be recognized and considered. Sometimes considered the "and what else" element, words or phrases that support the associated s/s element identify and describe any other pain, discomfort, or symptom the patient might currently be experiencing in addition to the CC.

associated signs and symptoms reports or observations of evidence of pathology or disease in the patient's physiology, such as blood in urine, and/or subjective observations of physical experience such as pain or discomfort

> **Examples of Words and Short Phrases That Support Associated Signs and Symptoms**
>
> - Pt has also been vomiting.
> - Pain does not radiate to any other part of body.
> - Head injury with no loss of consciousness (LOC)
> - Pain radiating to right shoulder
> - Pain in contiguous (neighboring) areas
> - Rash secondary to burning pain in neck
> - Headache began shortly after diarrhea.

As can be seen in the following examples, associated s/s reflect the interconnected nature of the patient's physiology.

> **Medical Documentation Examples of Associated Signs and Symptoms**
>
> 1. Pt is also complaining of significant nasal congestion.
> 2. Pt has not vomited but has diarrhea.
> 3. Pt also complains of pain radiating down right thigh.

When identifying the HPI elements, one must identify the specific finding that best supports a specific HPI element. In some clinical notes, several findings may be identified to support one HPI element, but only one HPI finding is required to support the HPI element. For example, a patient may experience more than one associated sign and symptom; however, in the clinical note, *only* one of the listed findings needs to be listed as an associated sign and symptom.

During the medical interview between clinician and patient, a complete description of the patient's CC is derived from the eight HPI factors:

1. Where does it hurt?
2. How badly does it hurt?
3. How often during the day does this occur?
4. Does anything make it better/worse?
5. How would you describe the CC?
6. How long has it been occurring?
7. Did something happen to cause this s/s?
8. Is the CC accompanied by any other s/s?

The HPI is so intimately related to the CC (the pain, discomfort, or symptom) that only the examining clinician can document the HPI findings.

Exercise 2.1 Identifying the Eight HPI Elements

Identify the eight HPI elements in the following medical documentation by underlining the supporting findings.

1. Face hurts, especially on the right cheek beneath eye. Face hurts so much, "I feel like I can't open my eyes all the way." The pain in face is constant. Alka-Seltzer Cold only helped in the morning. Stabbing pain beneath right eye. Face started hurting like this about 3 days ago. Pt had been caught in rain while camping a few days ago. Pt is also complaining of significant nasal congestion.

2. Stomach hurts, down low on the right side. Stomach hurts really, really badly. Stomach doesn't hurt all the time, but it's worst in the morning after getting up, an 8 on pain scale. Stomach feels better after pt eats breakfast. Pain is sharp and burning in lower stomach. The pain became really bad last week. Pt's child had stomach flu last week. Pt has not vomited but has diarrhea.

3. Low back hurts, down by beltline; pain is very severe. The pain in low back is sporadic, mostly when standing after sitting for a while. Ibuprofen used to help, but now it does not help back pain anymore. Low back pain is sharp and throbbing. Pt has had low back pain for about 20 years, since first in the service. Pain noticed shortly after pt played touch football with adult children at Thanksgiving. Pt also complains of pain radiating down right thigh.

Although not every one of the eight HPI elements may be documented in the clinical note, each one of the HPI elements reflects part of the nature of the presenting problem.

Number of Findings Required for Each HPI Element It is important to stress that only one HPI finding is required to support an HPI element. HPI findings *describe* the present illness: the severity, duration, quality, and so on. In some clinical notes, the documented HPI finding is a concise description whereas other clinical notes contain extensive descriptive language, which may provide several findings for the documented HPI element. However, no matter how many findings have been documented for an HPI element, only one HPI finding is required to support that specific HPI element.

Example: Johnny's Irritating Cough

Johnny presents with an irritating (*quality*) cough that has been bothering him for 4 months (*duration*). He has tried an **over-the-counter (OTC) medication** (cough syrup), gargling with salt water, drinking tea and honey (*modifying factors*), and has found no relief. His cough is worst in the morning and night (*timing*), but he reports no fever, no diarrhea, no chest pain or heart palpitations when coughing, yet reports that he hasn't gotten a good night's sleep (*associated s/s*) since his cough began this past April (*duration*). He remembers having a very (*severity*) stuffy nose (*associated s/s*) in April (*timing*) and reports postnasal drainage (*associated s/s*) throughout the spring and summer (*timing*).

over-the-counter medication any medication that does not require a prescription, such as Tylenol, Advil, or nonprescription allergy medication such as Benadryl

HPI findings from "Johnny's Irritating Cough"

Quality (1 finding):
irritating cough

Duration (2 findings):
for 4 months
since this past April

Modifying factor (3 findings):
cough syrup
gargling with salt water
drinking tea and honey

Timing (3 findings):
worst in morning and night
in April
throughout spring and summer

continued

Associated signs and symptoms (6 findings):

hasn't gotten good night's sleep

postnasal drainage

no fever

no chest pain

no heart palpitations

no diarrhea

Severity (1 finding):

very (stuffy nose)

In the previous example, the HPI elements duration, modifying factor, timing, and associated signs and symptoms all have more than one finding. However, since only one HPI finding is required to support each of these HPI elements, the person who is reviewing the clinical note has to determine which HPI finding is most clinically appropriate to support the HPI element and thus the chief complaint. Again, regardless of how many HPI elements are identified in the documentation, each element needs only one documented finding.

LEVELS OF HISTORY OF PRESENT ILLNESS

According to the 1995 and 1997 evaluation and management documentation guidelines, there are two different levels of documenting the HPI:

brief history of present illness documentation of one to three history-of-present-illness standardized descriptions

extended history of present illness documentation of four or more of the history-of-present-illness standardized descriptions

comorbidity a secondary or additional disease or illness that is separate from the presenting problem but that occurs at the same time as the presenting problem

- **Brief history of present illness:** 1–3 elements of HPI
- **Extended history of present illness:** 4+ elements of HPI *or* 3+ associated **comorbidity** (e.g., diabetes, hypertension, osteoporosis)

During the review of medical documentation, it is helpful to utilize efficient tools, which facilitate identification of the HPI elements. ■ FIGURE 2.1 presents the HPI levels in a format that enables easy review and will prove to be very helpful during future exploration of all four of the history elements in this text.

HPI is part of the first element of the content of service. Although Figure 2.1 presents HPI as one single element, it is important to remember that the HPI operates in synthesis with all of the content of service elements, which can be reviewed in one compiled worksheet in Appendix D.

Example of Brief HPI

Frankie's Sore Throat

Frankie complains of a sore throat (*location*) and barking cough (*quality*). No complaints of nasal drainage (*associated signs or symptoms*).

Three HPI Elements:

Location—sore throat; a specific location on the body or a place on the body that the patient can point to

Quality—barking cough; a term or phrase that subjectively describes how the patient experiences the sign or symptom

Associated sign or symptom—no complaints of nasal drainage; a report or observation of evidence of pathology or disease in the patient's physiology, such as blood in urine, *and/or* subjective observations of physical experience such as pain or discomfort

History of Present Illness Location, severity, timing, mod fact, quality, duration, context, assoc s/s	Brief (1)	Brief (2–3)	Ext. (4+, or 3 chronic problems)	Ext. (4+, or 3 chronic problems)

Figure 2.1 ■ Content of service element: history of present illness.

Example of Extended HPI

Johnny's Barking Cough

Johnny presents to the clinic with a very (*severity*) sore throat (*location*) and barking (*quality*) cough. No complaints of nasal drainage (*associated s/s*) during past week (*duration*).

    Four-plus HPI elements:

      Severity—very (sore throat); description of the pain or discomfort in degrees or on pain scale (1–10)

      Location—sore throat; identification of the pain, discomfort, or symptom at a specific location on the body, generally a place to which the patient can point

      Quality—barking cough; a term or phrase that subjectively describes how the patient experiences the sign or symptom

      Associated s/s—no complaints of nasal drainage; a report or observation of evidence of pathology or disease in the patient's physiology, such as blood in urine, *and/or* subjective observations of physical experience such as pain or discomfort

      Duration—during the past week; any specific starting or stopping point of the onset of the sign or symptom

Even though the documentation of the E/M service visit is the only record of what happened, more words do not necessarily provide any benefit. HPI elements are documented by words or brief phrases that provide an accurate and adequate description of the CC, and once again—each HPI element requires only one finding.

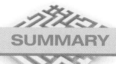

SUMMARY

- The CC is the first element of the history. Documented by the clinician, the CC presents the patient's own personalized description of the specific health issue, complaint, or disease for which the patient came to the clinician.

- The history of present illness describes the patient's CC, or the pain, discomfort, sign, or symptom the patient is currently experiencing. The eight HPI elements are sometimes considered the "empathy" elements because of the personalized detail each one presents. Some clinical notes may have as few as one HPI element, whereas others may contain six or more HPI elements. Only the performing physician may collect and document the HPI.

- HPI findings are most commonly found in the first section of the medical documentation. The HPI describes the patient's personal experience of the CC; therefore, the language tends to be past tense.

- The eight elements of the HPI are location, severity, timing, modifying factors, quality, duration, context, and associated signs and symptoms.

- Two levels of the HPI are brief and extended. A brief HPI documents between one and three HPI elements. An extended HPI documents four or more HPI elements or three or more comorbidities.

CHAPTER REVIEW

Multiple Choice

Choose the letter that best answers each question or completes each statement.

1. What does the acronym CC mean?
   a. Clinically conservative
   b. Consensual caregiving
   c. Chief complaint
   d. Comprehensive clinicopathology

2. What does the acronym HPI mean?
   a. Healthful plan of intervention
   b. Healthcare placement identifier
   c. Health preservation initiative
   d. History of present illness

3. Who may document the HPI?

   a. The front desk receptionist or appointment scheduler

   b. The medical assistant or registered nurse

   c. The performing physician

   d. The HPI is inherent to the E/M visit and doesn't need to be documented.

4. How many HPI elements must be documented to support a brief HPI?

   a. It does not matter how many elements are documented.

   b. Four or more HPI elements

   c. Six HPI elements

   d. One, two, or three HPI elements

5. How many HPI elements must be documented to support an extended HPI?

   a. Ten HPI elements

   b. One, two, or three HPI elements

   c. Four or more HPI elements

   d. Six HPI elements

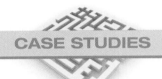

CASE STUDIES

Case Study 2-1

Read the following medical documentation, and then answer the questions that follow.

Patient presents with sharp upper abdominal pain that frequently burns. Pain has been present since November, about 5 months. Pain rated 7–8/10 between meals, and pain is constant. Antacids have provided some relief for several months, but pain has increased significantly during the past few weeks. Appetite greatly reduced, and patient reports feeling full after only a few bites of food.

1. In the phrase "sharp upper abdominal pain," which HPI element does the word sharp support?

   a. Location

   b. Quality

   c. Timing

   d. Modifying factor

2. In the phrase "sharp upper abdominal pain," which HPI element does the word upper support?

   a. Location

   b. Severity

   c. Associated signs and symptoms

   d. Timing

3. In the sentence "Pain has been present since November, about 5 months," which HPI element does the phrase "since November, about 5 months" support?

   a. Quality

   b. Timing

   c. Location

   d. Duration

4. In the phrase "Pain rated 7–8/10 between meals," which HPI element does the phrase "pain rated 7–8/10" support?

   a. Quality

   b. Severity

   c. Modifying factor

   d. Associated signs and symptoms

5. In the phrase "Pain rated 7–8/10 between meals," which HPI element does the phrase "between meals" support?

   a. Timing

   b. Location

   c. Duration

   d. Quality

6. In the sentence "Antacids have provided some relief for several months, but pain has increased significantly during the past few weeks," which HPI element does the phrase "antacids have provided some relief for several months" support?

   a. Location

   b. Quality

   c. Associated signs and symptoms

   d. Modifying factor

7. Which HPI element is supported by the sentence "Appetite greatly reduced, and patient reports feeling full after only a few bites of food"?

   a. Modifying factor

   b. Severity

   c. Associated signs and symptoms

   d. Timing

Case Study 2-2

Read the following case study, identify the appropriate findings for each of the HPI elements, and write the findings next to the HPI element listed.

Complaint: Franklin is well-known to me and presents for sharp left flank pain over the past 2 days, with dark-colored urine. His wife, Mary, accompanies Franklin. Three weeks ago, Franklin was involved in a minor ATV accident. Directly after the accident, Franklin's primary complaint involved injuries to his chin and chest, both of which suffered contusions and lacerations. At the subsequent visit 1 week after the accident, both chin and chest contusions and lacerations were healing well; however, his wife reported that Franklin was holding his abdomen carefully when he rose from a sitting position, and Franklin admits today that his abdominal pain has gradually moved to his left flank and increased in intensity. Two days ago, Franklin tripped on the computer cords in his home office, and his left flank pain became extreme in severity. Pain was not relieved after Excedrin and a hot bath. This morning Franklin vomited once, and his temperature was elevated to 101.6°F. Other than Excedrin, Franklin has taken no medications.

Location _____

Quality _____

Severity _____

Duration _____

Context _____

Timing _____

Modifying factor(s) _____

Associated signs and symptoms _____

Circle the appropriate level for the documented HPI:

    Brief

    Extended

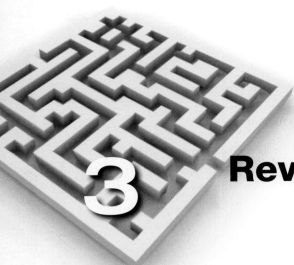

3. Review of Systems

Learning Objectives

After completing this chapter, you should be able to do the following:

- Spell and define the key terms and abbreviations presented in this chapter
- Recognize the purpose of the review of systems
- Distinguish the methods of collecting the review of systems information
- Identify the elements of the review of systems
- Describe the difference between the history of present illness and the review of systems
- List and define the four levels of the review of systems

Key Terms

allergic
cardiovascular
complete
constitutional
ears
endocrine
extended
eyes
gastrointestinal
genitourinary
hematologic
immunologic
integumentary
lymphatic
mouth
musculoskeletal
negative

neurological
none (or N/A)
nose
objective
organ system
pertinent
physical examination
psychiatric
respiratory
review of systems (ROS)
sign
subjective
symptom
throat

Abbreviations

ENT/M ears, nose, throat, and mouth
ROS review of systems

INTRODUCTION

Considered the first component of the E/M service, history pertains to a patient's medical background, specifically as it relates to the reason for the patient's current visit. The history component includes the patient's own personal description of the current problem, as well as a review of the patient's previous health and the circumstances of the patient's life that may, or may not, be related to the current problem. Four different elements comprise the history component: chief complaint, history of present illness, review of systems, and past, family, and social history. The chief complaint represents the reason, sign, or symptom for which the patient seeks clinical care, whereas the history of present illness describes the chief complaint in further detail. This chapter specifically addresses the review of systems, which provides a more in-depth glimpse of the patient's health.

Sometimes when a person experiences a specific discomfort or pain, other symptoms may be eclipsed by the intensity of that specific discomfort or pain. In other words, a patient's **objective** experience of an underlying disorder, complaint, or disease may be eclipsed by the **subjective** experience of the present illness. For instance, a patient suffering from painful sinus pressure may not notice a generalized pain in her chest when she coughs. When the chief complaint eclipses any other discomfort, pain, or symptom, a patient might forget about a different, possibly important symptom currently being experienced. The clinician may ask a series of questions that create an inventory of body systems currently affected by or having been impacted by different signs or symptoms. This inventory of body systems helps the clinician identify any other discomfort, pain, or symptom that may, or may not, be related to the chief complaint. These questions are known as the **review of systems (ROS)**, because the questions specifically review the patient's experience of health prior to the clinical visit.

Make a List

When preparing for a trip to the grocery store, making a list can make the shopping experience more efficient: eggs, facial tissues, carrots, bread, and canned beans. Each of these items is located in a different section of the store, identified by the category of items; for instance, carrots cannot be found in the bread section, and facial tissues will not be found in the dairy section with the eggs. However, having a list does not preclude a walk through the grocery store; in order to reach each of the items on the list, the shopper must walk through the aisles, past many different items, some of which may not be on the shopping list. While walking through the aisles, the shopper has the opportunity to review the other items in those sections and, perhaps, identify a needed item that is not written on the list, such as cheese, potatoes, or canned corn. Even though a grocery list makes a trip to the grocery store more efficient and effective, this walk through the organized aisles of the grocery store can provide a review of other important, needed items. Similarly, the review of systems is intended to identify **signs** and/or **symptoms** (s/s) that the patient might be experiencing but has overlooked because these symptoms may not seem as important as the chief complaint.

THE PURPOSE OF REVIEW OF SYSTEMS

The review of systems (ROS) can be considered a guided inventory of a patient's **organ systems** for the sole purpose of determining whether the patient has been, or is currently, experiencing any pain, discomfort, or other symptom prior to the beginning of the clinical visit.

Documentation Example: Lucy's Visit to the Doctor

Consider a patient named Lucy, who drives to her physician visit. She parks her car in the parking lot and, while walking toward the clinic, trips in a pothole and sprains her ankle.

Later, while she is in the physician's visit room, she recounts her clumsy accident in the parking lot and then mentions, "That's been happening a lot lately. I am getting hurt a lot more: tripping, bumping into things, banging my hands and knees. It's really irritating."

Her physician follows her comment with a question, "Do you find that you bruise easily?"

Lucy answers, "Oh yes, some nights I swear I have two or three new bruises, and I have to work hard to remember how I got them!"

ROS information is gathered through questions and answers that focus on the recent health of the patient. For the clinical interchange between Lucy and her clinician, the following organ systems were reviewed:

Musculoskeletal: sprained ankle

Hematologic: easy bruising

---

objective referring to any method of impartially measuring patient symptoms or signs; can be repeated with a variety of patients and will provide consistent results—for example, a numeric pain scale of 1–10

subjective a patient's personalized description or individualized measurement of a specific symptom, which is unique to a specific patient and may not be able to be accurately repeated with any other patient

review of systems (ROS) a patient's verbal or written responses to questions posed by the clinician or representative of the clinic; relates to the patient's status of health and the presence or absence of any signs and/ or symptoms prior to the clinical visit

sign objective evidence of an illness, condition, or pathology that can be scientifically observed and quantified

symptom a patient's subjective report of the discomfort, pain, illness, or disease currently experienced

organ system a specific set of anatomically interconnected tissues, structures, and organs that operate together to perform a specific physiological function within the human body

physical examination
the objective clinical assessment of a patient's current health status, performed by a physician during an E/M service visit; identifies the functions, performance, and structure of the patient's physiology and health

Sometimes the ROS may be confused with the physical exam. However, the difference between the ROS and the **physical examination** is very stark: the ROS information is gathered only through questions and answers, whereas the physical exam requires the clinician to physically touch the patient.

As with the HPI, language matters when reviewing the ROS documentation. The following list provides some examples of ROS language related to patient answers:

- ... denies any ...
- ... complains of ...
- ... has noticed ...
- ... has experienced ...

Notice that each of these examples indicates a review of a pain, discomfort, or symptom. Even when the language expresses an absence of pain, discomfort, or symptom, that specific organ system has been reviewed.

THE METHODS OF ACCOMPLISHING THE REVIEW OF SYSTEMS

There are two methods of obtaining the review of systems information: either a series of questions during a face-to-face interaction between clinician and patient or written answers to ROS questions on a preprinted questionnaire, such as in ■ FIGURE 3.1.

Whereas the performing clinician must document the HPI, the ROS information may be gathered by any member of the clinical staff, for example, a registered nurse (RN), medical assistant (MA), or licensed practical nurse (LPN). This distinction makes the collection of ROS information very different from the collection of HPI information.

An Example of One of the Two ROS Gathering Formats: Face-to-Face Interview

- **Clinician:** What brings you in today?
- **Patient:** I feel nauseous, and my stomach hurts.
- **Clinician:** Has anything helped you feel better?
- **Patient:** Yeah, eating saltines and drinking Sprite has helped a little.
- **Clinician:** Have you been able to drink water?
- **Patient:** Yes, water and Sprite are fine.
- **Clinician:** Before this most recent problem, how has your digestion been? Have you had any problems with diarrhea or constipation before this?
- **Patient:** No, everything's been normal.
- **Clinician:** How has your health been otherwise—any breathing problems?
- **Patient:** No.
- **Clinician:** Any chest pains?
- **Patient:** No.
- **Clinician:** What about any problems with urination: pain, burning, itchiness?
- **Patient:** No, . . . wait . . . last week it really hurt when I went to the bathroom. I figured I wasn't drinking enough water.
- **Clinician:** How long did the pain last?
- **Patient:** I don't know that it did go away. I noticed the pain when I urinated last Thursday, but I spent all weekend in bed because I felt so nauseous, but yeah, it still hurts when I go to the bathroom.
- **Clinician:** That's really good to know; perhaps a urine sample might be a good idea. Have you noticed any dizziness or ringing in your ears?
- **Patient:** I've been dizzy every time I stand up, and my vision goes all white.
- **Clinician:** Does this happen only when you stand after you've been lying down?
- **Patient:** No, it's all the time. My friend drove me today because I've gotten so dizzy during the past few days.
- **Clinician:** Any ringing in your ears?
- **Patient:** No, just the dizziness. However, I am thirsty all the time.
- **Clinician:** Really? Have you been drinking enough fluids?
- **Patient:** No, my mouth always seems to be dry, sandy.

Patient Name:_____ DOB: _____ ____ Date of Visit: _____

What brings you in today?

Review of Systems (Please circle):

Constitutional (general):   chills   fatigue   weight loss   weight gain

other _____

Cardiovascular (heart):   chest pain   chest pressure   rapid heartbeat   high blood pressure

other _____

Respiratory (breathing):   shortness of breath   asthma   bronchitis   pneumonia

other _____

Gastrointestinal (digestion):   heartburn   diarrhea   constipation   cramping

other _____

Urinary: painful urination   blood in urine   inability to urinate   frequent urination

other _____

Genital/Reproductive: genital itchiness   painful intercourse   rash   discomfort

other _____

Women: when did your last menstrual cycle begin _____

Neurological: headache   fainting   seizures   paralysis   dizziness

other _____

Eye (vision):   glasses: Yes   No   double/blurred   vision   redness   dryness

other _____

Ears (hearing):   hearing loss   ringing   deafness   discharge   earache   tinnitus

other _____

Nose and Throat: bleeding   dryness   discharge   obstruction   pain   sinusitis   hay fever

other _____

Musculoskeletal: sprains   strains   arthritis   swollen joints   stiffness

other _____

Skin: rash   itch   changes in hair/nails   infections   sores   hives

other _____

Psychological: anxiety   sleep disturbances   depression   memory loss   confusion

other _____

Endocrine: heat or cold intolerance   weight change   diabetes   excessive sweating

other _____

Hematologic: anemia   bleeding   bruising   transfusions   fatigue

other _____

Lymphatic: enlarged glands   tender lymph nodes   slow healing after cut(s)

other _____

Allergy/Immune: multiple colds and/or infections?   auto-immune disease?

other _____

Allergy: any known allergies to a specific food, animal, pollen, medication, etc. NO   YES _____

What is the reaction to this allergen?_____

MD initial & date signifying review of systems_____

Figure 3.1 ■ Sample of preprinted review of systems questionnaire.

The clinician asks questions of the patient and listens to the answers; the clinician then documents the responses to the questions in order for a record of these questions and answers to exist. The ROS is truly performed only when the clinician has recorded the patient's responses. During the exchange in the previous example, the clinician would have documented the organ systems that were reviewed during the ROS portion of the clinical visit:

Several Examples of Medical Documentation of the ROS

Gastrointestinal: negative (**Negative** is another way of documenting that the patient reports no identifiable problems. In this example, the patient reports that, before this most recent episode of stomach pain, there were no problems with digestion and no problems with diarrhea or constipation.)

Respiratory: negative (The patient reports that, before this most recent episode of stomach pain, there were no problems with breathing or respiration.)

Cardiovascular: negative (In other words, the patient noticed no chest pain.)

Genitourinary: dysuria (Patient identified painful urination in addition to the stomach pain.)

Neurological: dizziness, vision going white (Patient identified dizziness and problems with vision in addition to the stomach pain.)

Endocrine: polydipsia, or excessive thirst (Patient identified polydipsia in addition to the stomach pain.)

In the preceding documentation example, notice that the clinician reviewed six different organ systems during the ROS. Even though three of the organ systems reviewed were causing no pain, discomfort, or symptoms, every organ system that is reviewed gives the clinician more information on the health history of the patient.

Generally, when a patient makes an initial visit to a clinic, the patient is asked to complete some paperwork. Within this packet of paperwork, the patient may encounter a form that may ask a variety of questions about the patient's health. This form contains questions specifically designed to collect information about the patient's review of systems. The patient is to answer all pertinent questions.

An Example of a Patient's Completed Form

Have you experienced any of the following?

- Heart problems (chest pain, rapid heartbeat, high blood pressure, etc.): *Yes–chest pain*
- Respiratory problems (shortness of breath, asthma, bronchitis, pneumonia, etc.): *Bronchitis last year and shortness of breath for about 4 months after that*
- Digestive problems (heartburn, diarrhea, constipation, etc.): *No problems, but I'm never hungry anymore.*
- Urinary problems (painful urination, blood in urine, inability to urinate, etc.): *No problem; urine smelly though.*
- Bone/muscle problems (sprains, strains, fractures, arthritis, etc.): *No*

When the patient has completed the ROS questionnaire, the clinician reviews the completed form. Answers to these questions provide a review of the patient's organ systems that can give important insight into the patient's health and, perhaps, the CC. Notice in the previous example that the patient has provided information about four organ systems: heart, or **cardiovascular,** system; **respiratory** system; digestive, or **gastrointestinal,** system; and urinary, or **genitourinary,** system. The clinician's signature and date ensure that a clear record exists of the clinician's personal review of the completed form.

negative in the context of a review of systems, refers to the absence of any identifiable symptoms or signs of discomfort; considered to be interchangeable with "none" or "N/A"

cardiovascular the organ system related to the flow of blood from the heart to the lungs and through the body—including, but not limited to, the function of the heart, dispersal of oxygenated blood through the entire body and the return of deoxygenated blood to the lungs for reoxygenation, veins, arteries, and capillaries

respiratory the organ system related to the inspiration of air into the lungs, the oxygenation of blood in the lungs, and the exhalation of deoxygenated air, including, but not limited to, the lobes of the lungs, the trachea (windpipe), lungs, bronchioles, and alveoli

gastrointestinal the organ system related to the intake, digestion, and processing of food and the disposal of solid waste products; includes every part of the digestive system from the lips of the mouth to the anus

genitourinary any part of the human body relating to either the production of urine—such as kidneys, ureters, and urethra—or reproduction and the male/female genitalia—such as the uterus, ovaries, and vagina for women and the testicles, penis, and prostate for men

THE ELEMENTS OF THE REVIEW OF SYSTEMS

Whether the ROS information is collected via a personal conversation or the completion of a preprinted form, the review follows the anatomical distinctions of the body:

- **Constitutional**
- **Eyes**
- **Ears /Nose/Throat/Mouth (ENT/M)**
- **Cardiovascular**
- **Respiratory**
- **Gastrointestinal**
- **Genitourinary**
- **Musculoskeletal**
- **Integumentary** (skin)
- **Neurological**
- **Psychiatric**
- **Endocrine**
- **Hematologic/Lymphatic**
- **Allergic/Immunologic**

Each of these organ systems represents part of the entire human anatomy. The clinician's education, knowledge, wisdom, and professional experience afford an intimate understanding of the concerted efforts of these organ systems, a review of which can provide important clues into a patient's state of health (see ■ FIGURE 3.2).

DISTINGUISHING BETWEEN THE HPI AND THE ROS

The HPI identifies the history of the patient's present illness or complaint, whereas the ROS identifies the patient's health just prior to the present illness; thus, different aspects of the patient's health are portrayed by the HPI and the ROS. When seen from this perspective, both the HPI and the ROS provide complementary views of the patient's story of health. However, even though these two history elements address different aspects of the patient's health, these two distinct elements of history can be easily confused because of the similarity of language. Like interlocking fingers of two different hands, the elements of each hand might look very similar but are actually very different entities. Each hand is separate and distinct, even though the fingers may look very similar.

To help distinguish between the HPI and the ROS, imagine a left hand folded together with a right hand. One hand represents the HPI, which identifies the health history of the patient's present illness, whereas the other hand represents the ROS, which reviews the status and function of the patient's health prior to the present illness. The documented directions that follow illustrate how to distinguish between the HPI and the ROS:

1. Place the palms of your hands together.
2. Spread your fingers apart slightly.
3. Turn one hand slightly forward, allowing the fingers of one hand to fill the space between the fingers of the opposite hand.
4. Bend all of the fingers onto the back of the opposite hand, thereby folding your hands.

Which Fingers Belong to Which Hand?

Notice that the fingers of both hands form an interconnected, linking pattern of fingers. To an untrained eye, it may be difficult to identify the right index finger from the left middle finger. However, with practice and skill, one can easily identify the right fingers from the left fingers. No matter how complex the interlinking pattern of fingers may seem to be, each hand still has only one index finger, one middle finger, one pinkie, and so on.

The HPI and the ROS operate in a similar fashion to that of the previous example. In some clinical notes, the ROS findings are documented in a separate section from that of the HPI. In other clinical notes, the HPI and ROS are documented concurrently, in one section of the clinical note. Each provides important information, and each requires only one finding for each element.

constitutional referring to the anatomy and functions of the human body that provide the underlying sense and experience of health—such as body temperature, weight, height, pulse rate, paleness or flushed skin—any of which factors, if disturbed, may indicate ill health or disease

eyes the anatomic organ and tissue system within the human body related to vision, such as the eyeball, conjunctiva (white of the eye and inside of eyelids), the eyelids, eyelashes, tear ducts, and optic nerve

ears the anatomic organ and system within the human body related to hearing, such as the earlobe, ear canal, and eardrum; often documented in conjunction with the nose, throat, and mouth and abbreviated as ENT/M

nose the anatomic organ and structure related to the sense of smell, including the nasal cavity and septum; often documented in conjunction with the ears, throat, and mouth and abbreviated as ENT/M

throat the anatomic junction between the nasal cavity, mouth, and upper part of the throat visible in the back of the mouth, which is called the nasopharynx; often documented in conjunction with the ears, nose, and mouth and abbreviated as ENT/M

mouth the anatomic section of the body that identifies the beginning of digestion, is necessary for production of speech, and includes the tongue, gums, teeth, palate, and taste buds; often documented in conjunction with the ears, nose, and throat and abbreviated as ENT/M

- **Constitutional symptoms (Const):** good general health lately, has been fatigued, gained weight, weight loss/gain, has felt feverish, feels chilled, sweats profusely, increased/decreased appetite, syncope, headache, sleep habits, unusual symptoms/problems, weakness, exercise intolerance, impaired ability to carry out daily functions
- **Eyes:** vision, wears glasses, contact lenses, denies any (or complains of) eye pain, diplopia, itch, dryness, redness, infection, glaucoma, eye disease or injury, discharge, spots, retinal detachment, twitching, light sensitivity, date/results of last eye exam
- **Ears/Nose/Throat and Mouth (ENT/M):**
  - **Ears:** hearing loss/ringing, deafness, discharge, earache, vertigo, tinnitus, ringing, ear infections, excessive ear wax, date/results of last hearing test, noise sensitivity
  - **Nose, Sinuses:** decrease in sense of smell, bleeding, dryness, discharge, obstruction, pain, sinusitis, hay fever, impaired ability to smell, postnasal drip, sneezing, difficulty breathing, trauma
  - **Mouth, Throat:** soreness, pain, infection, sore tongue, ulcers, lip lesions, blisters, canker sores, teeth, swallowing, hoarseness, tonsillitis, bleeding gums, swollen glands in neck, voice change, bad breath, bad taste
- **Cardiovascular (CV):** heart trouble, angina, chest pain, dyspnea (on exertion) orthopnea, paroxysmal nocturnal dyspnea, murmur, palpitations, syncope, rheumatic fever, electrocardiogram results, phlebitis, varicosities, claudication, irregular pulse, hypertension, coldness/numbness of extremities, color change in fingers or toes, leg pain when walking, hair loss on legs, shortness of breath when walking or lying flat, swelling of feet, ankles, or hands
- **Respiratory (Resp):** chronic or frequent cough, chest pain, wheezing, hemoptysis, dyspnea, sputum (color, frequency), recurrent infection, exposure to tuberculosis, asthma, cyanosis, pneumonia, pleurisy, pneumonia, cyanosis, bronchitis, shortness of breath
- **Gastrointestinal (GI):** nausea, vomiting, diarrhea, belching, dysphagia, heartburn, hematemesis, food intolerance, change in bowel habits, incontinence (bowel), constipation, laxative or enema use, hematochezia, bloating, hernia, hemorrhoids, black stools, melena, ulcers, abdominal pain, indigestion, jaundice, abdominal swelling, ascites, burning sensation in esophagus, gall bladder disease, liver disease
- **Genitourinary (GU):** hematuria, frequency, burning, polyuria, inability to start stream, incontinence (urine), renal stones, infection, urgency, dysuria, flank pain, dribbling, renal calculi, decreased or increased urine output, sexual difficulty
  - **Male:** testicle pain, penile pain
  - **Female:** pain with periods, irregular periods, vaginal discharge, # of pregnancies/miscarriages/abortions, date of last pap smear
  - **Children:** toilet training, bed wetting, voiding schedule
- **Musculoskeletal:** muscle cramps/pain, weakness, atrophy, joint pain (nature of), fracture, kyphosis, scoliosis, lordosis, back injury, limitations on walking, joint stiffness/swelling, twitching, noise with joint movement, spinal deformity, cold extremities
- **Integumentary (skin and/or breast):** rash, itch, color change, moles and changes, hair and changes, nails and changes, infections, tumor, sores, hives, skin reactions to hot/cold, presence of scars
  - **Breast:** tenderness, swelling, breast feeding, nipple discharge, varicose veins, breast pain/lump
- **Neurological:** frequent/recurring headache, syncope, seizures, vertigo, blindness, diplopia, paralysis/paresis, dizziness, tremor, coordination, pain, memory loss, tremor, ataxia, dysesthesia, tics, blackouts, numbness, tingling, convulsions, stroke, head injury
- **Psychiatric:** anxiety, sleep disturbances, depression, nervousness, suicidal thoughts, emotional instability, delusions, hallucinations, memory loss, confusion, tension, psychiatric conditions/treatment
- **Endocrine:** heat or cold intolerance, weight change, diabetes, excessive sweating, hair changes/loss, voice change, polydipsia, polyuria, goiter, thyroid disease, adrenal problems, increased appetite, thirst, hormone therapy, pigmentation changes, height changes
- **Hematologic/Lymphatic:**
  - **Hematologic:** anemia, bleeding, bruising, malignancy, lymphadenopathy, transfusions, fatigue, low platelet count, phlebitis, past transfusion
  - **Lymphatic:** enlarged glands, tender lymph nodes, slow healing after cut(s)
- **Allergic and/or Immunologic:**
  - **Immunologic:** multiple colds and/or infections, autoimmune disease, syndrome or condition
  - **Allergic:** any known allergens—such as a specific food, animal, pollen—with the patient's typical allergic reaction to that specific allergen; any known allergies to medication—such as sulfa, penicillin—with the patient's typical allergic reaction to that specific medication; unlike other elements, must be documented (both allergen and allergic reaction)

Figure 3.2 ■ Examples of review of systems documentation.

> **Documentation Example: Johnny's Irritating Cough**
>
> Johnny presents with an irritating cough, which has been bothering him for 4 months. He has tried OTC cough syrup, gargling with salt water, and drinking tea and honey, none of which has brought relief. His cough is worst in the morning and at night, but he reports no fever and no diarrhea. He denies chest pain or heart palpitations when coughing but reports that he hasn't gotten a good night's sleep since his cough began this past April. He remembers having a very stuffy nose in April and reports having postnasal drainage throughout the spring and summer.

Given that each HPI element requires only one finding and each ROS element requires only one finding, medical documentation can show the HPI and ROS working together to present a thorough illustration of the history of a patient's present illness as well as the patient's prior state of health, as shown in ■ FIGURE 3.3.

Notice in Figure 3.3 that some of the ROS findings also include some of the so-called "empathy" elements. However, in Figure 3.3 the findings selected to support the HPI and ROS elements never overlap. When reviewing the HPI and the ROS findings, the reviewer must determine which findings are the most appropriate to support the HPI and which are most appropriate to support the ROS. Most importantly, each finding should be listed once, to support either the ROS or the HPI; a finding may be listed only as many times as it appears in the medical documentation. For example, if a patient's sore throat is

---

Johnny's Irritating Cough: HPI and ROS

Johnny presents with an irritating **(quality)** cough that has been bothering him for 4 months **(duration)**. He has tried OTC cough syrup **(modifying factor)**, gargling with salt water, drinking tea and honey, and has found no relief. His cough is worst in the morning and night **(timing)**, but he reports no fever **(const)**, no diarrhea **(GI)**, denies chest pain **(resp)** or heart palpitations **(CV)** when coughing, but reports that he hasn't gotten a good night's sleep **(assoc s/s)** since his cough began this past April. He remembers having a very stuffy nose in April and reports postnasal drainage **(ENT/M)** throughout the spring and summer.

HPI
(only 1 finding per element)

Quality: (irritating cough)

Duration: (for 4 months)

Modifying factor: (cough syrup)

Timing: (worst in morning and night)

Assoc s/s: (hasn't gotten good night's sleep)

ROS
(only 1 finding per element)

Const: (no fever)

GI: (no diarrhea)

Resp: (no chest pain)

CV: (no heart palpitations)

ENT/M: (reports postnasal drainage)

Figure 3.3 ■ HPI and ROS documentation for Johnny's irritating cough.

---

musculoskeletal the organ system responsible for the structure and movement of the human body, including, but not limited to, the bones, ligaments, tendons, muscles, cartilage, and vertebral discs

integumentary the organ system that covers the exterior of the human body in protective tissues, including, but not limited to, the epidermis, dermis, sweat glands, body hair, toenails, and fingernails; also known as skin

neurological the organ system responsible for the electric impulses that control the function and movement of the human body, including, but not limited to, the brain, spinal cord, and complex network of nerves extending throughout the entire body, even into the extremities

psychiatric the organ system responsible for the emotional and mental health of the human body and the human experience

endocrine the anatomic system of organs and tissues within the human body that relates to the excretion, or release, of hormones into the blood; influences growth, metabolism, and many other functions and includes the thyroid, pancreas, adrenals, and pituitary gland

hematologic the blood and blood-producing organs, structures, and anatomy of the human body, including, but not limited to, the bone marrow and the spleen; often documented in conjunction with the lymphatic system

documented only once, the sore throat can be listed only once, either to support the HPI or the ROS, but not both. Inappropriately listing one documented finding to support both the HPI and the ROS is known as double dipping and is strongly discouraged.

Exercise 3.1 | **Identifying the ROS Elements**

Identify the ROS elements listed in the following medical documentation by underlining the finding that best supports the ROS element. The first line of each medical documentation states the chief complaint.

1. Patient has presented for sinus pressure and cough. Patient's face hurts so much that she feels she cannot open her eyes all the way. She complains of a ringing in her right ear, and the right side of her throat hurts when she swallows. She has no appetite, complains of heartburn but no nausea. Nighttime has been interrupted by frequent urination; no pain with urination but very smelly urine. Patient denies joint pain other than a sore neck. Patient complains of heavy chest pressure and pain upon coughing. Patient states she can feel her heartbeat in her head as a throbbing but denies any heart palpitations.

Patient is dizzy upon standing and reports she has spent 3 days lying down due to the discomfort.

2. Patient presents for abdominal pain and diarrhea. Patient denies bloody stools and nausea. Patient states his urine is dark and odorous but denies painful urination. Patient complains of midback pain from last week, with some achy muscles; however, denies joint pain. Patient felt dizzy last week after walking upstairs; he felt out of breath and states his heartbeat felt very "heavy" at the top of the stairs. Patient denies any tingling in hands or feet, no problem with vision, and no unexplained bruises.

3. Patient presents for sprained ankle. Patient denies any other joint pain other than his right ankle. Denies double vision or dizziness. No chest pain or shortness of breath.

---

lymphatic the organ system responsible for the production, flow, and processing of lymphatic fluid, a clear fluid that contains white blood cells, circulates through the human body in lymphatic vessels, and is filtered by lymph nodes; significantly impacts a patient's immunity, as well as several other elements of health; often documented in conjunction with the hematologic system

allergic the internal, physiologic reaction to substances or factors that cause a heightened sensitivity within the human body; often documented in conjunction with the immunologic system

THE FOUR LEVELS OF THE REVIEW OF SYSTEMS

There are four different levels of documenting the ROS: none (otherwise known as N/A), pertinent, extended, and complete.

None (N/A)

At this level no systems were reviewed during the clinical visit. There is no documentation of any questions asked or answers given, no questionnaire completed and reviewed. Although this is not very common, it is very important for the proper level of documentation to be noted. When no systems have been reviewed, then **none (N/A)** is the appropriate ROS level (see ■ FIGURE 3-4).

> **Example of Documentation Supporting None (N/A) ROS**
>
> **Johnny's Irritating Cough**
>
> Johnny presents with a cough that has bothered him for 3 months.
>
> No review of systems documented; only the chief complaint (cough) and one HPI element (duration: 3 months) have been documented.
>
> The absence of any ROS elements supports this ROS level: none (N/A).

History of Present Illness Location, severity, timing, mod fact, quality, duration, context, assoc s/s	Brief (1)	Brief (2–3)	Ext. (4+, or 3 chronic problems)	Ext. (4+, or 3 chronic problems)
Review of Systems Constitutional, ENT/M, respiratory, GU, skin/breast, endocrine, all/imm, eyes, CV, GI, musculoskeletal, psychiatric, neurologic, hem/lymph	None	Pert. (1 system)	Extended (2–9 systems)	Complete (10+ systems)

Figure 3.4 ■ Content of service element: review of systems.

Pertinent (1 System)

A **pertinent** ROS level reflects a documented review of only one system and can be found in the history section of the clinical note, as in the following example:

Example of Documentation Supporting Pertinent ROS

Johnny's Irritating Cough

Johnny presents with a cough that has bothered him for 3 months. No chest pain when coughing.

One ROS element: Respiratory—no chest pain when coughing

One ROS element supports this ROS level: pertinent.

Extended (2–9 Systems)

An **extended** ROS reflects the documented review of at least two systems and no more than nine systems in the history section of the clinical note, as in the following example:

Example of Documentation Supporting Extended ROS

Johnny's Irritating Cough

Johnny presents with a cough, which has bothered him for 3 months. No chest pain or dizziness when coughing. Pt denies fever, abdominal pain, joint pains, sinus pressure, and heart palpitations.

Six ROS elements:

- *Respiratory*—no chest pain when coughing
- *Constitutional*—denies fever
- *Gastrointestinal*—denies abdominal pain
- *Musculoskeletal*—denies joint pains
- *ENT/M*—denies sinus pressure
- *Cardiovascular*—denies heart palpitations

Even though this patient didn't experience dizziness, it's useful to make a point about dizziness and other such generalized symptoms, which may be indications of a wide variety of organ involvement. For example, a number of different factors can cause dizziness: inner ear problems, lack of blood flow to the brain, neurologic problems, or general lightheadedness. Since dizziness is such a generalized symptom with broad origins, this finding should be used to support an ROS element appropriate to the chief complaint. Individuals with no clinical training should not claim that a finding supports an ROS element without documented evidence; for instance, this medical documentation includes no support of a neurologic problem, inner ear problems, or cardiovascular issues of the brain.

Six ROS elements support this ROS level: extended.

Complete (10–14 Systems)

A **complete** ROS reflects a documented review of 10–14 systems in the history section of the clinical note, as shown in the following example:

Example of Documentation Supporting Complete ROS

Johnny's Irritating Cough

Johnny presents with a cough, which has bothered him for 3 months. No chest pain or dizziness when coughing. Pt denies fever, abdominal pain, joint pains, sinus pressure, heart palpitations, and painful urination. Pt is allergic to shellfish with resultant hives upon exposure. Pt denies any rash, itching, or unusual redness of skin. Pt denies blurred vision, although complains of "fuzzy eyeballs."

continued

---

immunologic pertaining to the physiological reaction of a patient's immunity and any reactions to external or internal factors, pathologies, or substances; often documented in conjunction with the allergic system

none (or N/A) the level of review of systems that includes no organ systems in the medical documentation

pertinent the level of review of systems that includes one organ system in the medical documentation

extended the level of review of systems that includes between two and nine organ systems in the medical documentation

complete the level of review of systems that includes 10 or more organ systems in the medical documentation

Ten ROS elements:

- *Respiratory*—no chest pain when coughing
- *Constitutional*—denies fever
- *Gastrointestinal*—denies abdominal pain
- *Musculoskeletal*—denies joint pains
- *ENT/M*—denies sinus pressure
- *Cardiovascular*—denies heart palpitations
- *Genitourinary*—denies painful urination
- *Allergic/Immunologic*—allergic to shellfish with hives as reaction
- *Integumentary (skin)*—denies rash, itching, or unusual redness
- *Eyes*—denies blurred vision, although "fuzzy eyeballs"

Ten ROS elements support this ROS level: complete.

Special Circumstance for a Complete ROS   There may be circumstances during E/M service visits when a clinician reviews all 14 ROS elements with the patient in order to gain a more in-depth illustration of the prior health status of the patient. In the event that the patient reports a sign or symptom for each one of the 14 organ systems inventoried, the clinician should document each of the appropriate responses in order to provide a thorough documentation of the patient's history. However, there may be times when the patient denies any sign or symptom for some of the organ systems reviewed. In order to facilitate thorough documentation, physicians and other performing clinicians may utilize one of several time-saving expressions in order to convey the absence of signs or symptoms. Each of these time-saving expressions reflects a complete review of all 14 organ systems, for example:

- "The remainder of the ROS is unremarkable." This statement indicates that the remaining ROS revealed nothing worthy of clinical note and had no bearing on the patient's chief complaint or current pathology.
- "The remainder of the ROS is negative in detail." This statement indicates that the patient has denied any sign or symptom in the remaining ROS organ systems.

There is something that each person who reads medical documentation should keep paramount in his or her mind: the medical documentation should make sense and be logical. For instance, if a healthy 8-year-old child presents to a physician's clinic for a sprained ankle, it would be inappropriate for the ROS to include a review of the respiratory, neurologic, eye, and genitourinary systems unless the medical documentation supports a reason for review of these systems.

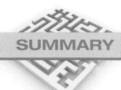

SUMMARY

- The review of systems can be considered a guided inventory of the patient's organ systems for the sole purpose of determining whether the patient has been, or is currently, experiencing any pain, discomfort, or other symptoms prior to the beginning of the clinical visit. The ROS assists the clinician in identifying any other health issues, concerns, symptoms, or complaints that may be related to the chief complaint or may provide insight into the nature of the presenting problem.
- There are two methods of collecting the ROS information:
  - The patient may be interviewed by any member of the clinical staff: registered nurse (RN), medical assistant (MA), licensed practical nurse (LPN). This interview should include questions from the clinician as well as the patient's responses regarding the patient's review of systems. The collection of ROS information is very different

from the collection of HPI information, since only the performing physician may collect the HPI information.
  - The patient may complete a preprinted questionnaire that lists the ROS inventory in a standardized series of questions. In order to document a thorough review of the patient's responses on this preprinted questionnaire, the performing physician must sign and date the form.
- The ROS is composed of 14 organ systems: constitutional, eyes, ears/nose/throat/mouth, cardiovascular, respiratory, gastrointestinal, genitourinary, musculoskeletal, integumentary (skin), neurological, psychiatric, endocrine, hematologic/lymphatic, and allergic/immunologic.
- When reviewing the HPI and the ROS findings, the reviewer must determine which findings are most appropriate to support the HPI and which are most appropriate to support the

ROS element. A finding from the history section of the medical documentation may be listed only as many times as it is documented; the findings selected to support the HPI and ROS elements never overlap. The ROS addresses the previous state of the patient's health, whereas the HPI describes the chief complaint.

- There are four levels of the ROS: none (N/A), which includes no documentation of any ROS element; pertinent, which includes the documentation of only 1 ROS element; extended, which supports the documentation of between 2 and 9 ROS elements; and complete, which supports the documentation of between 10 and 14 ROS elements.

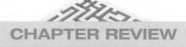

CHAPTER REVIEW

Multiple Choice

Choose the letter that best answers each question or completes each statement.

1. What does the acronym ROS mean?
   a. Review of symptoms
   b. Random order of systems
   c. Review of systems
   d. Redundancy of operative systems

2. Which of the following phrases best defines the ROS?
   a. Descriptive words or phrases that further explain the patient's chief complaint
   b. An inventory of the patient's organ systems that helps identify the state of the patient's health prior to the clinical visit
   c. The specific sign, symptom, or illness for which the patient presents to the clinician
   d. The system or protocol to which every clinician must adhere during a clinical visit with a patient

3. What distinguishes the ROS from the HPI?
   a. The HPI describes events in the patient's life, whereas the ROS addresses the current chief complaint.
   b. The HPI describes the patient's previous medical history, whereas the ROS describes only the treatments or medications the patient has taken in an attempt to alleviate the sign, symptom, or illness.
   c. The HPI describes only the onset of the chief complaint, whereas the ROS addresses only the reason for the clinical visit.
   d. The HPI describes the chief complaint, whereas the ROS describes the state of the patient's health before the clinical visit.

4. How many organ systems must be reviewed in the documentation to support an ROS level of extended?
   a. One
   b. Between two and nine
   c. Ten or more
   d. None

5. How many organ systems must be reviewed in the documentation to support an ROS level of complete?
   a. Between two and nine

   b. Ten or more
   c. None
   d. One

6. How many organ systems must be reviewed in the documentation to support an ROS level of pertinent?
   a. Ten or more
   b. Between two and nine
   c. One
   d. None

7. How many organ systems must be reviewed in the documentation to support an ROS level of none, or N/A?
   a. Ten or more
   b. Between two and nine
   c. One
   d. None

8. Which of the following phrases is not an appropriate example of ROS language?
   a. Patient denies . . .
   b. Patient complains of . . .
   c. Patient has experienced . . .
   d. Patient will be . . .

9. What are the levels of ROS?
   a. Brief, extended
   b. None (N/A), pertinent, extended, and complete
   c. Low, many, lots
   d. Regardless of how many organ systems are documented, the level is always extended.

10. When the physician performing the E/M service reviews the completed ROS questionnaire, that physician should
    a. give the reviewed form back to the patient to ensure patient privacy.
    b. sign and date the completed questionnaire, documenting that the performing physician has read the patient's answers.
    c. identify any areas of inconsistency between the patient's verbal and written answers to ensure that the correct patient is sitting in the room.
    d. destroy the completed questionnaire to ensure patient privacy.

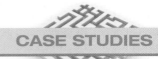

CASE STUDIES

Case Study 3-1

Read the following medical documentation, and then answer the questions that follow.

Patient presents with sharp upper abdominal pain that frequently burns. Pain has been present since November, about 5 months. Pain rated 7–8/10 between meals, and pain is constant. Antacids have provided some relief for several months, but pain has increased significantly during the past few weeks. Appetite greatly reduced, and patient reports feeling full after only a few bites of food. Patient denies any history of chest pain, heart palpitations, bloody diarrhea, or joint pain. The remainder of the ROS is negative in detail.

1. Which organ system is reviewed in the documented phrase "patient denies . . . heart palpitations"?
   a. Respiratory
   b. Musculoskeletal
   c. Cardiovascular
   d. Genitourinary

2. Which organ system is reviewed in the documented phrase "patient denies . . . bloody diarrhea"?
   a. Cardiovascular
   b. Gastrointestinal
   c. Respiratory
   d. Genitourinary

3. Which organ system is reviewed in the documented phrase "patient denies . . . joint pain"?
   a. Neurologic
   b. Musculoskeletal
   c. Endocrine
   d. Integumentary

4. The sentence "the remainder of the ROS is negative in detail" supports which level of ROS?
   a. None (N/A)
   b. Complete
   c. Pertinent
   d. Extended

Case Study 3-2

Read the following medical documentation, identify the documented ROS finding next to the ROS element listed, and select the appropriate ROS level.

Complaint: Franklin is well-known to me and presents for sharp left flank pain over the past 2 days, with dark-colored urine. Franklin is accompanied by his wife, Mary. Three weeks ago, Franklin was involved in a minor ATV accident. Directly after the accident, Franklin's primary complaint involved injuries to his chin and chest, both of which suffered contusions and lacerations. At the subsequent visit 1 week after the accident, both chin and chest contusions and lacerations were healing well; however, his wife reported that Franklin was holding his abdomen carefully when he rose from a sitting position, and Franklin admits today that his abdominal pain has gradually moved to his left flank and increased in intensity. Two days ago, Franklin tripped on the computer cords in his home office, and his left flank pain became extreme in severity. Pain was not relieved after Excedrin and a hot bath. This morning Franklin vomited once, and his temperature was elevated to 101.6°F. Other than Excedrin, Franklin has taken no medications.

The contusions and lacerations Franklin sustained in the ATV accident have healed appropriately. Other than his abdominal and flank pain and fever, Franklin has been in good health. He reports no loss of memory or dizziness since the accident and denies any joint, muscle, or bone pain. No shortness of breath reported, and patient denies any chest pain, heart palpitations, or tingling in arms or fingers. Bowel movements have been normal, regular, and painless. Franklin reports his painful urination has caused him to postpone urination at times; however, postponing urination does not relieve his flank pain or painful urination. Other than his fever this morning and one episode of vomiting, Franklin denies chills, night sweats, or any reported fever since the ATV accident.

Constitutional _____

Eyes _____

Ears, Nose, Mouth, Throat _____

Cardiovascular _____

Respiratory _____

Gastrointestinal _____

Genitourinary _____

Musculoskeletal _____

Integumentary (skin) _____

Neurological _____

Psychiatric _____

Hematologic/Lymphatic _____

Allergic/Immunologic _____

Circle the appropriate level for the documented ROS:

None (N/A)
Pertinent
Extended
Complete

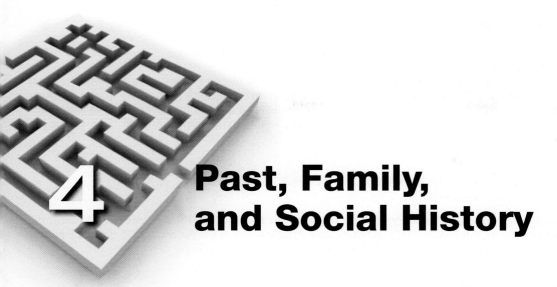

4 Past, Family, and Social History

Learning Objectives

After completing this chapter, you should be able to do the following:

- Spell and define the key terms and abbreviations presented in this chapter
- Identify the three elements of the past, family, and social history
- Distinguish the different methods of collecting the past, family, and social history
- List and define the two levels of past, family, and social history
- Recognize how the levels of past, family, and social history are impacted by the patient's status as a new or established patient

Key Terms

differential diagnosis

established patient complete PFSH

established patient pertinent PFSH

family history

hereditary

new patient complete PFSH

new patient pertinent PFSH

past, family, and social history (PFSH)

past history

plan of care

social history

Abbreviations

PFSH past, family, and social history

INTRODUCTION

Considered the first component of the E/M service, history pertains to the patient's medical background, specifically as it relates to the reason for the patient's current visit. The history component includes the patient's personal description of the current problem, as well as a review of the patient's previous health and the circumstances of the patient's life that may or may not be related to the current problem. Four different elements make up the history component: chief complaint, history of present illness, review of systems, and past, family, and social history. This chapter addresses one of the elements of history—past, family, and social history—which offers the clinician a holistic understanding of the patient's life before the E/M service visit.

Three different elements constitute the story of health for almost every human being: previous medical events or illnesses, the impact of genetic heredity and traits on the person's physical health, and the work, recreational, or other physical activities in which the individual chooses to engage. Each of these three elements influences the patient's healthcare story in a different way, and the knowledge of these three elements can help to complete that story.

THE MEANING OF PAST, FAMILY, AND SOCIAL HISTORY

Past, family, and social history (PFSH) illustrates the background of the patient's life. Whereas the other two history components, HPI and ROS, look into the health of the patient, PFSH allows the patient to be seen as a complex person with different facets providing a deeper sense of the individual.

Past History

past, family, and social history (PFSH) the third element of history, which is composed of the patient's past medical history, the medical history of the patient's family, and the patient's day-to-day social activities

past history the patient's past medical history that may be pertinent to the chief complaint; includes any childhood illnesses, surgeries or procedures, injuries, and prescribed medications or treatments

differential diagnosis the process by which a physician identifies a diagnosis through the elimination of different pathologies

plan of care the method of treatment, maintenance of health, or plan of therapy prescribed by the physician for the patient's symptoms, condition, diagnosis, or disease

In a global context, the word *past* may refer to the previous year or one thousand years ago; it provides a context for literature, socioeconomic developments, and political events of a specific country or section of the globe. In the life of a human being, the word *past* refers to the various events and circumstances of a person's life, beginning at birth, that have influenced or affected his or her current life. Within the context of an E/M service visit, *past* refers to the patient's **past history** of a medical nature, which includes childhood illnesses, previous surgeries or procedures, injuries, or prescribed medications or treatments the patient has used or undergone. Any of these findings may provide a context for the patient's chief complaint, **differential diagnosis**, or potential **plan of care**. Past medical events may or may not be related to a current condition; however, knowledge of a patient's past medical history improves communication between the clinician and the patient and can empower the clinician with a more holistic understanding of the patient. For example, a patient's past medical history of frequent lung infections in childhood bears no relevance to the chief complaint of a sprained ankle. However, the physician's education, knowledge, and experience allow the physician to discern the pertinence of past medical history.

The Difference between Past History and the Review of Systems   One of the most common causes of confusion about the past history is the difference between the ROS and the past history. After all, the ROS is an inventory of the patient's organ systems prior to the E/M service visit, which would be considered the past. However, the past history identifies any medical condition, illness, injury, or treatment that may be significant to the chief complaint, which is very different from an inventory of the patient's organ systems prior to the E/M service visit.

Documentation Example: A 9-Year-Old's Abdominal Pain

Consider a 9-year-old patient who presents with sharp, stabbing, periumbilical abdominal pain, which he states is a 9/10 on a pain scale. Mother and patient deny any intestinal illnesses in the family; no report of recent abdominal injury. Mother states that patient had appendectomy at age 5.

Notice in the previous example that "deny any intestinal illness in the family; no report of recent abdominal injury" represents an inventory of the gastrointestinal system, whereas the report of an appendectomy 4 years prior addresses the past medical surgery that is pertinent to the chief complaint.

Examples of Phrases That Support Past History

Surgeries:

* Hernia repair 25 years ago
* Tonsillectomy at age 6
* Appendectomy at age 14

Illnesses:

- Lifelong history of asthma
- Whooping cough at 10 months of age, followed by frequent lung infections until age 5

Injuries:

- Fractured femur 10 years ago
- Concussion at age 19, as a result of automobile accident
- Left ulna fractured at age 7

Prescribed medications:

- List of medications currently taken
- Identification of vaccination status
  - Vaccinations up-to-date
  - Vaccinations withheld by parent/guardian

Prescribed treatments:

- Chemotherapy
- Radiation therapy
- Physical therapy for 3 months after injury

Family History

The patient's **family history** addresses the medical history of the patient's immediate family, which may or may not be relevant to the health of the patient. Family history reviews any **hereditary** and/or lifestyle health factors of the patient's immediate family that could provide further insight into the physiology of the patient and any cause of the patient's current condition. Any medical history of these immediate family members—such as parents, siblings, and even grandparents—may inform the clinician's understanding of the patient's chief complaint. Even though the informational findings generated by family history questions tend to be hereditary in nature, some circumstances warrant a closer look at family history, such as a history of alcohol abuse or a situation involving domestic abuse, especially when this history is relevant to the chief complaint, such as depression, anxiety, or even certain physical ailments.

Regardless of where any person travels or resides in the world, the genetics of a person does not change. Family history recognizes that "you can choose your friends, but you can't choose your genetics" and provides a forum for highlighting any hereditary or familial influence on the patient's chief complaint.

family history the medical history of the patient's immediate family, which may or may not be relevant to the health of the patient; any hereditary and/or lifestyle health factors of the patient's immediate family that could provide further insight into the physiology of the patient and any cause of the patient's current condition

hereditary referring to an inherited condition, disease, or syndrome that is passed through bloodlines, or from parent to offspring or extended relative to descendant, such as grandparent to grandchild

Examples of Phrases That Support Family History

These examples relate to heredity:

- Mother died of Parkinson's disease.
- Brother has adult-onset diabetes.
- Sister is battling breast cancer.
- Brother lives in nearby memory-care assisted living.
- Grandmother lost sight due to diabetic retinopathy.

The following examples relate to nonhereditary factors:

- Grandfather has COPD (chronic obstructive pulmonary disease).
- Father is recovering alcoholic now but not during patient's childhood.
- Brother committed suicide 2 years ago.
- Sister was diagnosed with alcoholic liver disease.

Social History

The ancient Greek philosopher Aristotle stated, "Man is a social animal." Without delving into any socioeconomic or philosophical considerations, this quote should stand as a reminder that every patient is more than the chief complaint that brought him or her to the physician. Every patient is ultimately a person who lives a life full of interactions with co-workers, friends, entertaining pursuits, physical activity, and many other aspects of life that are integral to and fulfill the patient's life. Although the patient may be ill and have no energy or desire to engage in these social interactions or activities right now, these social elements may affect the patient's health in unexpected ways and are important considerations for the performing physician.

social history the patient's social activities, including employment or school attendance; use of cigarettes, cigars, or other tobacco; the amount of physical activity in which the patient regularly engages; alcohol consumption; sports activities; sexual activity; use of any illicit drugs or substances; and the patient's living situation

The patient's **social history** addresses the patient's social activities. These social elements or activities could include the patient's job or occupation; use of cigarettes, cigars, or other tobacco; the amount of physical activity in which the patient regularly engages; alcohol consumption; sports activities; sexual activity; use of any illicit drugs or substances; and the patient's living situation. If the patient is under 18 years of age, the patient's social history would also include school attendance, grade, and any extracurricular activities.

The social interaction in which the patient engages has an effect on his or her life and health in unexpected ways. The nature of the patient's work bears a certain influence; for example, night shifts in a manufacturing company have a different effect on a patient than a typical 8–5 office job does. Similarly, use of alcohol and/or tobacco could change the focus of a clinician's perspective on a patient's chief complaint; the fact that a patient with a persistent cough happens to live with a smoker presents a very different consideration from that of a patient with a persistent cough who does not. Likewise, a patient's overall living situation informs the clinician of the environment in which the patient currently lives; a patient who has recently moved into the area would be experiencing a different set of stressors than a patient who has lived in the area for 35 years.

As with past history and family history, the pertinence of the finding should be the guiding factor in the documentation. In other words, common sense is important with regard to social history: it would be inappropriate to document that a 2-year-old child is not currently married. However, it may be appropriate to document that a 2-year-old child is currently living with its father while its mother is on military duty overseas because this living situation impacts a 2-year-old patient in a unique way.

Examples of Phrases That Support Social History

- Works two jobs
- Smokes four cigarettes a day
- Drinks approximately one glass of wine daily
- Heavy coffee drinker
- Has missed varsity volleyball practice because of illness
- Sexually active
- Lives with grandmother, mother, and stepfather
- Travels extensively for work
- Attends church regularly, although not since illness began
- Admits use of marijuana
- Recently moved to area and started new job
- Divorced for 3 years, abusive relationship with former spouse

---

THE METHODS OF COLLECTING THE PAST, FAMILY, AND SOCIAL HISTORY

As with the ROS, there are two methods of obtaining the PFSH information: either a series of questions during a face-to-face interaction between clinician and patient or written answers to specific questions about the patient's past medical history, family medical history, and social history on a preprinted questionnaire, such as in ■ FIGURE 4.1.

One of the most important aspects of the PFSH is the method of documentation; however, the collection of the PFSH is similar to that of the ROS. Whereas the performing clinician must document the HPI, the PFSH information, like the ROS, may be gathered by any member of the clinical staff, such as an RN, MA, or LPN.

The clinician asks questions of the patient, listens to the answers, and then documents the responses to the questions. This means that the PFSH is truly performed only when the clinician has recorded the patient's responses. Therefore, during the following exchange, the clinician must document any PFSH information that has been reviewed during this portion of the clinical visit.

Patient Name: _____ **DOB:** _____ ____ **Date of Visit:** _____

Reason for visit:

Past Medical History (Please circle all that apply):

Eyes: Glaucoma   LASIX   Other _____

Neurologic: Seizures   ADD/Hyperactivity   Other _____

Endocrine (gland):   Diabetes   Adrenal Disease   Other _____

Pulmonary (breathing):   Asthma/Wheezing   Pneumonia   Other _____

Cardiac (heart):   High Blood Pressure   Congenital Heart Disease Other _____

Gastrointestinal: Crohn's/UC   GE Reflux   Other _____

Infections: Hepatitis   Tuberculosis (Tb)   Other _____

Surgeries: _____

Injuries:_____

Female: Pregnancies _____   Surgeries _____   Male: Prostate problems _____   Surgeries _____

Family Medical History:

History of Cancer: No   Yes: Relation _____

Respiratory/Lung Diseases: No   Yes: Relation _____

Cardiovascular/Heart Disease: No   Yes: Relation _____

Diabetes: No   Yes: Relation _____   Bleeding disorders: No   Yes: Relation_____

Other: _____

Social History:

Currently working: No   Yes: Where?_____

In school: No   Yes: Where/year in school? _____

Number of people living in home: _____

Activities/Interests:_____

    Alcohol/tobacco/drugs: Yes   No

    Sexually active: Yes   No

    Recent travel: _____

    Other _____

MD Notes: _____

_____

MD Initial & Date signifying Review of PFSH _____

Figure 4.1 ■ Preprinted past, family, and social history questionnaire.

- **Clinician:** What brings you in today?
- **Patient:** I feel nauseous, and my tummy hurts.
- **Clinician:** Where does your tummy hurt?
- **Patient:** Right here . . . just below my belly button.
- **Clinician:** How much does your tummy hurt?
- **Patient:** This weekend my belly hurt so much I couldn't get out of bed.
- **Clinician:** How bad was your nausea?
- **Patient:** I never threw up, but I wished I had . . . maybe it might have helped.
- **Clinician:** How long has your tummy hurt?
- **Patient:** All weekend.
- **Clinician:** Did anything happen last week, maybe on Thursday or Friday? Were you around anyone who was sick?
- **Patient:** No, no one was sick at the office all week, and there was a potluck party at work Friday afternoon.
- **Clinician:** What kind of food was at the potluck party?
- **Patient:** Chips and this really good spinach dip . . .
- **Clinician:** Do you know who made the dip?
- **Patient:** No one made it; it came from the grocery store. Come to think of it, Judy went crazy over the dip, and she went home early throwing up.
- **Clinician:** Have you been drinking enough fluids?
- **Patient:** No, my mouth always seems to be dry, sandy.
- **Clinician:** Is there any history of diabetes in your family?
- **Patient:** My grandfather, my mom's dad, has diabetes, but it was diagnosed when he was 60. He's 75 now, and he's good; does that count?
- **Clinician:** That sounds like type II diabetes, and that counts. Anyone else in your family?
- **Patient:** No.
- **Clinician:** What about any intestinal issues in your family?
- **Patient:** My dad's mom died of colon cancer 2 years ago.
- **Clinician:** I'm sorry to hear that.
- **Patient:** Thanks. My mom's mom has diving-tickle-itis.
- **Clinician:** Diverticulitis?
- **Patient:** Yes, that's it. Diverticulitis. I don't know what it is, but she gets pretty sick every once in a while, like just before my grandpa was diagnosed with diabetes.
- **Clinician:** Have you had any history of intestinal problems?
- **Patient:** I had an ulcer when I was in college, 10 years ago, but I transferred to a different school, and between the change and the antacids the doc gave me, it went away in a couple months.
- **Clinician:** Do you smoke?
- **Patient:** No, not any more. I smoked when I was in college, but my ulcer put a stop to that.
- **Clinician:** Do you drink alcohol?
- **Patient:** A little; maybe one-beer-on-a-weekend type of thing.

> **Examples of Medical Documentation of PFSH**
>
> **Past medical history:** ulcer during college years, 10 years ago, which resolved after lifestyle change and antacid use
>
> **Family medical history:** maternal grandmother's diverticulitis; paternal grandmother died of colon cancer; paternal grandfather's type II diabetes
>
> **Social history:** patient works; potluck lunch the day prior to the patient's illness; drinks approximately one beer a week; does not smoke anymore but did years ago

Notice in the medical documentation example that the clinician reviewed all three of the past, family, and social histories during this interchange, and each provided insight into the patient's life.

Generally, on an initial visit to a clinic, a patient is asked to complete some paperwork. Within this packet of paperwork, the patient may encounter a form that asks a variety of questions about the patient's life. Depending on the focus of the healthcare setting, different kinds of questions may be asked. For instance, a gerontology clinic may not ask questions about school attendance, whereas in a pediatric clinic this question may be pertinent. Regardless of the nature or specialty of the clinical setting, however, the preprinted questionnaire will address the patient's past medical history, family medical history, and any social history that may be pertinent to the patient's health, as shown in ■ FIGURE 4.2.

The patient reads the questions and answers any that are pertinent, as shown in ■ FIGURE 4.3.

Past History *Have you experienced any of the following?*

    Injuries:

    Significant illnesses:

    Surgery or anesthesia:

    Medications:

    Allergies:

    Immunizations:

Family History *Has any member of your immediate family experienced any of the following?*

    Disease similar to problem you're currently encountering:

    Bleeding disorder:

Social History *To help us understand your current complaint, please share the following:*

    Are you currently working?   No   Yes

        If yes, does your job require physical labor?

    Activities/hobbies:

    Do you drink alcohol?   No   Yes

        (If yes, identify the number of drinks per week: 0-1   2-3   4+)

    Do you smoke tobacco?   No   Yes

        (If yes, identify the number of packs per week: 0   1-2   3+)

    How many people reside in your home?

    Recent travel:

Figure 4.2 ■ PFSH gathering format: sample from a preprinted questionnaire.

Past History *Have you experienced any of the following?*

    Injuries: *No*

    Significant illnesses: *Ulcer 10 years prior; antacids helped.*

    Surgery or anesthesia: *No*

    Medications: *prescription antacid for ulcer*

    Allergies: *No*

    Immunizations: *No*

Family History *Has any member of your immediate family experienced any of the following?*

    Disease similar to problem you're currently encountering: *grandmother—colon cancer (died); grandmother–diving-tickle-itis; grandfather—diabetes (adult)*

    Bleeding disorder: *No*

Social History *To help us understand your current complaint, please share the following:*

    Are you currently working?   No   *Yes*

    If yes, does your job require physical labor?   *No*

    Activities/hobbies: *knitting; watching roller derby*

    Do you drink alcohol?   No   *Yes*

    (If yes, identify the number of drinks per week: *0-1*   2-3   4+)

    Do you smoke tobacco?   *No*   Yes **(used to 10+ years ago)**

    (If yes, identify the number of packs per week: 0   1-2   3+)

    How many people reside in your home?   *only me*

    Recent travel: *None*

Figure 4.3 ■ PFSH gathering format: sample from a completed preprinted questionnaire.

After the patient has completed the questionnaire, the clinician reviews the form. Answers to these questions offer a more holistic insight into the patient's life and more detail about how his or her lifestyle, environment, and heredity could influence the chief complaint. The clinician who reviews the completed PFSH answers written by the patient should sign and date the reviewed form to document that he or she has read the patient's answers, thus verifying that the clinician personally reviewed the patient's responses on that specific date. As with the ROS responses, the clinician's signature and date ensures that a clear record exists of the clinician's personal review of the completed prewritten form.

Exercise 3.1   **Identifying the PFSH Elements**

Identify the PFSH elements in the following medical documentation by underlining the finding that supports the past, family or social elements. The first line of each medical documentation states the chief complaint.

1. Patient has presented for sinus pressure and cough.

   Patient is dizzy upon standing and reports she has spent 3 days lying down because of discomfort. No report of sick contact at work; however, her husband had the flu last month. Neither patient nor husband smokes.

2. Patient presents for abdominal pain and diarrhea.

   Patient denies any tingling in hands or feet, no problem with vision, no unexplained bruises. Patient is 12th grader at Hardy Oaks High School and active on football team. Recently heavily tackled with sharp abdominal pain; patient reports domestic incident between parents at practice. Patient's primary residence is with father, with joint custody with mother. Per patient, visitation with mother is occasional with stressful transitions. Patient denies tobacco use; denies alcohol use when living with father.

3. Patient presents for lower back pain.

   Patient denies tobacco or alcohol use. Pain has not affected patient's work as a fifth-grade teacher.

LEVELS OF THE PAST, FAMILY, AND SOCIAL HISTORY

A patient's past medical history does not change from year to year; it can only be added to. The fractured tibia at age 7 will always remain a part of the patient's past medical history, regardless of how the patient's health may change over time. Likewise, the patient's family medical history does not change: the grandmother who fought and conquered breast cancer will remain an inspiration to the patient; the grandmother's medical history will not change depending on the patient's health. Of the three PFSH elements, only social history is likely to change over the course of a patient's life: the patient who did smoke might quit; the patient who used to play football in high school may choose not to play any team sports in later life. Because of these differences, the requirements for the PFSH levels are more complex than the levels for the HPI or the ROS.

There are just two levels of the PFSH: pertinent and complete; however, the documentation requirements for both are complicated by another factor—the clinician's familiarity with the patient. For instance, a patient's very first E/M service visit in a physician's clinic office is considered a new patient visit. During this new patient visit, the physician must learn about the patient's past, family, and social histories in order to gain an in-depth understanding of the PFSH factors in the patient's life. When that same patient returns to the physician's clinic 1 year later, that subsequent visit is known as an established patient visit. During this established patient visit, the patient's past and family histories will not have changed much, and the physician will not need to acquire as much information for a thorough documentation of the patient's PFSH. The following example shows the impact of patient type on the documentation requirements for a complete PFSH.

Examples of The Two Types of Complete PFSH

New Patient Complete PFSH

For the new patient complete PFSH, at least one finding supporting each of the three PFSH elements must be documented for the following categories of E/M service:

- Office or other outpatient service: new patient
- Hospital observation service
- Hospital inpatient service, initial care
- Consultation
- Comprehensive nursing facility assessment
- Domiciliary care: new patient
- Home care: new patient

Established Patient Complete PFSH

For the established patient complete PFSH, at least one finding supporting two of the three PFSH elements must be documented for the following categories of E/M services:

- Office or other outpatient service: established patient
- Emergency department
- Domiciliary care: established patient
- Home care: established patient

Thorough documentation is essential to determine whether a visit is categorized as that of an established or a new patient. Although a healthcare facility should have a specific protocol for identifying a patient's status, it is still prudent for the clinician to accept some responsibility for ensuring the documentation of the patient's status.

Examples of Clinical Documentation Identifying New and Established Patients

Examples of New Patient Documentation

- Patient has been referred to me . . .
- This new patient presents . . .
- Patient is new to the area . . .
- Patient has not received any health care in the past 10 years . . .

Examples of Established Patient Documentation

- Patient is well known to me . . .
- Patient is a long-time patient of my partner Dr. G . . .
- Patient's condition has not improved since last week . . .
- Patient's condition has improved since last year's visit . . .

Since the documentation requirements for the PFSH levels include the specification of the type of E/M visit, an inclusive representation of the PFSH levels makes these distinctions: new patient pertinent and new patient complete, as well as established patient pertinent and established patient complete.

NEW PATIENT PFSH

As shown in the previous example, the phrase "new patient" refers to an initial visit between a patient and physician, that is, a visit during which the physician must become familiar with not only the patient's current complaint, but also the patient's past medical history, any pertinent hereditary concerns, and the patient's social history. By virtue of the unfamiliarity of a new patient, more thorough documentation is required for the PFSH, as shown in ■ FIGURE 4.4.

History of Present Illness Location, severity, timing, mod fact, quality, duration, context, assoc s/s	Brief (1)	Brief (2–3)	Ext. (4+, or 3 chronic problems)	Ext. (4+, or 3 chronic problems)
Review of Systems Constitutional, ENT/M respiratory, GU, skin/breast, endocrine, all/imm, eyes, CV, GI, musculoskeletal, psychiatric, neurologic, hem/lymph	None	Pert. (1 system)	Extended (2–9 systems)	Complete (10+ systems)
Past, Family, and Social History New/initial/consults	Pertinent (1–2 elements)	Pertinent (1–2 elements)	Pertinent (1–2 elements)	Complete (3 elements)
Past, Family, and Social History Established patient/subsequent hospital	Pertinent (1 element)	Pertinent (1 element)	Pertinent (1 element)	Complete (2–3 elements)

Figure 4.4 ■ Content of service element: past, family, and social history—new patient.

New Patient Pertinent: Documentation Supporting One or Two of the Three PFSH Elements

The **new patient pertinent PFSH** level reflects documentation that is directly related and specifically pertinent to the chief complaint, without any additional information about the patient's past, family, and social history.

> ### Examples of New Patient Pertinent PFSH Documentation
>
> #### Johnny's Irritating Cough
>
> Johnny is a new patient who presents with a cough that has bothered him for 3 months. Johnny recently moved in with his girlfriend, who smokes. He also recently started work as a bartender at Smoky's Sports Bar, where the patrons are allowed to smoke in the bar. Grandfather died last year of lung cancer after a long history of cigar use.
>
> The phrase "Johnny is a new patient" defines this E/M visit as that of a new patient.
>
> #### Family and Social History Documentation
>
> **Family history:** paternal grandfather's lung cancer
>
> **Social history:** moved in with girlfriend (*living situation*); girlfriend smokes, and there's smoke in the bar where he works (*tobacco use or exposure*); started working as bartender (*employment*)
>
> Although three different findings of the patient's social history have been documented—employment, tobacco use (or exposure), and living situation—these three findings still support only one PFSH element: social history. Regardless of the number of findings supporting a PFSH element, the element is counted only once.

New Patient Complete: Documentation Supporting All Three of the PFSH Elements

The **new patient complete PFSH** level reflects documentation that not only is pertinent to the chief complaint, but also holistically illustrates the patient's life outside the chief complaint. Documentation supporting a new patient complete PFSH provides insight into the patient's past medical history, the patient's family medical history, and the social factors of the patient's life.

> ### Example of New Patient Complete PFSH Documentation
>
> #### Johnny's Irritating Cough
>
> Johnny is a new patient who presents with a cough that has bothered him for 3 months. Johnny recently moved in with his girlfriend, who smokes. Johnny also recently started work as a bartender at Smoky's Sports Bar, where the patrons are allowed to smoke in the bar. Paternal grandfather died last year of lung cancer after a long history of cigar use. Other than his recent cough, Johnny has never had any respiratory issues, even as a child.
>
> The phrase "Johnny is a new patient" defines this E/M visit as that of a new patient.
>
> #### Past, Family, and Social History Documentation
>
> **Past history:** no childhood respiratory issues
>
> **Family history:** paternal grandfather's lung cancer
>
> **Social history:** moved in with girlfriend (*living situation*); girlfriend smokes, and there's smoke in the bar where he works (*tobacco use or exposure*); started working as bartender (*employment*)

ESTABLISHED PATIENT PFSH

The phrase "established patient" suggests that a patient is well-known to the physician. Generally, in such a situation, the patient's past medical history is familiar, any hereditary or family medical history has been discussed, and the patient's social history has also been discussed. In recognition of the familiarity between a physician and an established patient, the documentation requirements for **established patient pertinent PFSH** are less stringent, as shown in ■ FIGURE 4.5.

History of Present Illness Location, severity, timing, mod fact, quality, duration, context, assoc s/s	Brief (1)	Brief (2–3)	Ext. (4+, or 3 chronic problems)	Ext. (4+, or 3 chronic problems)
Review of Systems Constitutional, ENT/M, respiratory, GU, skin/breast, endocrine, all/imm, eyes, CV, GI, musculoskeletal, psychiatric, neurologic, hem/lymph	None	Pert. (1 system)	Extended (2–9 systems)	Complete (10+ systems)
Past, Family, and Social History New/initial/consults	Pertinent (1–2 elements)	Pertinent (1–2 elements)	Pertinent (1–2 elements)	Complete (3 elements)
Past, Family, and Social History Established patient/subsequent hospital	Pertinent (1 element)	Pertinent (1 element)	Pertinent (1 element)	Complete (2–3 elements)

Figure 4.5 ■ Content of service element: past, family, and social history—established patient.

Established Patient Pertinent: Documentation Supporting One of the Three PFSH Elements

Although the established patient pertinent PFSH reflects documentation pertinent to the chief complaint, the documentation requirements are less rigorous than the new patient pertinent requirements because of the high probability that the patient's PFSH has already been reviewed and documented during previous E/M service visits.

> **Examples of Established Patient Pertinent PFSH Documentation**
>
> Johnny's Irritating Cough
>
> Johnny is well-known to me and presents with a cough that has bothered him for 3 months. He recently moved in with his girlfriend, who smokes, and also started work as a bartender at Smoky's Sports Bar, where the patrons are allowed to smoke in the bar.
>
> The phrase "Johnny is well-known to me" defines this E/M visit as that of an established patient.
>
> Social History Documentation
>
> > **Social history:** moved in with girlfriend (*living situation*); girlfriend smokes, and there's smoke in the bar where he works (*tobacco use or exposure*); started working as bartender (*employment*)
>
> Since Johnny is an established patient, his past medical history may already be known to the performing physician and will not have changed since his last visit; however, the change in the patient's social life is pertinent to the patient's chief complaint and bears great significance for this E/M service visit.

Established Patient Complete: Documentation Supporting Two or Three of the Three PFSH Elements

It is said that the only constant in life is change. Given the reality of change in the human experience, it would be unlikely for a patient's life to remain constant and stagnant throughout the years: jobs change, different health concerns develop, and family members develop unexpected health conditions. Accordingly, the **established patient complete PFSH** reflects documentation pertinent to the chief complaint, as well as documentation of one other element of past, family, or social history.

established patient complete PFSH documentation supporting two or three of the three PFSH elements for an established patient of the clinician or facility

> **Examples of Established Patient Complete PFSH Documentation**
>
> Johnny's Irritating Cough
>
> Johnny is an established patient who presents with a cough that has bothered him for 3 months. Johnny recently moved in with his girlfriend, who smokes. He also recently started work as a bartender at Smoky's Sports Bar, where the patrons are allowed to smoke in the bar. Paternal grandfather died last year of lung cancer after a long history of cigar use.
>
> *continued*

The statement "Johnny is an established patient" defines this E/M visit as that of an established patient.

Past and Family History Documentation

Family history: paternal grandfather's lung cancer

Social history: moved in with girlfriend (*living situation*); girlfriend smokes, and there's smoke in the bar where he works (*tobacco use or exposure*); started working as bartender (*employment*)

As an established patient, there is a high likelihood that the performing physician has reviewed some of Johnny's past medical history. Even though some parts of Johnny's distant past medical history may not have changed since his last visit, a more recent aspect of his past medical history may be pertinent. The element of Johnny's PFSH that has the greatest impact for this current E/M visit is the change in his social life and the lung cancer death of his grandfather. These recent changes in Johnny's history are both very pertinent to his chief complaint, which gives his family and social histories great significance for this E/M service visit.

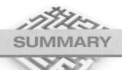

SUMMARY

- Past, family, and social history (PFSH) is the element of history that is composed of the patient's past medical history. This may include childhood illnesses, previous surgeries or procedures, injuries, and prescribed medications or treatments the patient has undergone. This also includes the medical history of the patient's immediate family—parents, siblings, grandparents—as well as any of the family's hereditary and/or lifestyle health factors that could provide further insight into the physiology of the patient and any cause of the patient's current condition. PFSH also encompasses the patient's day-to-day social activities, which could include employment, or educational status if the patient is a minor; tobacco or alcohol use; sports or other physical activity in which the patient regularly engages; sexual activity; use of any illicit drugs or substances; and the patient's living situation.

- There are two methods of gathering PFSH information. It may be gathered during a face-to-face interaction between the patient and a representative of the healthcare facility, such as a registered nurse (RN), medical assistant (MA), or licensed practical nurse (LPN). The PFSH information may also be gathered by having the patient complete a preprinted questionnaire about past medical history, family medical history, and social interactions. If the PFSH is gathered on a pre-printed questionnaire, the clinician should sign and date the completed questionnaire after reviewing it in order to ensure proper medical documentation.

- There are two levels of PFSH—pertinent and complete—which are complicated by the new or established status of the patient. There are new patient pertinent and complete PFSH levels and established patient pertinent and complete PFSH levels.

  - The new patient pertinent PFSH level requires documentation supporting one or two of the three PFSH elements for a patient who is new to the clinician or facility. A new patient complete PFSH requires documentation supporting all three of the PFSH elements for a patient who is new to the clinician or facility.

  - The established patient pertinent PFSH level requires documentation supporting one of the three PFSH elements for a patient who is established with the clinician or facility. An established patient complete PFSH requires documentation supporting two or three of the PFSH elements for a patient who is established with the clinician or facility.

CHAPTER REVIEW

Multiple Choice

Choose the letter that best answers each question or completes each statement.

1. In the acronym PFSH, what does the *S* stand for?
   a. Symptom
   b. Sickness
   c. Social
   d. Science

2. Which of the following best describes the past history?
   a. Any reference to a specific illness the patient has experienced regardless of the time period
   b. Childhood illnesses, previous surgeries or procedures, injuries, and prescribed medications or treatments the patient has undergone
   c. The measures taken by the patient to alleviate or change the symptoms of the current medical problem
   d. Childhood experiences with healthcare providers

3. What is the most important difference between the ROS and the past history?

   a. Any gathered information related to the ROS must be asked before the patient begins the clinical visit, whereas the past history information may be gathered during the clinical visit.

   b. Past history identifies any medical condition, illness, injury, or treatment that may be significant to the chief complaint, whereas the ROS is an inventory of the patient's organ systems prior to the E/M service visit.

   c. There is no discernible difference between the ROS and the past history.

   d. Past history addresses only the events of the patient's health since the most recent E/M service visit.

4. Which of the following best describes the family history?

   a. Frequency of family visits, such as holidays and birthdays

   b. Whether the patient gets along with his or her family

   c. Medical history of the patient's immediate family, including any hereditary and/or lifestyle health factors that could provide further insight into the physiology of the patient and any cause of the patient's current condition

   d. Family history should document the presence of a family member at the E/M service visit because medical knowledge or support provided by the patient's family member at the E/M service visit can help the clinician identify the patient's education level and indicate the family member's willingness to participate in the patient's process of health

5. Which of the following best describes the social history?

   a. The patient's interpersonal skills, which provide the clinician with helpful insight into the patient's psychiatric and emotional health

   b. The patient's social activities, including, but not limited to, employment or school attendance, tobacco use, sexual activity, use of any illicit drugs or substances, and living situation

   c. The patient's ability to determine and describe his or her own level of social awkwardness when asked about using illicit drugs

   d. The patient's presentation of a valid photo identification and submission to a police record search

6. Which of the following does NOT support the social history?

   a. Watched father physically abuse mother during childhood

   b. Recently moved to area and started new job

   c. Drinks one to two beers a week

   d. Works as waitress at two separate restaurants, averaging 70 hours a week

7. Which of the following influences the level of past, family, and social history?

   a. The clinician's familiarity with the patient and the requirements for the specific E/M service visit

   b. How thoroughly the patient can answer the questions

   c. The level of the ROS

   d. Whether the questions were asked by the performing physician or a supporting staff member

8. Which of the following phrases best describes a new patient?

   a. The patient has never experienced this specific chief complaint before.

   b. The patient has never before received any professional or clinical care from the clinician or facility, or has not within the previous 3 years

   c. The patient has engaged in a different social activity since the patient's most recent healthcare encounter

   d. The patient has requested a new clinician in the healthcare facility because he or she was unhappy with the previous clinician

9. Which of the following phrases best describes an established patient?

   a. The patient has been experiencing a chronic condition and has an established plan of care.

   b. The patient has established a standard of care to which the clinician is expected to perform.

   c. The patient has received previous healthcare services from the specific clinician or facility within the last 3 years.

   d. The patient has experienced this chief complaint before.

10. The levels of past, family, and social history are

   a. none, pertinent, extended, comprehensive.

   b. brief, extended.

   c. pertinent, extended.

   d. pertinent, complete.

CASE STUDIES

Case Study 4-1

Read the following documentation, and then answer questions 1–3 by identifying the response that best supports the PFSH element; answer questions 4–7 by identifying the best description of the PFSH level.

Patient is well-known to me and presents with sharp upper abdominal pain that frequently burns. Patient states his job has become increasingly stressful at Comico Oil Company, and he has been working a lot of weekends. His wife has a history of breast cancer, although, per patient, she is now cancer free, which has relieved his personal stress; however, he is increasingly anxious about the number of hours he spends traveling for work. Patient denies any gastrointestinal problems in his life, although he remembers having heartburn around the time his father died of colon cancer.

1. Which of the following selections from the documentation best supports past history?
   a. Patient states his job has become increasingly stressful at Comico Oil Company, and he has been working a lot of weekends.
   b. His wife has a history of breast cancer, although, per patient, she is now cancer free, which has relieved his personal stress; however, he is increasingly anxious about the number of hours he spends traveling for work.
   c. Patient denies any gastrointestinal problems in his life, although he remembers having heartburn . . . .
   d. His father died of colon cancer.

2. Which of the following selections from the documentation best supports family history?
   a. Patient denies any gastrointestinal problems in his life, although he remembers having heartburn . . . .
   b. His father died of colon cancer.
   c. Patient states his job has become increasingly stressful at Comico Oil Company, and he has been working a lot of weekends.
   d. His wife has a history of breast cancer, although, per patient, she is now cancer free, which has relieved his personal stress; however, he is increasingly anxious about the number of hours he spends traveling for work.

3. Which of the following selections from the documentation best supports social history?
   a. His wife has a history of breast cancer, although, per patient, she is now cancer free, which has relieved his personal stress; however, he is increasingly anxious about the number of hours he spends traveling for work.
   b. Patient denies any gastrointestinal problems in his life, although he remembers having heartburn . . . .
   c. His father died of colon cancer.
   d. Patient states his job has become increasingly stressful at Comico Oil Company, and he has been working a lot of weekends.

4. Which of the following best describes the new patient pertinent PFSH level?
   a. Documentation supporting one or two of the three PFSH elements for a patient who is new to the clinician or facility
   b. Documentation supporting all three of the three PFSH elements for a patient who is new to the clinician or facility
   c. Documentation supporting one of the three PFSH elements for a patient who is established with the clinician or facility
   d. Documentation supporting two or three of the three PFSH elements for a patient who is established with the clinician or facility

5. Which of the following phrases best describes the established patient pertinent PFSH level?
   a. Documentation supporting all three of the three PFSH elements for a patient who is new to the clinician or facility
   b. Documentation supporting one of the three PFSH elements for a patient who is established with the clinician or facility

   c. Documentation supporting two or three of the three PFSH elements for a patient who is established with the clinician or facility
   d. Documentation supporting one or two of the three PFSH elements for a patient who is new to the clinician or facility

6. Which of the following best describes the established patient complete PFSH level?
   a. Documentation supporting two or three of the three PFSH elements for a patient who is established with the clinician or facility
   b. Documentation supporting all three of the three PFSH elements for a patient who is new to the clinician or facility
   c. Documentation supporting one of the three PFSH elements for a patient who is established with the clinician or facility
   d. Documentation supporting one or two of the three PFSH elements for a patient who is new to the clinician or facility

7. Which of the following phrases best describes the new patient complete PFSH level?
   a. Documentation supporting two or three of the three PFSH elements for a patient who is established with the clinician or facility
   b. Documentation supporting one of the three PFSH elements for a patient who is established with the clinician or facility
   c. Documentation supporting one or two of the three PFSH elements for a patient who is new to the clinician or facility
   d. Documentation supporting all three of the three PFSH elements for a patient who is new to the clinician or facility

Case Study 4-2

Identify the documented PFSH findings in this case, and then write them next to the appropriate PFSH elements listed. Also answer the two questions.

Complaint: Franklin is well-known to me and presents for sharp left flank pain over the past 2 days, with dark-colored urine. Franklin is accompanied by his wife, Mary. Three weeks ago, Franklin was involved in a minor ATV accident. Directly after the accident, Franklin's primary complaint involved injuries to his chin and chest, both of which suffered contusions and lacerations. At the subsequent visit 1 week after the accident, both chin and chest contusions and lacerations were healing well; however, his wife reported that Franklin was holding his abdomen carefully when he rose from a sitting position, and Franklin admits today that his abdominal pain has gradually moved to his left flank and increased in intensity. Two days ago, Franklin tripped on the computer cords in his home office, and his left flank pain became extreme in severity. Pain was not relieved after Excedrin and a hot bath. This morning, Franklin vomited once, and his temperature was elevated to 101.6°F. Other than Excedrin, Franklin has taken no medications.

The contusions and lacerations Franklin sustained in the ATV accident have healed appropriately. Other than his abdominal and flank pain and fever, Franklin has been in good health. He reports no loss of memory or dizziness since the accident and denies any joint, muscle, or bone pain. No shortness of breath reported, and patient denies any chest pain, heart palpitations, or tingling in arms or fingers. Bowel movements have been normal, regular, and painless. Franklin reports pain in his penis and urethra during urination has caused him to postpone urination at times; however, postponing urination does not relieve his flank pain or painful urination. Other than his fever this morning and one episode of vomiting, Franklin denies chills, night sweats, or any reported fever since the ATV accident. There is no history of kidney disease, pyelonephritis, or diabetes in Franklin's past or Franklin's family. He has never had a urinary tract infection.

Is Franklin a new patient or an established patient? _____

Past medical history _____

Family medical history _____

Social history _____

Please circle the appropriate level of this documented PFSH:

New patient pertinent
New patient complete
Established patient pertinent
Established patient complete

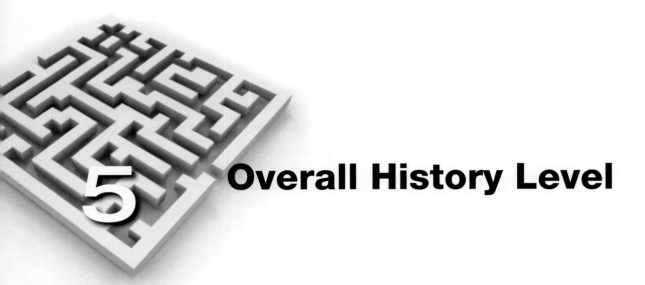

5 Overall History Level

Learning Objectives

After completing this chapter, you should be able to do the following:

- Spell and define the key terms and abbreviations presented in this chapter
- Identify the requirements for the overall level of history
- List and define the four levels of overall history

Key Terms

comprehensive history
detailed history
expanded problem-focused history
overall history
problem-focused history
selecting overall history

Abbreviations

Comp comprehensive
Det detailed
EPF expanded problem-focused
PF problem-focused

INTRODUCTION

Whether *history* refers to the pharaohs of Egypt or the American Civil War, the concept is composed of certain elements recorded in chronological terms: certain people in a particular place during a specified time undergoing specific events. If any of these elements are not recorded, then the story of that unique history becomes ambiguous and imprecise. As the first component of the E/M service, history pertains to the patient's medical background, specifically as it relates to the reason for the patient's current visit. Four different elements make up the history component: chief complaint, history of present illness, review of systems, and past, family, and social history. This chapter specifically focuses on the overall history level that brings together the history of present illness, the review of systems, and the past, family, and social history.

REQUIREMENTS FOR THE OVERALL HISTORY

As the first component of an E/M service, the overall history documents a specific person, during a certain period of time, who is experiencing unique signs or symptoms that cause him or her to seek professional healthcare. During an E/M service visit, four elements must be documented in order to effectively record the history of the patient's health: the chief complaint, history of present illness, review of systems, and the past, family, and social history. As with any other record of history, if any of these elements are not recorded, then the history of the patient's health remains incomplete.

Known as **selecting the overall history**, the process of identifying the level of history requires analysis of the documented elements that constitute the overall history component: the chief complaint, the history of present illness, the review of systems, and the past, family, and social history. **Overall history** describes the combination of HPI, ROS, and PFSH, which make up the total history. Since the history of the patient represents such an important piece of information for the promotion of health, the absence of any of the three history elements—HPI, ROS, or PFSH—significantly affects the overall history. Therefore, the level of overall history is determined by the lowest level of the history elements. For instance, if no HPI has been documented, then the HPI level determines the overall history level, regardless of the extent of documented findings for the ROS or the PFSH.

selecting overall history the process by which the levels for each of the individual history elements—HPI, ROS, and PFSH—are reviewed to determine the level of total history

overall history the combined levels of HPI, ROS, and PFSH

| Exercise 5.1 | **Identifying the Documented Levels for HPI, ROS, and PFSH** |

In each of the following medical documentations, identify the documented level for each of the three history elements—HPI, ROS, and PFSH—by underlining the respective findings that support each of these three history elements.

1. Patient has presented for sinus pressure and cough. Patient's face hurts so much on the right cheek beneath eye that she feels she cannot open her eyes all the way because of the stabbing pain. She complains of a ringing in her right ear, and the right side of her throat hurts when she swallows. She has no appetite, complains of heartburn but no nausea. Nighttime has been interrupted by frequent urination without pain but very smelly urine. Patient denies joint pain other than a sore neck. Patient complains of heavy chest pressure and pain upon coughing. Patient states she can feel her heartbeat in her head as a throbbing but denies any heart palpitations. Patient is dizzy upon standing and reports she has spent 3 days lying down because of the discomfort. No report of sick contact at work; however, her husband had the flu last month. Neither patient nor her husband smokes tobacco.

2. Timmy is an established patient and presents for abdominal pain and diarrhea. Timmy says his stomach hurts, down low on the right side, and it hurts really, really badly, but not all the time. Timmy's father reports his son complains most about the pain in the morning after getting up, and Timmy describes that pain as an 8 on pain scale. Per father's report, Timmy feels better after eating breakfast, but the pain became bad last week. Per father's report, Timmy had stomach flu last month with no vomiting but explosive diarrhea. Timmy's father denies bloody stools but states that Timmy's urine is dark and odorous but that Timmy denies painful urination. Upon query, Timmy complains of some pain in his back during the last week, placing his hands on his midback. Timmy states he felt dizzy during the past week after walking upstairs at school and home. Patient is second grader at Hardy Oaks Elementary and active in peewee Soccer as a goalie; per father, Timmy was recently involved in a goal-side tackle with resultant sharp abdominal pain. Timmy reported domestic incident between his parents at practice; father corroborates Timmy's report. Patient's primary residence is with father, with joint custody with mother; Timmy states visitation with mother is very occasional with stressful transitions. Timmy's father denies use of tobacco or alcohol.

3. New patient presents for lower back pain. Low back hurts, down by beltline, and pain is very severe. The pain is sporadic, mostly when standing up after sitting in one place for an extended period. Ibuprofen used to help, but now it does not. Low back pain is sharp and throbbing. Patient has had occasional back pain for about 20 years, since first in the service. Patient first noticed this particular low back pain shortly after playing touch football with adult children this past Thanksgiving. Patient also complains of pain radiating down the back of his right thigh. Patient denies any other joint pain. Denies double vision or dizziness. No chest pain or shortness of breath. Patient denies tobacco or alcohol use. Pain has not affected patient's work as a fifth-grade teacher.

HISTORY (chief complaint included)	Problem-Focused	Expanded Problem-Focused	Detailed	Comprehensive
History of Present Illness Location, severity, timing, mod fact, quality, duration, context, assoc s/s	Brief (1)	Brief (2–3)	Ext. (4+, or 3 chronic problems)	Ext. (4+, or 3 chronic problems)
Review of Systems Constitutional, ENT/M, respiratory, GU, skin/breast, endocrine, all/imm, eyes, CV, GI, musculoskeletal, psychiatric, neurologic, hem/lymph	None	Pert. (1 system)	Extended (2–9 systems)	Complete (10+ systems)
Past, Family, and Social History New/initial/consults	Pertinent (1–2 elements)	Pertinent (1–2 elements)	Pertinent (1–2 elements)	Complete (3 elements)
Past, Family, and Social History Established patient/subsequent hospital	Pertinent (1 element)	Pertinent (1 element)	Pertinent (1 element)	Complete (2–3 elements)

Figure 5.1 ■ Content of service: overall history (CC, HPI, ROS, and PFSH).

THE FOUR LEVELS OF OVERALL HISTORY

The structure of the overall history requires that the individual history elements function together as a whole in order to properly reflect the extent of the patient's overall history. The identified level of that history describes the combination of HPI, ROS, and PFSH, which produce the total level of history. The chief complaint, the reason for the patient's presence at the E/M visit, is considered an inherent part of the E/M medical documentation and therefore is not a contributing factor in the selection of the overall history. The four levels of overall history are problem-focused (PF), expanded problem-focused (EPF), detailed (Det), and comprehensive (Comp). ■ FIGURE 5.1 illustrates the four levels of history, which, again, are based on the HPI, ROS, and PFSH.

SELECTING THE OVERALL HISTORY LEVEL

Remember that the CC, as the symptomatic reason for the patient's E/M visit, does not contribute to the overall level of history. However, each of the other history elements—HPI, ROS, and PFSH—provides an essential perspective on a patient's overall history. The absence of any one of the individual history elements could affect the physician's understanding of the others—the history of the patient's present illness, the review of the patient's organ systems, or the patient's past medical history, family medical history, or social factors—in relation to the presenting problem. As a result, each overall history level must reflect the documented HPI, ROS, and PFSH levels.

Problem-Focused History

problem-focused history the lowest level of documented history, requiring a brief HPI, no ROS, and no PFSH

Problem-focused history requires a brief HPI, no documented ROS findings, and no documented PFSH findings. The following example of problem-focused history reflects the documented HPI, ROS, and PFSH; see ■ FIGURE 5.2 for the documentation requirements in a comparative format.

Example: Problem-Focused History

Johnny's Irritating Cough

Johnny is a new patient who presents with a very sore throat and barking cough. Patient has no complaints of nasal drainage. Cough lozenges and cough suppressants have not helped his throat or cough. Johnny recently moved in with his girlfriend, who smokes. He also recently started work as a bartender at Smoky's Sports Bar, where the patrons are allowed to smoke in the bar. Grandfather died last year of lung cancer.

HPI—extended (4—severity, quality, associated s/s, modifying factor)

ROS—none (N/A)

New patient PFSH—pertinent (social & family Hx)

Level of history: problem-focused, determined by the ROS level

History (chief complaint included)	Problem-Focused	Expanded Problem-Focused	Detailed	Comprehensive
History of Present Illness Location, severity, timing, mod fact, quality, duration, context, assoc s/s	Brief (1)	Brief (2–3)	Ext. (4+, or 3 chronic problems)	Ext. (4+, or 3 chronic problems)
Review of Systems Constitutional, ENT/M, respiratory, GU, skin/breast, endocrine, all/imm, eyes, CV, GI, musculoskeletal, psychiatric, neurologic, hem/lymph	None	Pert. (1 system)	Extended (2–9 systems)	Complete (10+ systems)
Past, Family, and Social History New/initial/consults	Pertinent (1–2 elements)	Pertinent (1–2 elements)	Pertinent (1–2 elements)	Complete (3 elements)
Past, Family, and Social History Established patient/subsequent hospital	Pertinent (1 element)	Pertinent (1 element)	Pertinent (1 element)	Complete (2–3 elements)

Figure 5.2 ▪ Content of service element: overall history, problem-focused.

Expanded Problem-Focused History

An **expanded problem-focused history** requires a brief HPI, a pertinent ROS, and a pertinent PFSH. The following example of an expanded problem-focused history reflects the documented HPI, ROS, and PFSH; see ▪ FIGURE 5.3 for the documentation requirements in a comparative format.

expanded problem-focused history the second level of documented history, requiring a brief HPI, pertinent ROS, and no PFSH

Example: Expanded Problem-Focused History

Johnny's Irritating Cough

Johnny is a new patient who presents with a very sore throat and barking cough. Patient has no complaints of nasal drainage. Cough lozenges and cough suppressants have not helped his throat or cough. Patient denies chest pain when he coughs. Johnny recently moved in with his girlfriend, who smokes. He also recently started work as a bartender at Smoky's Sports Bar, where the patrons are allowed to smoke in the bar. Grandfather died last year of lung cancer.

HPI—extended (4—severity, quality, associated s/s, modifying factor)

ROS—pertinent (respiratory)

New patient PFSH—pertinent (social & family Hx)

Level of history: expanded problem-focused, determined by the level of ROS

History (chief complaint included)	Problem-Focused	Expanded Problem-Focused	Detailed	Comprehensive
History of Present Illness Location, severity, timing, mod fact, quality, duration, context, assoc s/s	Brief (1)	Brief (2–3)	Ext. (4+, or 3 chronic problems)	Ext. (4+, or 3 chronic problems)
Review of Systems Constitutional, ENT/M, respiratory, GU, skin/breast, endocrine, all/imm, eyes, CV, GI, musculoskeletal, psychiatric, neurologic, hem/lymph	None	Pert. (1 system)	Extended (2–9 systems)	Complete (10+ systems)
Past, Family, and Social History New/initial/consults	Pertinent (1–2 elements)	Pertinent (1–2 elements)	Pertinent (1–2 elements)	Complete (3 elements)
Past, Family, and Social History Established patient/subsequent hospital	Pertinent (1 element)	Pertinent (1 element)	Pertinent (1 element)	Complete (2–3 elements)

Figure 5.3 ▪ Content of service element: overall history, expanded problem-focused.

History (chief complaint included)	Problem-Focused	Expanded Problem-Focused	Detailed	Comprehensive
History of Present Illness Location, severity, timing, mod fact, quality, duration, context, assoc s/s	Brief (1)	Brief (2–3)	Ext. (4+, or 3 chronic problems)	Ext. (4+, or 3 chronic problems)
Review of Systems Constitutional, ENT/M, respiratory, GU, skin/breast, endocrine, all/imm, eyes, CV, GI, musculoskeletal, psychiatric, neurologic, hem/lymph	None	Pert. (1 system)	Extended (2–9 systems)	Complete (10+ systems)
Past, Family, and Social History New/initial/consults	Pertinent (1–2 elements)	Pertinent (1–2 elements)	Pertinent (1–2 elements)	Complete (3 elements)
Past, Family, and Social History Established patient/subsequent hospital	Pertinent (1 element)	Pertinent (1 element)	Pertinent (1 element)	Complete (2–3 elements)

Figure 5.4 ■ Content of service element: overall history, expanded problem-focused.

What happens if the documented findings for the HPI, ROS, and PFSH do not meet the specific levels listed here? It is important to remember to think critically about the documentation requirements for each of the overall history levels. The following example reveals the identification of the HPI, ROS, and PFSH elements in a slightly different manner; see ■ FIGURE 5.4 for a comparative visual format.

Example: Expanded Problem-Focused History

Johnny's Irritating Cough

Johnny is a new patient who presents with very sore throat. Cough lozenges and cough suppressants have not helped his throat or helped him sleep. Patient denies chest pain or dizziness when he coughs. Denies fever, abdominal pain, joint pains, sinus pressure, heart palpitations, and painful urination. Patient is allergic to shellfish, with hives upon exposure. Reports no rash, itching, or unusual redness of skin. Patient denies blurred vision, although he complains of "fuzzy eyeballs." Johnny recently moved in with his girlfriend, who smokes. He also recently started work as a bartender at Smoky's Sports Bar, where the patrons are allowed to smoke in the bar. Grandfather died last year of lung cancer.

HPI—brief (2—severity, modifying factor)

ROS—complete (10—respiratory, constitutional, gastrointestinal, musculoskeletal, ENT/M, cardiovascular, genitourinary, allergic/immunologic, integumentary [skin], eyes)

New patient PFSH—pertinent (social & family Hx)

Level of history: expanded problem-focused, determined by the level of HPI

Detailed History

detailed history the third level of documented history, requiring an extended HPI, extended ROS, and pertinent PFSH

Detailed history requires an extended HPI, extended ROS, and a pertinent PFSH. In contrast with the previous illustrations in Figures 5.3 and 5.4, which reflect two different examples of expanded problem-focused history. ■ FIGURE 5.5 reflects the simplified documentation requirements for a detailed overall history, shown in a now-familiar format.

Example: Detailed History

Johnny's Irritating Cough

Johnny is a new patient who presents with a very sore throat and barking cough. Patient has no complaints of nasal drainage. Cough lozenges and cough suppressants have not helped his throat or cough. Patient reports no fever and denies chest pain when he coughs. Johnny recently moved in with his girlfriend, who smokes. He also recently started work as a bartender at Smoky's Sports Bar, where the patrons are allowed to smoke in the bar. Grandfather died last year of lung cancer.

HPI—extended (4—severity, quality, associated s/s, modifying factor)

ROS—extended (2—respiratory, constitutional)

New patient PFSH—pertinent (social & family Hx)

Level of history: detailed, determined by the level of ROS

History (chief complaint included)	Problem-Focused	Expanded Problem-Focused	Detailed	Comprehensive
History of Present Illness Location, severity, timing, mod fact, quality, duration, context, assoc s/s	Brief (1)	Brief (2–3)	Ext. (4+, or 3 chronic problems)	Ext. (4+, or 3 chronic problems)
Review of Systems Constitutional, ENT/M, respiratory, GU, skin/breast, endocrine, all/imm, eyes, CV, GI, musculoskeletal, psychiatric, neurologic, hem/lymph	None	Pert. (1 system)	Extended (2–9 systems)	Complete (10+ systems)
Past, Family, and Social History New/initial/consults	Pertinent (1–2 elements)	Pertinent (1–2 elements)	Pertinent (1–2 elements)	Complete (3 elements)
Past, Family, and Social History Established patient/subsequent hospital	Pertinent (1 element)	Pertinent (1 element)	Pertinent (1 element)	Complete (2–3 elements)

Figure 5.5 ■ Content of service: overall history, detailed.

Comprehensive History

Comprehensive history requires an extended HPI, complete ROS, and complete PFSH. The comprehensive history example reflects the documented HPI, ROS, and PFSH; see ■ FIGURE 5.6 for the documentation requirements in a familiar format.

comprehensive history the fourth level of documented history, requiring an extended HPI, complete ROS, and complete PFSH

> **Example: Comprehensive**
>
> **Johnny's Irritating Cough**
>
> Johnny is a new patient who presents with very sore throat and barking cough. Patient states his cough keeps him up at night. Cough lozenges and cough suppressants have not helped his throat or helped him sleep. Patient denies chest pain or dizziness when he coughs. Denies fever, abdominal pain, joint pains, sinus pressure, heart palpitations, and painful urination. Patient is allergic to shellfish, with hives upon exposure. Reports no rash, itching, or unusual redness of skin. Patient denies blurred vision, although he complains of "fuzzy eyeballs." Johnny recently moved in with his girlfriend, who smokes. He also recently started work as a bartender at Smoky's Sports Bar, where the patrons are allowed to smoke in the bar. Grandfather died last year of lung cancer. Other than his recent cough, Johnny has never had any respiratory issues, even as a child.
>
> HPI—extended (4—severity, quality, associated s/s, modifying factor)
>
> ROS—complete (10—respiratory, constitutional, gastrointestinal, musculoskeletal, ENT/M, cardiovascular, genitourinary, allergic/immunologic, integumentary [skin], eyes)
>
> New patient PFSH—complete (past, family, & social Hx)
>
> Level of history: comprehensive

History (chief complaint included)	Problem-Focused	Expanded Problem-Focused	Detailed	Comprehensive
History of Present Illness Location, severity, timing, mod fact, quality, duration, context, assoc s/s	Brief (1)	Brief (2–3)	Ext. (4+, or 3 chronic problems)	Ext. (4+, or 3 chronic problems)
Review of Systems Constitutional, ENT/M, respiratory, GU, skin/breast, endocrine, all/imm, eyes, CV, GI, musculoskeletal, psychiatric, neurologic, hem/lymph	None	Pert. (1 system)	Extended (2–9 systems)	Complete (10+ systems)
Past, Family, and Social History New/initial/consults	None	None	Pertinent (1–2 elements)	Complete (3 elements)
Past, Family, and Social History Established patient/subsequent hospital	None	None	Pertinent (1 element)	Complete (2–3 elements)

Figure 5.6 ■ Content of service element: overall history, comprehensive.

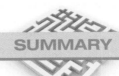

SUMMARY

- The patient's history tells an important part of the patient's story of health. During an E/M service visit, the extent of documented findings for each of the elements—HPI, ROS, and PFSH—determines the level of overall history.

- There are four levels of history: problem-focused, expanded problem-focused, detailed, and comprehensive. Each of these represents a combination of HPI, ROS, and PFSH documen-

tation; the lowest level of HPI, ROS, or PFSH documentation determines the level of overall history. Therefore, in order to select the overall history level, the levels for each of the three individual history elements must be determined. Only when the levels for HPI, ROS, and PFSH have been determined can the overall history level be selected.

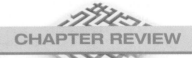

CHAPTER REVIEW

Multiple Choice

Choose the letter that best answers each question or completes each statement.

1. What does the acronym HPI mean?
   a. Hypertension prevention ideas
   b. History of present illness
   c. Headache pain index
   d. Healthcare to patient initiative

2. What does the acronym ROS mean?
   a. Review of surgery
   b. Review of scenarios
   c. Review of symptoms
   d. Review of systems

3. What does the acronym PFSH mean?
   a. Past, family, and social history
   b. Preventive fungal scrubbing hand cream
   c. Patient fatigue screening handbook
   d. Prenatal fetal stressed heartbeat

4. How is the chief complaint related to the overall history?
   a. The chief complaint is completely different from the history.
   b. The chief complaint is the same as the nature of the presenting problem.
   c. The chief complaint is considered to be private information that cannot be documented or shared.
   d. The chief complaint is included in the overall history.

5. In referring to the problem-focused level of overall history, which of the following is most descriptive?

   a. HPI, brief; ROS, pertinent; PFSH, none
   b. HPI, brief; ROS, none; PFSH, none
   c. HPI, extended; ROS, complete; PFSH, complete
   d. HPI, extended; ROS, extended; PFSH, pertinent

6. In referring to the expanded problem-focused level of history, which of the following is most descriptive?
   a. HPI, brief; ROS, pertinent; PFSH, N/A
   b. HPI, extended; ROS, complete; PFSH, complete
   c. HPI, brief; ROS, N/A; PFSH, N/A
   d. HPI, extended; ROS, extended; PFSH, pertinent

7. In referring to the detailed level of history, which of the following is most descriptive?
   a. HPI, brief; ROS, pertinent; PFSH, None
   b. HPI, extended; ROS, extended; PFSH, pertinent
   c. HPI, brief; ROS, N/A; PFSH, none
   d. HPI, extended; ROS, complete; PFSH, complete

8. In referring to the comprehensive level of overall history, which of the following is most descriptive?
   a. HPI, extended; ROS, extended; PFSH, pertinent
   b. HPI, brief; ROS, none; PFSH, N/A
   c. HPI, brief; ROS, pertinent; PFSH, none
   d. HPI, extended; ROS, complete; PFSH, complete

9. In selecting the level of history
   a. the highest level of the three history elements—HPI, ROS, PFSH—determines the level of history.
   b. the lowest level of the three history elements—HPI, ROS, PFSH—determines the level of history.

c. the highest level of the three history elements—HPI, ROS, PFSH—must be dropped to determine the level of history.

d. the lowest level of the three history elements—HPI, ROS, PFSH—can be dropped to determine the level of history.

10. Marianne Munroe presents to her primary care physician because she has experienced some dizziness in the past month. Her physician, who is very familiar with Marianne

because she visits her physician annually, documents an extended HPI, a pertinent ROS, but does not document any PFSH. What should the level of history be for this visit?

a. Detailed

b. Problem-focused

c. Comprehensive

d. Expanded problem-focused

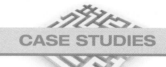

CASE STUDIES

Case Study 5-1

Read the following documentation, and then answer questions 1–5 by identifying the response that best supports the level of overall history.

George presents with sharp upper abdominal pain that frequently burns. George is well-known to me, has been my patient for the past 20 years. George rates pain at 7–8/10 between meals. Antacids have provided some relief for several months, but the antacids have not provided any relief in the past few weeks. George states his job has become increasingly stressful at Comico Oil Company, and he has been working many weekends. Frances, George's wife, is present at visit, and George expresses relief that she is now cancer free after 2 years of treatment. George repeats that this has relieved his personal stress; however, he is increasingly anxious about the number of hours he spends traveling for work. Frances remembers that George had heartburn around the time his father died of colon cancer 10 years ago.

1. The level of documented HPI is best described as
   a. Brief: 1 HPI element (location)
   b. Brief: 2 HPI elements (location and timing)
   c. Brief: 3 HPI elements (location, timing, severity)
   d. Extended: 4 HPI elements (location, timing, severity, modifying factor)

2. The level of documented ROS is best described as
   a. None (N/A): no review of systems having been documented
   b. Pertinent: 1 review of system
   c. Extended: between 2 and 9 systems reviewed
   d. Complete: more than 10 systems reviewed.

3. The PFSH would be considered
   a. new patient because this is a new problem for the physician.
   b. new patient because the patient's wife is present.
   c. established patient because the patient has been seen by the physician within the last 3 years.
   d. established patient because the patient's wife is now cancer free.

4. The level of documented PFSH is best described as
   a. pertinent new patient because only family and social history have been documented for this visit.
   b. pertinent established patient because only social history has been documented for this visit.
   c. complete new patient because past, family, and social history have been documented for this visit.
   d. complete established patient because past, family, and social history have been documented for this visit.

5. The level of history for the medical documentation of George's sharp upper abdominal pain is best described as
   a. problem-focused.
   b. expanded problem-focused.
   c. detailed.
   d. comprehensive.

Case Study 5-2

For the following medical documentation, identify the documented HPI, ROS, and PFSH levels by underlining the finding that support the respective history elements, and then identify the documented level of overall history.

Complaint: Franklin is well-known to me and presents for sharp left flank pain over the past 2 days, with dark-colored urine. Franklin is accompanied by his wife, Mary. Three weeks ago, Franklin was involved in a minor ATV accident. Directly after the accident, Franklin's primary complaint involved injuries to his chin and chest, both of which suffered contusions and lacerations. At the subsequent visit 1 week after the accident, both chin and chest contusions and lacerations were healing well; however, his wife reported that Franklin was holding his abdomen carefully when he rose from a sitting position, and Franklin admits today that his abdominal pain has gradually moved to his left flank and increased in intensity. Two days ago, Franklin tripped on the computer cords in his home office, and his left flank pain became extreme in severity. Pain was not relieved after Excedrin and a hot bath. This morning Franklin vomited once, and his temperature was elevated to 101.6°F. Other than Excedrin, Franklin has taken no medications.

The contusions and lacerations Franklin sustained in the ATV accident have healed appropriately. Other than his abdominal and flank pain and fever, Franklin has been in good health. He reports no loss of memory or dizziness since the accident and denies any joint, muscle, or bone pain. No shortness of breath reported, and patient denies any chest pain, heart palpitations, or tingling in arms or fingers. Bowel movements have been normal, regular, and painless. Franklin reports his painful urination has caused him to postpone urination at times; however, postponing urination does not relieve his flank pain or painful urination. Other than his fever this morning and one episode of vomiting, Franklin denies chills, night sweats, or any reported fever since the ATV accident. There is no history of kidney disease, pyelonephritis, or diabetes in Franklin's past or his family. He has never had a urinary tract infection.

Physical Exam: T, 101.3; BP, 126/86; P, 78. Eyes clear without jaundice. Head is atraumatic without tenderness, nodules, or swelling. Neck is soft without masses. Auscultation of lungs is clear without wheezes or rub. Auscultation of heart reveals regular rate and rhythm with no abnormal sounds noted. No cervical, thoracic, or lumbar spine tenderness; however, costovertebral tenderness noted upon palpation. Palpation of abdomen reveals guarding, tenderness with rebound. Franklin expressed nausea upon palpation and vomited immediately after abdominal exam. His face became quite flushed. Although palpation of lower abdomen caused significant pain, bladder was palpable even though Franklin provided copious urine specimen before examination. No rashes noted during abdominal exam, along groin, or on penis. Urinary meatus clear, without redness or inflammation.

1. Identify the appropriate level of the documented HPI:
   _____

2. Identify the appropriate level of the documented ROS:
   _____

3. Identify the appropriate level of the documented PFSH:
   _____

4. Circle the level of overall history:

   Problem-focused
   Expanded problem-focused
   Detailed
   Comprehensive

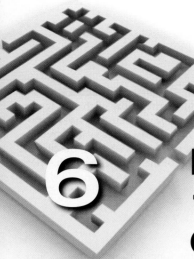

6

Physical Examination— 1995 Documentation Guidelines

Learning Objectives

After completing this chapter, you should be able to do the following:

- Spell and define the key terms and abbreviations presented in this chapter
- Locate the physical examination findings in the medical documentation
- Define the specific characteristics of the physical examination in the medical documentation
- Recognize and identify organ systems and body areas
- List and identify the requirements for the physical examination in the "1995 Documentation Guidelines for Evaluation and Management Services"
- List and define the four levels of physical examination documentation as defined in the "1995 Documentation Guidelines for Evaluation and Management Services"

Key Terms

abdomen

anatomy

auscultation

back

body area

bruit

carotid

chest

conjunctivae

edema

extremity

genitalia

groin

head

nature of the presenting problem

neck

organ system

palpation

percussion

physical examination

thyroid

tympanic membrane

varicosities

Abbreviation

PE physical examination

INTRODUCTION

An examination requires an investigation or analysis of a current situation. For instance, when a student prepares to take a written examination on study material, that test examines the status of the student's knowledge and understanding of the material at the time of the test—not whatever the student has forgotten or what the student will learn in the future. Similarly, the examination in an E/M service visit addresses the status of the patient's health at the time of the visit. Within the story of the patient's health, the physical examination tells the story of what's happening right now, at the moment of the E/M service visit—not what has happened or what might yet occur in the patient's health.

LOCATING THE PHYSICAL EXAMINATION IN THE MEDICAL DOCUMENTATION

physical examination the objective clinical assessment of the patient's current health status, performed by the physician during the E/M service visit; identifies the functions, performance, and structure of the patient's physiology and health

The **physical examination (PE)** is a snapshot of the patient's health: the functions, performance, and structure of the patient's body at the moment of the physical examination. With this in mind, the structure of the medical documentation of an E/M service reveals a certain sublime logic: the documentation of the history is usually found before the documentation of the PE. In other words, what has happened before the visit precedes what is happening right now. The verb tense and use of language also provide help in identifying the documented physical examination. Whereas history happened in the past, which suggests the use of past tense language, the physical examination is occurring at the time of the visit, which would be present tense language.

Example of History Language and Physical Examination Language

This 25-year-old woman presents to the clinic with complaints of chest congestion, nasal discharge, and "feeling cruddy." Patient reports an extreme headache for the past 3 days, which she rates at its worst as an 8/10 on a pain scale. She has been very lethargic, with a heavy, productive cough and fever. She states that OTC cough syrup has not helped her cough but has increased her nausea and "cruddiness." Her appetite has been greatly decreased over the past week. However, she reports no change in bowel or bladder patterns in the past 3 days except that she has urinated more than usual. Patient reports she has experienced racing heart and pounding head when she stands up or leans over, with episodes of excruciating pain. Ill contact probable as, per patient, several people at work have been ill; she works for Pinequist Public Housing as a grant writer.

Patient is pale and appears very tired. Her clothes are rumpled, but she appears well groomed. **Conjunctivae** are clear without swelling. Nasal passages are quite congested and very swollen. Fluid is noted within inner ear bilaterally. However, **tympanic membrane** does not appear significantly pressured. Throat appears mottled with yellow and white patches, and tonsils significantly red and swollen. **Palpation** of neck reveals very tender, swollen lymph nodes. Patient expresses extreme discomfort when asked to swallow during exam.

The same medical documentation with language highlighted, Hx in yellow and PE in green:

This 25-year-old woman presents to the clinic with complaints of chest congestion, nasal discharge, and "feeling cruddy." Patient reports an extreme headache for the past 3 days, which she rates at its worst as an 8/10 on a pain scale. She has been very lethargic, with a heavy, productive cough and fever. She states that OTC cough syrup has not helped her cough but has increased her nausea and "cruddiness." Her appetite has been greatly decreased over the past week. However, she reports no change in bowel or bladder patterns in the past 3 days except that she has urinated more than usual. Patient reports she has experienced racing heart and pounding head when she stands up or leans over, with episodes of excruciating pain. Ill contact probable as, per patient, several people at work have been ill; she works for Pinequist Public Housing as a grant writer.

Patient is pale and appears very tired. Her clothes are rumpled, but she appears well groomed. Conjunctivae are clear without swelling. Nasal passages are quite congested and very swollen. Fluid is noted within inner ear bilaterally. However, tympanic membrane does not appear significantly pressured. Throat appears mottled with yellow and white patches, and tonsils significantly red and swollen. Palpation of neck reveals very tender, swollen lymph nodes. Patient expresses extreme discomfort when asked to swallow during exam.

---

conjunctivae the inner surface of the eyelids and the surface of the eyeball

tympanic membrane the eardrum

palpation determining the status of an organ by pressing, gently pushing, or touching with fingertips, fingers, or palm of hand; for example, palpating the upper left quadrant of the abdomen to determine the size of the spleen

Notice in the previous example that the present tense of the language documenting the physical examination findings is accompanied by clinical terms used to define the clinician's findings during the physical examination.

CHARACTERISTICS OF THE PHYSICAL EXAMINATION IN THE MEDICAL DOCUMENTATION

Whereas the history requires a verbal exchange between the clinician and the patient, the physical examination requires physical interaction between the physician and the patient. During an E/M service visit, a transition occurs between the collection of history and the shift into the physical examination. Some people may be able to identify a certain turn of phrase or a shift in attention signaling the beginning of the physical examination. This shift of attention may occur when the patient is given a robe to change into while the physician discreetly leaves the room. Or the clinician may ask the patient, "Is it all right if I listen to your chest?" This shift of attention does not indicate that further conversation about any history is prohibited, because many physicians are able to continue the collection of history findings during this shift into the physical examination.

As a nonsurgical, noninvasive medical procedure, the physical examination assesses the health of the patient at the time of the E/M service visit. Since the exam allows the physician to systematically investigate and/or inspect the patient's status of health, there is a standardized order in which the physician will review the patient's **anatomy**.

anatomy the physical structure of the human body

In order to perform the physical examination, the physician must physically interact with the patient—for example, to examine the patient's eyes and ears, the physician must look into the patient's eyes and ears. In order to examine the patient's throat, the physician must ask the patient to open wide and say, "Ahhhh," to allow the physician to look into the patient's mouth and throat with the aid of a tongue depressor and light.

Examples: Characteristics of the Physical Examination

In order to examine …

- the patient's eyes and ears, the physician must look into the patient's eyes and ears.
- the patient's throat, the physician must ask the patient to open wide and say, "Ahhhh," to allow the physician, with the aid of a tongue depressor and light, to actually look at the condition of the patient's throat, tonsils, etc.
- the patient's respiration, the clinician must place the stethoscope on the patient's chest.
- the patient's bowels, the clinician must palpate the patient's abdomen.
- the patient's **thyroid**, the clinician must palpate the patient's neck.

thyroid the endocrine gland located in the neck

Anatomy of the Physical Examination

The human body is made up of many different parts or anatomical sections. Identifying the different anatomical sections can be as simple as the children's song, "The foot bone's connected to the ankle bone; the ankle bone's connected to the leg bone . . . ," or as complicated as an intricate anatomical medical textbook. For those without clinical training, the physical examination can be confusing. After all, how does a clinician examine a patient?

Every clinician undergoes extensive training in performance of the physical examination, including what to look for, what to examine, how to examine the patient, even why certain sections of the body should be examined. Identifying only one specific style of performing the physical examination would not effectively represent or duly respect the talent and skill of the hundreds of thousands of trained, practicing physicians performing physical examinations every day. However, to facilitate consistency in the discussion of the physical examination, one specific style will be referenced in this text to provide a basis for the discussion: the examination of the patient's entire body from the top of the head all the way down to the feet. This simplified description we will call the "head to heel." Before proceeding with a "head to heel" examination, the physician may initially examine what the overall appearance or demeanor of the patient is, how the patient appears to be feeling, and whether the patient appears ill or uncomfortable or in pain. The findings made by the physician during the physical examination must then be documented to ensure that the patient's medical record is complete.

Reading the Physical Examination Documentation

Understanding human anatomy helps facilitate reading about the documented physical examination. Human anatomy is composed of different tissues, organs, and systems that work in concert to promote the efficient functioning and health of the body. Some of the different parts of human anatomy are limited to specific anatomical territories, such as the ear or the eye, which are both located in the head. Other parts of human anatomy are spread throughout the human body, such as the network of arteries, veins, vessels, and organs that make up the cardiovascular system. Understanding the documentation of a physical examination sometimes requires a synthesis of the documented findings and the anatomical locations of the findings.

Legibility and the Documented Physical Examination   Nonclinically trained support staff—such as medical coders, billers, and others who work in a healthcare setting—will be exposed to a variety of documentation styles for the physical examination. Navigating these different styles requires an understanding of the guidelines for documenting the physical examination.

The 1995 and 1997 "Documentation Guidelines for Evaluation and Management Services" list seven principles of medical documentation, with the most important principle listed first: "The medical record should be complete and legible."[1] Legibility often refers to the quality of handwriting, yet with the advent of electronic medical records, legibility also refers to coherent and understandable documentation. Without guiding principles and standards, medical documentation could become as individualized as the various physicians and clinicians who perform the E/M services. Therefore, the documentation of a physical examination is guided by the need for clarity and transparency, to ensure that any clinician providing continuing care for the patient is able to read and understand the medical documentation. For the purposes of the physical examination, this clarity and transparency may be achieved through effective documentation of the performed physical examination and clear communication of the findings.. Consider the following example, which presents the documentation of a patient's cardiovascular findings during a cardiologist's physical examination.

> **Example: Documented Physical Examination Findings**
>
> Pulse rate 45; **carotid** upstrokes are symmetrical and without **bruits**; heart regular rate and rhythm; heart normal in size and location; no **edema** or **varicosities** in extremities.

carotid one of two large arteries that carry blood from the chest to the head

bruit a murmur or other unusual sound identified in the heart, most commonly identified by listening with a stethoscope

Notice that, although these documented findings may not provide specific anatomical locations for the findings, the documentation of the physical examination is legible. However, without specific, advanced clinical knowledge of anatomy, it might be difficult to identify the specific locations for these findings. Consider the same physical examination findings, documented in a head-to-heel format.

> **Example: Documented Physical Examination Findings in Head-to-Heel Format**
>
> **Constitutional:** pulse rate 45
> **Neck:** carotid upstrokes symmetrical and without bruits
> **Heart:** regular rate and rhythm; normal in size and location
> **Extremities:** no edema or varicosities

edema an abnormal collection of fluids between the cells of an organ or in intercellular tissues, a body cavity, or an extremity

varicosities enlarged or swollen veins that are commonly identified in the extremities but may be identified in any other part of the human body

Notice that both of these examples present legible documentation of the cardiovascular findings, regardless of the style used to document them.

ORGAN SYSTEMS AND BODY AREAS

Documenting the physical examination could prove problematic without specific guidelines. After all, describing the anatomy "above the shoulders" could include the head, neck, ears, eyes, mouth, brain, spinal cord, musculoskeletal system, veins, arteries, and more. Consistency in documentation provides clarity for all involved. The 1995 Documentation Guidelines define two distinct categories: **organ systems** and body areas. (The directions for accessing these guidelines can be found in Appendix A.) An organ system is a series of interconnected tissues, structures, and organs that operate together to perform a specific physiological function. The musculoskeletal organ system is composed of bones, tendons, ligaments, cartilage, muscles, and other tissues such as bursas and intervertebral disks, which operate in concert for optimal function. Twelve organ systems are listed in the 1995 DGs:

organ system a specific set of anatomically interconnected tissues, structures, and organs that operate together to perform a specific physiological function within the human body

- Constitutional
- Eyes

---

[1]Centers for Medicare and Medicaid Services, "1995 Documentation Guidelines for Evaluation and Management Services," "1997 Documentation Guidelines for Evaluation and Management Services."

- Ears, Nose, Throat, and Mouth
- Cardiovascular
- Respiratory
- Gastrointestinal
- Genitourinary
- Musculoskeletal
- Skin (integumentary)
- Neurologic
- Psychiatric
- Hematologic/Lymphatic/Immunologic

A **body area** is one of seven specific anatomic regions that make up the entire human body. The seven body areas are these:

- **Head,** including face
- **Chest,** including breasts and armpits
- **Genitalia,** including **groin** and buttocks
- **Back,** including spine
- **Extremities**
- **Neck**
- **Abdomen**

These categories provide the basis of the 1995 guidelines for a physical examination, which initially addresses an affected body area or organ system. For instance, consider a patient who presents because of a sore throat. According to the 1995 DGs, that examination begins with the patient's throat. If any other body areas or organ systems are also symptomatic or related to the affected organ system, then those additional organ systems or body areas should also be examined. The sore throat—which is part of the ears, nose, throat, and mouth organ systems—is related to two different organ systems, respiratory and gastrointestinal.

What Is the Difference between Organ Systems and Body Areas?

The difference between body areas and organ systems comes down to a category difference. The body area category divides the entire human structure into geographic sections, and each section contains several different systems (see ■ FIGURE 6.1). The organ system category divides the human body into separate anatomical systems, each of which operates for one specific physiologic function (see ■ FIGURE 6.2).

body area one of seven specific anatomic regions that make up the entire human body

head the body area above the chin; includes, but is not limited to, the head hair, brain, eyes, eyelids, ears, nose, sinuses, oropharynx, nostrils, teeth, gums, tongue, lips

chest the body area between the collarbone and the lowest rib; encompasses, but is not limited to, the lungs, heart, ribs, trachea, bronchioles, mediastinal cavity, including the thoracic diaphragm, which is the sheet of muscle that separates the organs within the chest cavity from the organs within the abdominal cavity

genitalia the body area related to the male and female sex organs; includes, but is not limited to, the male penis and testicles and the female vagina, uterus, and fallopian tubes

groin a triangular area of the body between the pelvic bones, including, but not limited to, the pelvic muscles, tendons, and hip bones

back the body area extending from the lowest part of the neck down to the top of the buttocks, including, but not limited to, the spinal cord and the bones, muscles, tendons, and other connective tissue of the back

extremity the body area of the arms and legs, including the joints of the arms and legs; the muscles, tendons, and connective tissue; phalanges (fingers and toes); the circulatory veins, arteries, and vessels; the lymphatic vessels and nodes

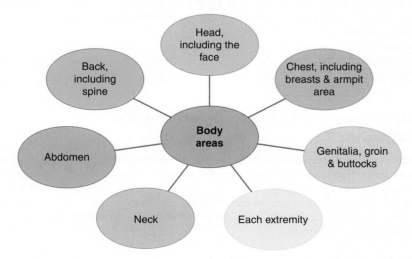

Figure 6.1 ■ Body areas.

- **Head, including the face** (brain, bone, eyes, nose, etc.)
- **Neck** (trachea, esophagus, thyroid, larynx, arteries, veins, bones or muscles, etc.)
- **Chest, including breasts and armpit area** (lungs, heart, armpits, breast tissue, sternum, lymph, etc.)
- **Abdomen** (large and small intestine, pancreas, bladder, arteries, etc.)
- **Genitalia, groin, and buttocks** (male and female genitals, musculoskeletal anatomy of groin, pelvis, etc.)
- **Back, including spine** (bone, tendon, nerve, veins, etc.)
- **Each extremity** (bone, muscle, tendon, veins, etc.)

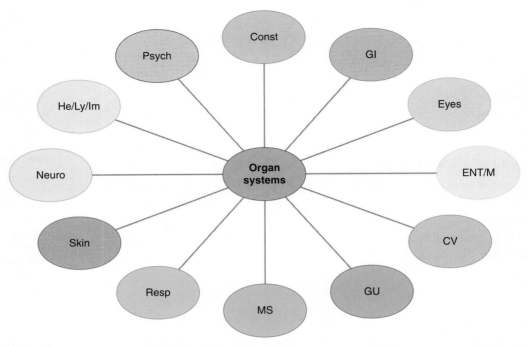

Figure 6.2 Organ systems.

- **Constitutional (Const)**: vital signs (temperature, height, weight, blood pressure, pulse, etc.), general appearance (attention to grooming), body habitus (or physical and/or constitutional characteristics of the individual), etc.
- **Eyes**: eyeball, conjunctivae (inner surface of eyelids), eyelids, pupils, irises, eyeball, retina, etc.
- **Ears, nose, throat, & mouth (ENT/M)**: **Ears**: outer ear (earlobe, ear canal, surface of eardrum), middle ear, inner ear; **Nose**: nasal passages, sinuses, septum; **Throat & Mouth**: tongue, palate, tonsils, pharynx, epiglottis, larynx, etc.
- **Cardiovascular (CV)**: heart auscultation, palpation, pulse, amplitude; bruits in arteries; aorta; veins; edema in extremities; varicosities in extremities; etc.
- **Respiratory (Resp)**: lungs auscultation, percussion, palpation, etc.
- **Gastrointestinal (GI)**: auscultation, percussion, palpation of abdomen; liver; stomach; small and large intestines; rectum; anus; etc.
- **Genitourinary (GU)**: genitals (male testicles, spermatic cord, penis, etc.; female ovaries, vagina, uterus, mammary glands, etc.), urinary (kidneys, ureters, urethra, bladder, meatus, etc.)

- **Musculoskeletal (MS)**: gait (ability to walk, step, skip, etc.), joints, bones, muscles, ligaments, range of motion, etc.
- **Skin or Integumentary (Integ)**: dermis, epidermis, subcutaneous tissue, hair, nails, sweat glands, etc.
- **Neurologic (Neuro)**: concentration skills, language ability (dysphasia, aphasia, dysarthria, apraxia, etc.), cranial nerve function via reflex, sensation, coordination testing, etc.
- **Psychiatric (Psych)**: speech patterns (volume, rate, coherence, speed/rate, etc.), thought processes (logical vs. illogical, etc.), computation ability, abnormal or psychotic thoughts (hallucinations, delusions, homicidal or suicidal ideation, obsessions, etc.), orientation to time, place, and person, etc.
- **Hematologic/Lymphatic/Immunologic (He/Ly/Im)**: **Hematologic**: blood or blood-producing agents (spleen, etc.); **Lymphatic& Immunologic**: lymph nodes, lymph vessels, etc.

neck the body area between the chin and the collarbone; includes, but is not limited to, the trachea, larynx (voice box), thyroid, upper esophagus, lymph nodes, neck (cervical) vertebrae, muscles, tendons

abdomen the body area extending from the lowest rib to the pelvic bones, encompassing the small and large intestines; liver; spleen; bladder; muscles, tendons, and connective tissue of the abdomen; veins and arteries of the abdomen (including the aorta)

Can Body Areas and Organ Systems Be Listed Together?

Recognizing when specific documentation reflects a body area or an organ system requires critical thinking and common sense. Body areas refer to geographic sections of the body, whereas organ systems refer to systemic tissues, organs, vessels, or other specific anatomical parts. The anatomical references in the documentation must be reviewed to determine whether the findings reflect a general body area or a specific organ system. The following example reflects a physical examination of the respiratory organ system and the cardiovascular organ system.

> **Example: Documentation of Organ Systems**
>
> Lungs clear on **auscultation**. Heart sounds normal without murmur.

The next example reflects a physical examination of the body area of the chest and the cardiovascular organ system.

> **Example: Documentation of Organ Systems and Body Area**
>
> Lungs clear on auscultation. Breasts symmetrical without lumps or nodules.

auscultation listening to the sounds produced in an organ or body cavity

CMS recognized something very important about every clinical encounter: every patient is unique and has a different chief complaint. This means that every physical examination will be different. The 1995 DGs provide clarity and consistency across the medical industry without imposing too many limitations; clinicians are free to document the physical examination using body areas or organ systems.

Exercise 6.1 Identifying Organ Systems and Body Areas in the Physical Examination

Underline the organ systems and body areas that are documented in each of the following examinations and identify the specific body area and organ system findings in the spaces below.

1. History: Patient has presented for sinus pressure and cough. Patient's face hurts so much on the right cheek beneath eye that she feels she cannot open her eyes all the way because of the stabbing pain. She complains of a ringing in her right ear, and the right side of her throat hurts when she swallows. She has no appetite, complains of heartburn but no nausea. Nighttime has been interrupted by frequent urination without pain but very smelly urine. Patient denies joint pain other than a sore neck. Patient complains of heavy chest pressure and pain upon coughing. Patient states she can feel her heartbeat in her head as a throbbing but denies any heart palpitations. Patient reports she has spent 3 days lying down because of the discomfort and feels dizzy upon standing up. No report of sick contact at work; however, her husband had the flu last month. Neither patient nor her husband smokes tobacco.

   Exam: Patient is pale and appears very tired, appears well groomed. Conjunctivae clear without swelling. Nasal passages quite congested and very swollen. Fluid noted within inner ear bilaterally; however, tympanic membrane does not appear significantly pressured. Throat mottled with yellow and white patches, and tonsils significantly red and swollen. Palpation of neck reveals very tender, swollen lymph nodes. Patient expresses extreme discomfort when swallowing.

   Documented body areas:

   _____

   _____

   _____

   Documented organ systems:

   _____

   _____

   _____

2. Timmy is an established patient and presents for abdominal pain and diarrhea. Timmy says his stomach hurts, down low on the right side, and that it hurts really, really badly, but not all the time. Timmy's father reports his son complains most about the pain in the morning after getting up, and Timmy describes that pain as an 8 on pain scale. Per father's report, Timmy feels better after eating breakfast, but the pain became bad last week. Per father's report, Timmy had stomach flu last month with no vomiting but explosive diarrhea. Timmy's father denies bloody stools but states that Timmy's urine is dark and odorous but that Timmy denies painful urination. Upon query, Timmy complains of some pain in his back during the last week, placing his hands on his midback. Timmy states he felt dizzy during the past week after walking upstairs at school and home. Patient is second grader at Hardy Oaks Elementary and active in peewee soccer as a goalie; per father, Timmy was recently involved in a goal-side tackle with resultant sharp abdominal pain. Timmy reported domestic incident between his parents at practice; father corroborates Timmy's report. Patient's primary residence is with father, with joint custody with mother; Timmy states visitation with mother is occasional with stressful transitions. Timmy's father denies use of tobacco or alcohol.

   PE: Timmy appears pale but without fever, pulse 130. Eyes clear with no jaundice. Lungs clear to auscultation. Heart: normal but rapid heartbeat without murmur. Timmy complains of pain during palpation of costovertebral angle. Abdomen firm with rebound; however, bladder full upon palpation, although Timmy provided urinary specimen and claims he emptied his bladder. Urinary meatus appears red and inflamed.

   Documented body areas:

   _____

   _____

   _____

   Documented organ systems:

   _____

   _____

   _____

3. Joan is an established patient who presents for lower back pain. Her lower back hurts, down by beltline, and pain is sometimes very severe. The pain is sporadic, mostly when standing up after sitting in one place for an extended period. Ibuprofen used to help, but now it does not help back pain anymore. At its worst, low back pain is sharp and throbbing. Joan has had occasional back pain for about 20 years, since

continued

first in the service, but she first noticed this particular low back pain shortly after playing touch football with adult children this past Thanksgiving. Patient denies any other joint pain. Denies double vision or dizziness. No chest pain or shortness of breath. Patient denies tobacco or alcohol use. Pain has not affected her work as a fifth-grade teacher.

Exam: Back is soft to the touch; palpation revealed no obvious lumps or masses. Lower back tender to applied pressure, but no costovertebral tenderness. She finds leaning forward painful and is unable to touch her toes, but the pain is localized to her lower back and does not radiate down legs or up her back.

Documented body areas:

_____

_____

_____

_____

Documented organ systems:

_____

_____

_____

_____

DOCUMENTATION REQUIREMENTS

The chief complaint is a simple, direct statement relating the reason for the patient's presence in the physician's office—for example, a sore stomach, sinus pressure and cough, or back pain. However, this chief complaint is only a starting point. From the time the physician documents the chief complaint, he or she proceeds to collect a wide range of information about the patient's health: a history of present illness, review of systems, and past, family, and social history. The physician executes mental gymnastics to synthesize the information provided by the patient, as well as the physician's own personal observation of the patient. This synthesis allows the physician to posit the underlying cause of the patient's chief complaint, known as the nature of the presenting problem.

Nature of Presenting Problem

The chief complaint is defined as the patient's description of the specific health issue, complaint, or disease for which the patient presents to the clinician for care. Sometimes the patient presents with only the CC, such as a headache. However, when an additional sign or symptom, such as thick, greenish brown phlegm, accompanies the headache, the CC becomes more complex. At other times, a combination of signs or symptoms—such as thick, greenish brown phlegm, a productive cough, and a high fever—accompany the headache. Other factors also increase the complexity of the CC, as evidenced when the headache is accompanied by thick, greenish brown phlegm, a productive cough, and a high fever in a patient who also happens to smoke cigarettes.

Whereas the chief complaint is the patient's description of the specific health issue, complaint, or disease for which the patient seeks care, the **nature of the presenting problem** is the physician's holistic view of the patient's illness, symptom, CC, disease process, or other reason for care before the definition of a diagnosis. Consider the following example of four patients, each of whom presented to the clinic for a headache.

nature of the presenting problem the physician's clinical identification of the severity of and risk posed by the condition, disease, illness, injury, complaint, or other medical reason for which the patient has presented to the healthcare facility for the E/M service

Four Different Examples for the Nature of Presenting Problem

Patient A came to the clinic because of a headache.

Patient D came to the clinic because of a headache and thick, greenish brown phlegm draining from the nose and down the throat.

Patient G came to the clinic because of a headache, thick, greenish brown phlegm draining from the nose and down the throat, a high fever, juicy cough, and neck pain.

Patient J came to the clinic because of a headache, thick, greenish brown phlegm draining from the nose and down the throat, a high fever, juicy cough, and neck pain. Patient J smokes one pack of cigarettes a day.

Notice that the nature of the presenting problem for Patient A did not seem as severe as that for Patient J. At the time of the E/M service visit, the physician must weigh the nature of the presenting problem with his or her own clinical judgment when deciding how to proceed with the physical examination. The documentation of the physical examination reflects the effort, knowledge, skill, and clinical judgment of the physician.

The "1995 Documentation Guidelines for Evaluation and Management Services" defines different types of physical examination documentation. Each of the different types represents a different level of complexity in the physical examination. The categories of body areas and organ systems help to organize the documentation of the physical examination by quantifying the physical examination. The 1995 DGs establish specific parameters for physicians to follow when documenting the physical examination, specifically addressing abnormal, unexpected, and normal, or negative, findings.

Documentation Requirements for Abnormal Physical Examination Findings

The phrase "symptomatic body area or organ system" suggests that a specific organ system or body area is experiencing symptoms of the chief complaint. In the physical examination documentation, the word *abnormal* suggests that a specific part of the patient's body is not functioning as it should, that is, something is wrong. When the physician identifies an aspect of the patient's physiology or anatomy that is abnormal, the documentation must indicate specifically what is abnormal. For instance, "the patient's temperature is abnormal" would be insufficient documentation of the body temperature of a 3-year-old patient who presents with a fever of 102°F. Therefore, the 1995 DGs require elaboration about any physical examination findings that the physician identifies as abnormal.

Documentation Requirements for Unexpected Findings in an Asymptomatic Organ System/Body Area

The phrase "asymptomatic body area or organ system" suggests that a specific organ system or body area is unaffected by the chief complaint. Occasionally, however, the physician may notice something abnormal or unexpected in an organ system or body area that is unaffected by the CC. For example, a woman might present for sinus pain and congestion, but the physical examination might reveal a pea-sized lump under her right armpit. The lump might be unrelated to the sinus pain and congestion but would constitute an abnormal and unexpected finding in an unaffected body area. In such a situation, the physician must explain what is abnormal or unexpected about this asymptomatic organ system or body area.

> **Example: Unexpected Findings in an Asymptomatic Organ System/Body Area**
>
> A 32-year old woman presents for sinus pain and congestion that has continued for two weeks. The patient denies abdominal pain, painful urination or muscle aches. During the physical examination, the physician identifies a pea sized lump under the right armpit that is painful to palpation.
>
> The lump under the armpit may be unrelated to the sinus pain and congestion, however, this is an abnormal and unexpected finding.

Documentation Requirements for Normal Physical Examination Findings

The word *normal* suggests that something is expected and of no concern. In the context of the physical examination, the word *negative* also suggests that the physician has found nothing of concern in that specific organ system or body area. Physicians spend a lot of time documenting the healthcare provided, and documentation is hard work. Therefore, the 1995 DGs provided physicians an opportunity for abbreviating the documentation of physical examination findings of unaffected organ systems or asymptomatic body areas that are functioning properly and posing no concern for the physician. A short phrase or a brief account specifying that the individual organ system or body area is normal or negative is sufficient. Given the number of physical examinations performed throughout the country on any given day, consistency in documenting the physical examination provides continuity across the country and ensures accountability within the medical field.

LEVELS OF PHYSICAL EXAMINATION

The 1995 DGs define four types of physical examination: problem-focused, expanded problem-focused, detailed, and comprehensive. Each of these four types reflects a different level of examination in relation to the affected body area or organ system and to any inclusion of other symptomatic or related organ systems (see ■ TABLE 6.1).

■ **TABLE 6.1** **THE FOUR TYPES OF PHYSICAL EXAMINATION**

- **Problem-focused**—a limited examination of the affected body area or organ system
- **Expanded problem-focused**—a limited examination of the affected body area or organ system and other symptomatic or related organ systems
- **Detailed**—an extended examination of the affected body area(s) or organ system(s) and other symptomatic or related body areas or organ systems
- **Comprehensive**—a general multisystem examination or a complete examination of a single organ system and other symptomatic or related body areas or organ systems, including about 8 or more of the 12 organ systems

Source: Centers for Medicare and Medicaid Services, "1995 Documentation Guidelines for Evaluation & Management Services," pp. 9–10, www.cms.gov/Outreach-and-Education/Medicare-Learning-Network-MLN/MLNEdWebGuide/Downloads/95Docguidelines.pdf.

These guidelines help to define the types of physical examination; however, there are no numeric guidelines for each specific type. This lack of specifically defined requirements has been the subject of intense discussion for many years among those in the medical documentation community, and some suggestions have been made by certifying organizations, such as the American College of Emergency Physicians, the American Association of Professional Coders, the American Health Information Management Association, as well as others. It is important to remember that any suggested quantifiable definitions of the four types of physical examination found in the 1995 DGs are not supported by the CMS but are merely suggestions that may be informally accepted as industry standards. This text recognizes that there are widely accepted numerical levels associated with the four types of physical examination found in the 1995 DGs, and these appear in ■ TABLE 6.2, as well as in ■ FIGURE 6.3 in a familiar format.

Remember that the numbers for each physical examination type refer only to the physical examination documentation, not to the actual physical examination. This reflection can be only as thorough as the physician's documentation of the physical examination actually performed.

■ **TABLE 6.2** **TYPES OF PHYSICAL EXAMINATION**

- **Problem-focused**—reflected in the documentation of one organ system or body area that has been examined by the clinician
- **Expanded problem-focused**—reflected in the documentation of between two and four organ systems and/or body areas that have been examined by the clinician
- **Detailed**—reflected in the documentation of between five and seven organ systems and/or body areas that have been examined by the clinician
- **Comprehensive**—reflected in the documentation of eight or more organ systems OR body areas that have been examined by the clinician

Physical Examination	Problem-Focused	Expanded Problem-Focused	Detailed	Comprehensive
1995 PE	A limited examination of affected body area or organ system (1 body area/organ system)	A limited examination of the affected body area or organ system and other symptomatic or related organ systems (2–4 body areas/organ systems)	An extended examination of the affected body area(s) or organ system(s) and other symptomatic or related body areas or organ systems (5–7 body areas/organ systems)	A general multisystem examination or complete examination of a single organ system and other symptomatic or related body areas or organ systems; should include 8 or more of the 12 organ systems (8+ body systems OR organ systems, but they cannot be mixed)

Figure 6.3 ■ Content of service element: 1995 physical examination.

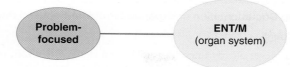

Figure 6.4 ■ Graphic example of problem-focused physical examination.

Problem-Focused

The problem-focused type of physical examination is reflected in the documentation of only one organ system or body area that has been examined. The following example shows documentation that supports a problem-focused physical examination, whereas ■ FIGURE 6.4 uses a bubble chart to represent this type graphically.

Example: Reviewing Documentation of Problem-Focused Physical Examination

Johnny's Irritating Cough

Serous fluid is apparent behind tympanic membrane. Patient is uncomfortably congested with significant mucus production via nares. Patient's cough produces thick, white phlegm upon expectoration and solid, white exudates apparent on tonsils and along back of pharynx.

The anatomical specificity of the documentation reflects **one organ system,** rather than the body area of the head.

Ears, Nose, Throat, and Mouth—

Ears: fluid behind tympanic membrane (eardrum)

Nose: congested with significant mucus via nares

Throat: white exudates apparent on tonsils and along back of pharynx

---

Expanded Problem-Focused

The expanded problem-focused physical examination is reflected in the documentation of between two and four organ systems and/or body areas that have been examined by the clinician. The 1995 DGs state that organ systems and body areas may be combined to support this type of physical examination. The following example shows documentation that supports an expanded problem-focused type of physical examination, whereas ■ FIGURE 6.5 represents this type graphically.

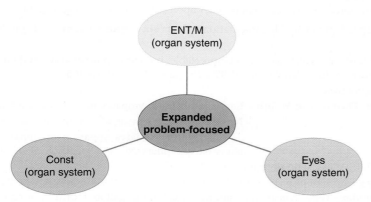

Figure 6.5 ■ Graphic example of expanded problem-focused physical examination.

Example: Reviewing Documentation of Expanded Problem-Focused Physical Examination

Johnny's Irritating Cough

Patient is alert, however clearly uncomfortable. Vital signs: T, 99.32F; pulse, 120; BP, 100/65. Eyes: conjunctivae clear. ENT/M: serous fluid apparent behind tympanic membrane. Patient is uncomfortably congested with significant mucus production via nares. Patient's cough produces thick, white phlegm upon expectoration and solid, white exudates apparent on tonsils and along back of pharynx.

The anatomical specificity of the documentation reflects **three organ systems,** rather than the body area of the head. Even though the eyes and ears, nose, and throat are all located in the head, the specific findings documented suggest physical examination of organ systems rather than geographical areas.

Constitutional—patient is alert, however clearly uncomfortable; vital signs: temperature, 99.32F; pulse, 120; blood pressure, 100/65

Eyes—conjunctivae clear

Ears, Nose, Throat, and Mouth—Ears: fluid behind tympanic membrane (eardrum)

Nose: congested with significant mucus via nares
Throat: white exudates apparent on tonsils and along back of pharynx

Detailed

The detailed physical examination is reflected in the documentation of between five and seven organ systems and/or body areas that have been examined. These include the affected body area(s) or organ system(s) and any other symptomatic or related body area(s) or organ system(s). The 1995 DGs state that organ systems and body areas may be combined to support a detailed type of physical examination. The following example shows documentation that supports a detailed type of physical examination, whereas ■ FIGURE 6.6 shows visual representation of this type of physical examination, indicating how the organ systems and body areas may be combined.

Example: Reviewing Documentation of Detailed Physical Examination

Johnny's Irritating Cough (and Stomachache)

Patient is clearly uncomfortable, but alert, in no distress, and curious about his surroundings. Vital signs: T, 99.32F; pulse, 120; BP, 100/65. Eyes: conjunctivae clear. ENT/M: serous fluid apparent behind tympanic membrane. Patient is uncomfortably congested with significant mucus production via nares. Patient's cough produces thick, white phlegm upon expectoration and solid, white exudates apparent on tonsils and along back of pharynx. Neck is soft, no masses; no thyromegaly. Chest: no sign of respiratory distress; lungs clear without crackles, wheezes. Regular heart rate and rhythm, without gallop, murmur, or rub. Abdomen: soft, mild tenderness noted in left lower quadrant with palpable stool. Patient states he has not passed BM for 3 days; no hepatosplenomegaly noted, but patient reports pain upon palpation of left upper quadrant.

The anatomical specificity of the documentation reflects **six organ systems** and **one body area**.

Constitutional—patient is clearly uncomfortable; but alert, in no distress, and curious about his surroundings. Vital signs: T, 99.32F; pulse, 120; BP, 100/65.

Eyes—conjunctivae clear

Ears, Nose, Throat, and Mouth—Ears: fluid behind tympanic membrane (eardrum)

Nose: congested with significant mucus via nares
Throat: white exudates apparent on tonsils and along back of pharynx

Neck—soft, no masses; no thyromegaly.

Respiratory—no sign of respiratory distress; lungs clear without crackles, wheezes.

Cardiovascular—regular heart rate and rhythm, without gallop, murmur, or rub.

Gastrointestinal (or Abdomen)—soft abdomen, mild tenderness noted in left lower quadrant with palpable stool. Patient states he has not passed BM for 3 days; no hepatosplenomegaly noted, but patient reports pain upon palpation of left upper quadrant.

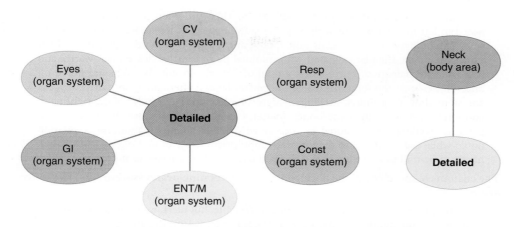

Figure 6.6 ■ Graphic example of detailed physical examination listing six organ systems and only one body area.

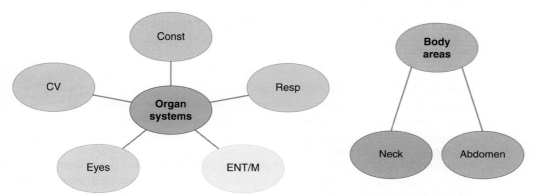

Figure 6.7 ■ Another version of a detailed physical examination listing five organ systems and two body areas.

In this example, the gastrointestinal findings of the physical examination could be listed as **either** organ system (GI) **or** body area (abdomen). The documentation requirements for a detailed physical examination (PE) state only that between five and seven body areas and/or organ systems must be documented. Remember, however, that there is a stark difference between an organ system and a body area in the 1995 DGs. ■ FIGURE 6.7 presents the documented findings as five organ systems and two body areas.

Comprehensive

The comprehensive physical examination is reflected in the documentation of eight or more organ systems OR body areas that have been examined. Notice the difference between the requirements for a comprehensive physical examination and the requirements for the other three types of physical examination. The comprehensive physical examination is the only type that prohibits combining the documented findings of organ systems and body areas; the requirements stipulate that eight organ systems **or** eight body areas may be counted, but not a combination of eight organ systems and body areas together. The following two examples reflect one documented comprehensive physical examination in two different formats to help illustrate the unique requirements of the separation of body areas and organ systems.

Example: Reviewing Documentation of Comprehensive Physical Examination Utilizing Organ Systems

Johnny's Irritating Cough (and Stomachache after a Bad Fall)

Patient is clearly uncomfortable, but alert, in no distress, and curious about his surroundings. Vital signs: T, 99.32F; pulse, 120; BP, 100/65. Head: atraumatic, nontender. Eyes: conjunctivae clear. ENT/M: serous fluid apparent behind tympanic membrane. Patient is uncomfortably congested with significant mucus production via nares. Patient's cough produces thick, white phlegm upon expectoration and solid, white exudates apparent on tonsils and along back of pharynx. Neck is soft, no masses; no thyromegaly. Chest: no sign of respiratory distress; lungs clear without crackles, wheezes.

continued

Regular heart rate, without gallop, murmur, or rub. Abdomen: soft, mild tenderness noted in left lower quadrant with palpable stool. Patient states he has not passed BM since fall; no hepatosplenomegaly noted, but patient reports pain upon palpation of left upper quadrant. Bladder palpated with minimal pain; testicles descended, warm, and nontender to palpation. Extremities: a total of four significant abrasions are noted on knees, lower legs, and forearms where the patient landed after falling onto driveway; the abrasions show no redness, swelling, or signs of infection. The wound of the right palm and forearm shows significant foreign matter. Patient is able to move all joints without pain; no swelling or pain noted in knee or wrist joints upon palpation; no crepitation noted when patient asked to demonstrate appropriate range of motion; patient seemed happy to be told to move freely and skipped back and forth across exam room.

The anatomical specificity of the documentation reflects **nine organ systems** and **two body areas**.

Constitutional—patient is clearly uncomfortable, but alert, in no distress, and curious about his surroundings. Vital signs: T, 99.32F; pulse, 120; BP, 100/65.

Head—atraumatic, nontender

Eyes—conjunctivae clear

Ears, Nose, Throat, and Mouth—Ears: fluid behind tympanic membrane (eardrum)

Nose: congested with significant mucus via nares

Throat: white exudates apparent on tonsils and along back of pharynx

Neck—neck soft, no masses; no thyromegaly

Respiratory—no sign of respiratory distress; lungs clear without crackles, wheezes

Cardiovascular—regular heart rate, without gallop, murmur, or rub

Gastrointestinal (or Abdomen): soft abdomen, mild tenderness noted in left lower quadrant with palpable stool. Patient states he has not passed BM since fall; no hepato-splenomegaly noted, but patient reports pain upon palpation of left upper quadrant.

Genitourinary—bladder palpated with minimal pain; testicles descended, warm, and nontender to palpation

Skin—four significant abrasions are noted on knees, lower legs, and forearms where the patient landed after falling onto driveway; the abrasions show no redness, swelling, or signs of infection. The wound of the right palm and forearm shows significant foreign matter.

Musculoskeletal—patient is able to move all joints without pain; no swelling or pain noted in knee or wrist joints upon palpation; no crepitation noted when patient asked to demonstrate appropriate range of motion; patient seemed happy to be told to move freely and skipped back and forth across exam room.

▧ FIGURE 6.8 gives a graphic representation of the organ systems and body areas documented in this example.

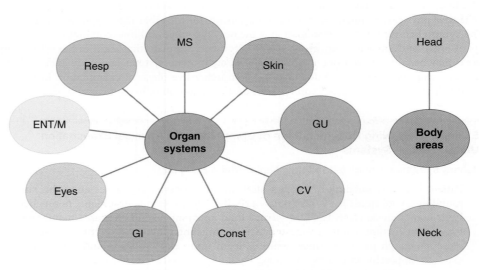

Figure 6.8 ▧ Graphic example of a comprehensive physical examination.

That same documentation of a comprehensive examination could be reviewed in a slightly different manner, identifying **nine body areas** and **one organ system.**

Example: Reviewing Documentation of Comprehensive Physical Examination Utilizing Body Areas

Johnny's Irritating Cough (and Stomachache after a Bad Fall)

Constitutional—patient is clearly uncomfortable, but alert, in no distress, and curious about his surroundings. Vital signs: T, 99.32F; pulse, 120; BP, 100/65.

Head—atraumatic, nontender. Eyes: conjunctivae clear. ENT/M: serous fluid apparent behind tympanic membrane. Patient is uncomfortably congested with significant mucus production via nares.

Neck—patient's cough produces thick, white phlegm upon expectoration and solid, white exudates apparent on tonsils and along back of pharynx. Neck soft, no masses; no thyromegaly.

Chest—no sign of respiratory distress; lungs clear without crackles, wheezes. Regular heart rate and rhythm, without gallop, murmur, or rub.

Abdomen—soft, mild tenderness noted in left lower quadrant with palpable stool. Patient states he has not passed BM since fall; no hepatosplenomegaly noted, but patient reports pain upon palpation of left upper quadrant. Bladder palpated with minimal pain.

Genitalia, groin, buttocks—testicles descended, warm, and nontender to palpation.

Extremities (a total of four)—a total of four significant abrasions are noted on two lower extremities (knees, lower legs) and two upper extremities (forearms) where the patient landed after falling onto driveway; the abrasions show no redness, swelling, or signs of infection. The wound of the right palm and forearm shows significant foreign matter. Patient is able to move all joints without pain; no swelling or pain noted in knee or wrist joints upon palpation; no crepitation noted when patient asked to demonstrate appropriate range of motion; patient seemed happy to be told to move freely and skipped back and forth across exam room.

To provide a visual aid, ■ FIGURE 6.9 shows these body areas and organ systems graphically.

Every physician who performs a physical examination follows a certain logic and reason in that examination. As a result, the documented type of physical examination informs the reviewer about the physician's logic and process. For instance, it may not be reasonable for the documented physical examination to include examination of the breast and axillary tissues of an 8-year-old boy with a sprained ankle, since breasts are not a common physiology for an 8-year-old boy.

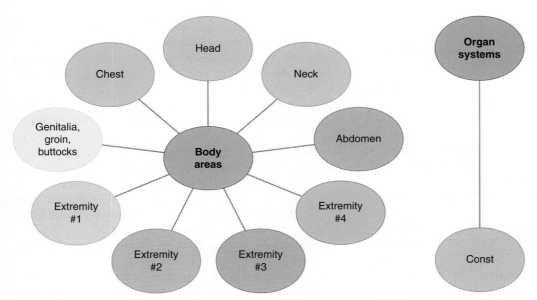

Figure 6.9 ■ Comprehensive organ system and body area graphic representation.

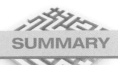

SUMMARY

- As a snapshot of a patient's health, the physical examination can often be found after the documented history. The verb tense helps to identify the documented physical examination, which reflects the state of the patient's health at the time of the EM service visit. The documented physical examination reveals clinical findings that would be identified by the performing physician, such as distinct vital signs and clinical terms.

- The physical examination requires physical interaction between the physician and the patient, which allows the physician to identify specific findings. These findings require the performing physician to actually touch the patient while palpating the abdomen, actually listen to the patient's heart with the help of a stethoscope, or actually look at the patient's throat with the help of a small light. The findings for the physical examination should be legibly documented to facilitate coordination of care and clarity within the patient's medical record.

- The 1995 DGs define two distinct categories: organ systems and body areas. There are twelve organ systems, each of which represents a series of interconnected tissues, structures, and organs that operate together to perform a specific physiological function. Seven body areas represent specific anatomic regions that comprise the entire human body.

- The 1995 DGs define different types of physical examination and identify the amount of documentation necessary to represent each type that is performed by a physician. The four types reflect the differing levels of complexity inherent in the physical examinations. The categories of body areas and organ systems help to organize the documentation of the physical examination.

- The 1995 DGs define four types of physical examination: problem-focused, expanded problem-focused, detailed, and comprehensive. Each of the four types reflects a different level of documented physical examination. The DGs do not specifically define a numerical equivalent for each of the types. For purposes of consistency, this text has assigned a specific numerical guide to each of the types. A problem-focused physical examination is reflected in the documentation of one organ system or body area that has been examined by the clinician. An expanded problem-focused physical examination is reflected in the documentation of between two and four organ systems and/or body areas. A detailed physical examination is reflected in the documentation of between five and seven organ systems and/or body areas. A comprehensive physical examination is reflected in the documentation of eight or more organ systems OR body areas. The comprehensive type is the only one that cannot combine both organ systems and body areas in determining the type of physical examination.

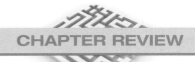

CHAPTER REVIEW

Multiple Choice

Choose the letter that best answers each question or completes each statement.

1. In the medical documentation of the E/M service visit, the physical examination reflects which of the following?
   a. The past medical history, family medical history, and day-to-day activities of the patient
   b. A snapshot of the patient's health at the time of the E/M service visit, including the functions, performance, structure, and health of the patient's body
   c. An inventory of the patient's status of health prior to the E/M service visit
   d. Descriptions provided by the patient that provide a personalized illustration of the symptom the patient is currently experiencing

2. Which of the following phrases best represents "organ systems"?
   a. Categories dividing the entire human structure into geographic sections

   b. Eight standardized descriptions that provide a personalized illustration of the patient's current symptom or condition
   c. Division of the human body into separate anatomical systems that each operate for one specific physiologic function
   d. A holistic view of the patient's illness, symptom, chief complaint, disease process, or other reason for care before the definition of a diagnosis

3. Which of the following phrases best represents "body areas"?
   a. Division of the human body into separate anatomical systems that each operate for one specific physiologic function
   b. A holistic view of the patient's illness, symptom, chief complaint, disease process, or other reason for care before the definition of a diagnosis
   c. Categories dividing the entire human structure into geographic sections
   d. Eight standardized descriptions that provide a personalized illustration of the patient's current symptom or condition

4. How many types of physical examination are listed in the "1995 Documentation Guidelines for Evaluation and Management Services"?

    a. Two

    b. Three

    c. Four

    d. Five

5. Which of the following represents the problem-focused type of physical examination?

    a. A limited examination of the affected body area or organ system

    b. A limited examination of the affected body area or organ system and other symptomatic or related organ systems

    c. An extended examination of the affected body area(s) or organ system(s) and other symptomatic or related body areas or organ systems

    d. A general multisystem examination or complete examination of a single organ system and other symptomatic or related body areas or organ systems

6. Which of the following represents an expanded problem-focused type of physical examination?

    a. A general multisystem examination or complete examination of a single organ system and other symptomatic or related body areas or organ systems

    b. A limited examination of the affected body area or organ system

    c. An extended examination of the affected body area(s) or organ system(s) and other symptomatic or related body areas or organ systems

    d. A limited examination of the affected body area or organ system and other symptomatic or related organ systems

7. Which of the following represents a detailed type of physical examination?

    a. An extended examination of the affected body area(s) or organ system(s) and other symptomatic or related body areas or organ systems

    b. A limited examination of the affected body area or organ system

    c. A general multisystem examination or complete examination of a single organ system and other symptomatic or related body areas or organ systems

    d. A limited examination of the affected body area or organ system and other symptomatic or related organ systems

8. Which of the following represents a comprehensive type of physical examination?

    a. A limited examination of the affected body area or organ system and other symptomatic or related organ systems

    b. A limited examination of the affected body area or organ system

    c. A general multisystem examination or complete examination of a single organ system and other symptomatic or related body areas or organ systems

    d. An extended examination of the affected body area(s) or organ system(s) and other symptomatic or related body areas or organ systems

9. In order to perform the physical examination, what must the physician do?

    a. Introduce him- or herself to the patient, using eye contact and a handshake

    b. Ensure the patient has signed a privacy agreement in the patient's medical documentation, either by asking whether the patient remembers signing the privacy agreement or actually finding the signed privacy agreement

    c. Physically interact with the patient, such as by touching or palpating, listening to, or looking at or inspecting different parts of the patient's body

    d. Ensure the stethoscope or any other instruments to be used on the patient are warm

10. Which of the following types of physical examinations does not allow the combination of body areas and organ systems?

    a. Problem-focused

    b. Expanded problem-focused

    c. Detailed

    d. Comprehensive

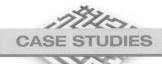

CASE STUDIES

Case Study 6-1

Read the following documentation, and then answer questions 1–11 by identifying the organ system or body area documented in the physical examination according to the 1995 Documentation Guidelines.

Light head contusion along lateral hairline with no pain upon examination. Extra-ocular movements are intact. Neck soft without masses. No cervical spine tenderness. No thoracic spine tenderness and no lumbar spine tenderness. Patient does have a dark, category 3 contusion along entire URQ, and patient expresses significant pain upon any palpation. Entire abdomen tense with no rebound, patient "holding breath against pain." Patient expressed nausea upon palpation and vomited immediately after abdominal exam; face flushed with temperature of 101.2. Palpation of lower abdomen reveals a full bladder; patient tolerated lower abdominal exam much better with only moderate pain. Inguinal hernia incision site is well healed with no redness, pain, or other s/s of infection or dehiscence.

1. Which organ system or body area is documented in the words "neck soft without masses"?

    a. Head

    b. ENT/M

    c. Neck

    d. Musculoskeletal

2. Which body area or organ system is documented in the words "palpation of lower abdomen reveals a full bladder"?
   a. Genitourinary
   b. Respiratory
   c. Cardiovascular
   d. Constitutional

3. Which organ system or body area is documented in these words: "No cervical spine tenderness . . . no thoracic spine tenderness and no lumbar spine tenderness"?
   a. Hematologic/Lymphatic/Immunologic
   b. Abdomen
   c. Extremities
   d. Musculoskeletal

4. Which body area or organ system is documented in the phrase "face flushed with temperature of 101.2"?
   a. Head
   b. Constitutional
   c. Abdomen
   d. Genitalia, groin, buttocks

5. Which organ system or body area is documented in the words "extra-ocular movements are intact"?
   a. Eyes
   b. Head
   c. Neurologic
   d. Ears, Nose, Throat, and Mouth

6. Which body area or organ system is documented in the phrase "light head contusion along lateral hairline with no pain upon examination"?
   a. Ears, Nose, Throat, and Mouth
   b. Head
   c. Neurologic
   d. Extremity

7. Which organ system or body area is documented in this selection: "Patient does have a dark, category 3 contusion along entire URQ, and patient expresses significant pain upon any palpation. Entire abdomen tense with no rebound, patient 'holding breath against pain.' Patient expressed nausea upon palpation and vomited immediately after abdominal exam"?
   a. Genitalia, groin, buttocks
   b. Psychiatric
   c. Gastrointestinal
   d. Constitutional

8. Which body area or organ system is documented in these words: "Inguinal hernia incision site is well healed with no redness, pain, or other s/s of infection or dehiscence"?
   a. Abdomen
   b. Skin (Integumentary)
   c. Cardiovascular
   d. Genitourinary

9. How many organ systems have been identified in this medical documentation?
   a. One
   b. Three
   c. Six
   d. Twelve

10. How many body areas have been identified in this medical documentation?
    a. One
    b. Two
    c. Six
    d. Twelve

11. What type of physical examination best reflects this documented physical examination?
    a. Problem-focused
    b. Expanded problem-focused
    c. Detailed
    d. Comprehensive

Case Study 6-2

Read the following documentation, then identify the documented level of overall history, the documented organ systems and/or body areas, and the level of physical examination according to the 1995 Documentation Guidelines.

Complaint: Frank is well-known to me and presents for sharp left flank pain and dark-orange-colored urine after a fall resulting in blunt abdominal trauma on Saturday afternoon, 2 days ago. He tripped on his dog and fell against the patio railing, striking his upper left abdomen against the decorative wrought iron. Patient reports experiencing immediate stabbing pain across his upper abdomen and down his left flank, which subsided quickly without recurrence. Upon rising on Sunday morning, Frank noticed sharp stabbing pain across ULQ abdomen, accompanied by dark, painful bruising in the area of his URQ where he was struck by the railing. The pain is most severe when he breathes deeply, rating pain at 8/10, and Frank cannot bend his torso without significant pain. He reports his urine sample to be very dark and odorous but denies painful urination. He denies any chest pain or racing heartbeat. No reports of tingling of extremities, dizziness, nausea, bloody stool. All other reviews of systems pertinent to this problem are negative. No report of ill contact at work or family, although Frank reports a higher stress level than usual, as budget cuts at work have caused many layoffs and he is anxious about his employment status. There is no history of gastrointestinal disease in family or past medical history.

Physical Exam: Frank appears without distress, gregarious with an appropriate sense of humor about his fall. Eyes clear without jaundice; pupils equal, round, reactive to light. Head is atraumatic without tenderness or rashes. Neck is soft without masses. Auscultation of lungs clear without wheezes or rub. Heart: regular rate and rhythm with no abnormal sounds noted. No cervical spine tenderness. No thoracic or lumbar spine tenderness or costovertebral tenderness noted upon palpation. No referred pain in left shoulder. Palpation of lower abdomen reveals soft, nontender abdomen, and no hepatomegaly or tenderness upon upper right quadrant palpation or **percussion.** Upper left abdomen mildly inflamed with dark circular bruise where patient identifies blow to abdomen. Very tender upper left quadrant upon palpation, and patient's pain precludes deep palpation of spleen. No dullness noted upon percussion of left or right flank.

Laboratory: CBC reveals white blood count normal, hemoglobin and hematocrit are normal. A FAST scan abdominal CT scan was reviewed with radiologist. Review of KUB revealed significant stool within sigmoid and rectum. Occult blood test negative.

Assessment: It is quite probable that at least one of the lower left ribs has been fractured, although the patient's pain makes specific rib identification impossible. A splenic injury should be ruled out through CT scan. In my opinion, it would be prudent to begin oral Augmentin treatment at 875 mg twice a day for 7 days and increase fluid intake. Follow up in 10 days for recheck.

1. Identify the level of overall history documented in this case study.

   Level of overall history: _____

   _____

   _____

   _____

   Please include your rationale. _____

   _____

   _____

   _____

2. Identify the documented body areas and organ systems in the physical examination in this case study.

   Documented body areas: _____

   _____

   _____

   _____

   _____

   _____

   Documented organ systems: _____

   _____

   _____

   _____

   _____

   _____

3. Identify the level of physical examination, according to the 1995 Documentation Guidelines: _____

   _____

percussion tapping to determine resonance in or around an organ or body cavity

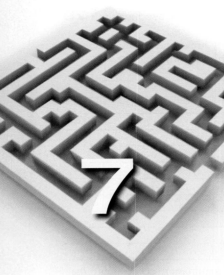

7 Physical Examination— 1997 Documentation Guidelines

Learning Objectives

After completing this chapter, you should be able to do the following:

- Spell and define the key terms and abbreviations presented in this chapter
- Define the specific characteristics of the general multisystem physical examination
- Recognize and identify elements identified by a bullet in the 1997 Documentation Guidelines
- List and identify the requirements for the general multisystem physical examination in the "1997 Documentation Guidelines for Evaluation and Management Services"
- List and define the four types of general multisystem physical examination documentation in the 1997 Documentation Guidelines

Key Terms

abrasion

accessory muscles

ankle jerk reflex

aorta

atrophy

auricle

Babinski test

bilaterally

bronchi

cog wheel

complicating pneumonia

contracture

costovertebral angle

cranial nerves

crepitation

deep tendon reflexes

dislocation

effusion

evidentiary checklist

examination of gait

examination of station

expectoration

extra-ocular movements

exudates

femoral arteries

femur

finger rub test

flaccid

forward flexion

fremitus

gallop

general multisystem physical examination

hard palate

hemorrhages

hepatosplenomegaly

induration

intercostal muscles

jaundice

laxity

luxation

murmur

nasal mucosa

normal visual field test

odorous

oral mucosa

orientation to person

orientation to place

orientation to time

otoscope

patellar reflex

pedal pulse

pertussis

plantar flexion

plantar reflexes

posterior

proprioception

pulmonologist

pupils equal, round, reactive to light (and accommodation)

quadriceps tendon

rebound

regular rate and rhythm

respiration

rhonchi

rub

septum

serous fluid

side-to-side flexion

soft palate

spastic

subluxation

systems/body areas

tibia

tibial tuberosity

tonsils

turbinates

urinary meatus

uvula

wheeze

Abbreviations

PERRL(A) pupils equal, round, reactive to light (and accommodation)

RRR regular heart rate and rhythm

INTRODUCTION

A student takes a variety of different types of examinations during the course of his or her entire education; the nature of those examinations changes according to the material covered, the experience of the student, and the student's comprehension of the material. Similarly, the branch of healthcare known as evaluation and management covers a wide range of services, experiences, and specificity, and the physical examination changes according to the nature of the clinical circumstance. Although the physical examination of any given E/M service visit always addresses the status of the patient's health at the time of the visit, not every physical examination is the same.

Within the story of the patient's health, the physical examination tells the story of what's happening right now, at the moment of the E/M service visit, not what has happened, nor what might yet occur in the patient's health. The circumstances surrounding certain E/M services may warrant a higher degree of specificity than other E/M services.

The 1995 Documentation Guidelines provide parameters for the documentation of the performed physical examination by distinguishing between body areas and organ systems. However, the 1995 Documentation Guidelines do not stipulate the amount of clinical specificity required in the documentation of any examined body area or organ system. Therefore, according to the 1995 Documentation Guidelines, documentation of "Lungs: clear" will support the documentation of a respiratory examination. Although this particular style of documentation may appropriately reflect a general physical examination of the lungs, it may not reflect a more in-depth respiratory physical examination performed by a **pulmonologist**, which may include more clinical elements than the 1995 Documentation Guidelines recognize.

pulmonologist a physician specializing in the health of the pulmonary, or respiratory, system, as well as the prevention and treatment of diseases related to the respiratory system

THE 1997 GENERAL MULTISYSTEM PHYSICAL EXAMINATION

Every clinician undergoes extensive training in performance of the physical examination, including what to look for, what to examine, how to examine the patient, even why certain sections of the body should be examined. After the publication of the 1995 Documentation Guidelines, it became clear that those guidelines for documentation of the physical examination would not effectively represent or offer due respect to the talent and skill of the thousands of trained, practicing physicians performing physical examinations every day. Therefore, to provide greater specificity for performing physicians, as well as to facilitate consistency in the discussion of the physical examination, the 1997 Documentation Guidelines were published. Some of the core aspects of the physical examination guidelines remained the same; for example, the nature of the presenting problem remains one of the foundations of the context of the physical examination, along with the clinical judgment of the performing physician and the patient's history. Also, specific abnormal or unexpected findings within a physical examination should still include elaboration, whereas normal findings may be accompanied by a brief statement documenting the normal or negative physical examination findings.

The most significant difference between the 1995 and 1997 Documentation Guidelines is found in the guidelines for the documentation of the physical examination. Whereas documentation of body areas and/or organ systems is required by the 1995 Documentation Guidelines, the 1997 Documentation Guidelines define requirements for a general multisystem physical examination and a single organ system physical examination.

When a performed physical examination addresses more clinical elements than the 1995 Documentation Guidelines support, the 1997 Documentation Guidelines provide specific parameters for a **general multisystem physical examination**, which is reflected in a more exhaustive documentation of the performed physical examination. The general multisystem physical examination documentation requirements address the status of the patient's health at the time of the E/M visit through the identification of specific clinical elements identified during an examination of multiple organ systems and/or body areas.

It is well-known that the human body is made up of many different parts or anatomical sections; identifying the different anatomical sections can be as simple as the children's song "The foot bone's connected to the ankle bone; the ankle bone's connected to the leg bone. . . ." However, if the 1997 general multisystem physical examination were put to music in this well-known children's song, the song might sound a little bit more like this: "The **tibia** is connected to the tibial tuberosity, the **tibial tuberosity** is connected to the **quadriceps tendon**, the quadriceps tendon is connected to the **femur**. . . ."

Even as a photograph reveals something different about the subject being photographed and the person taking the photograph, the documentation of the physical examination reveals a lot of information about the physician who performed the physical examination. For the 1997 Documentation Guidelines, the documented elements of the physical examination provide specific insight into the functions, performance, structure, and health of the patient's body at the moment of the physical examination. By the nature of the professional focus, a pediatrician's physical examination of a child with a sprained ankle will be different from the same physician's physical examination of a child with **pertussis** and **complicating pneumonia**. As a result, the documentation of the physical examination must reflect the specificity of the performed physical examination.

With this in mind, let us compare the documentation of the 1995 body area/organ system physical examination and the 1997 general multisystem physical examination. Each of these two different examinations has been performed by qualified, skilled physicians, and each reflects a different snapshot of the patient's state of health at the time of the visit.

general multisystem physical examination physical examination that follows the requirements listed in the 1997 Documentation Guidelines for documentation; includes an evidentiary checklist of anatomic, physiologic, and pathologic findings identified by bullets in the guidelines

tibia the larger of the two lower leg bones between the knee and the ankle

tibial tuberosity the rounded protuberance at either end of the tibia

quadriceps tendon the tendon that runs along the back of the thigh, from the hip to the knee

femur the large bone located in the thigh that extends from the hip bone to the knee

pertussis whooping cough

complicating pneumonia opportunistic pneumonia that develops as a result of an illness, often a secondary infection

bilaterally on both sides

Medical Documentation Example A: 1995 Organ System/Body Area Physical Examination

This 25-year-old woman presents to the clinic with complaints of chest congestion, nasal discharge, and "feeling cruddy." Patient is pale and appears very tired. Her clothes are rumpled, but she appears well groomed. Conjunctivae are clear without swelling. Nasal passages are quite congested and very swollen. Fluid is noted within inner ear **bilaterally**. However, tympanic membrane is not significantly pressured. Throat appears mottled with yellow and white patches, and tonsils significantly red and swollen. Palpation of neck reveals very tender, swollen lymph nodes. Patient expresses extreme discomfort when asked to swallow during exam.

Medical Documentation Example B: 1997 General Multisystem Physical Examination

This 25-year-old woman presents to the clinic with complaints of chest congestion, nasal discharge, and "feeling cruddy." T, 101.2; pulse, 70; BP, 120/69. Patient is pale and appears very tired. Her clothes are rumpled, but she appears well groomed. Conjunctivae are clear without swelling. External skin surface covering nostrils and upper lip are red and chapped.

Nasal passages are quite congested, patient unable to inhale through either nostril during patency test. Fluid is noted within inner ear **bilaterally**. However, tympanic membrane does not appear significantly pressured. Throat appears mottled with yellow and white patches, and tonsils significantly red and swollen. Palpation of neck reveals very tender, swollen cervical and postauricular lymph nodes. Patient expresses extreme discomfort when asked to swallow during exam. Lungs: auscultation reveals no **wheezes** or **rhonchi**, percussion resonant. Heart: innocent heart murmur, otherwise normal heart sounds.

Notice that Medical Documentation B, which records a 1997 general multisystem physical examination, includes specific clinical elements that are not documented in Medical Documentation A, which follows the 1995 organ system/body area physical examination. The presence or absence of these clinical elements may not be a reflection of the skill of the physician, but rather an indication of the physician's specialty and professional focus.

1997 GENERAL MULTISYSTEM ELEMENTS IDENTIFIED BY A BULLET

As a nonsurgical, noninvasive medical procedure, the physical examination assesses the health of the patient at the time of the E/M service visit. For the performance of a general multisystem physical examination, the physician examines the patient's state of health through some, or all, of the following organ systems and body areas, which are known as **systems/body areas**:

- Constitutional
- Eyes
- ENT/M
- Neck
- Respiratory
- Cardiovascular
- Chest (Breasts)
- Gastrointestinal (Abdomen)
- Genitourinary
- Lymphatic
- Musculoskeletal
- Skin
- Neurologic
- Psychiatric

The 1997 general multisystem physical examination guidelines describe requirements for the documentation and the content of that examination. These requirements are presented in the form of specific clinical elements, and each element is identified by a bullet (•). Each of these elements provides a different point of examination to produce specific, clinical findings; every element identified by a bullet requires the physician's performance of a specific portion of the physical examination. The following example illustrates different elements identified by bullets.

Example of Different Elements Identified by Bullets

The patient's tympanic membrane—the physician must use the otoscope to visually inspect the tympanic membrane.

- The patient's throat—the physician must ask the patient to say, "Ahh," and, with the aid of a light, visually inspect the oropharynx, which usually includes some or all of the following: the **oral mucosa**, **hard** and/or **soft palates**, tongue, **tonsils**, and/or **uvula**.
- The patient's respiratory effort—the clinician must inspect how the patient's **intercostal muscles** and **accessory muscles** respond to the process of **respiration**, as well as how the diaphragm moves.
- The patient's liver and spleen—the clinician must palpate the upper quadrants of the patient's abdomen by applying slow, steady pressure while determining the shape and structure of the patient's liver and spleen.
- The patient's thyroid—the clinician must gently palpate the midline of the patient's neck to determine any presence of abnormal thyroid tissue.

---

wheeze whistling sound that can be heard during auscultation of the lungs

rhonchi the plural form of *rhonchus*; an abnormal sound, similar to loud snoring or whistling, that is heard during lung auscultation and is caused by air rushing through mucosal secretions or swollen tissues of the bronchioles

systems/body areas the phrase used to identify the 14 different recognized body areas and organ systems that are included in the general multisystem physical examination in the 1997 Documentation Guidelines

oral mucosa the layer of moist tissue that covers the inside of the mouth, including the gums, tongue, and roof of the mouth

hard palate the hard part of the roof of the mouth

soft palate the soft section of the roof of the mouth

tonsils lymphatic tissue located at the back of the throat

uvula the tear-drop-shaped fleshy tissue that can be seen dangling in the back of the throat

intercostal muscles the muscles between the ribs that contract during respiration

accessory muscles supplemental muscles that provide support or aid to essential organs, tissues, or structures

respiration the act of breathing air, which is made up of inspiration and exhalation; requires the functioning of the lungs, diaphragm, intercostal muscles, and other parts of the anatomy

Name of System/Body Area	The elements that <u>may be examined</u> during the general multisystem physical exam (each individual element identified by an individual bullet): • Anatomic location of specific clinical finding
Example: Cardiovascular	Example: • Auscultation of heart with notation of abnormal sounds and murmurs

Figure 7.1 ■ 1997 General multisystem checklist example.

ELEMENTS AS EVIDENCE

The 1997 general multisystem physical examination description provides a lengthy list of the many different systems/body areas that may be examined during a physical examination. These listed elements identified by a bullet constitute an **evidentiary checklist** of the documented physical examination. ■ FIGURE 7.1 is an example of the 1997 general multisystem exam checklist.

The checklist for the general multisystem physical examination appears on pages 14–18 of the "1997 Documentation Guidelines for Evaluation and Management Services." (The directions for accessing these guidelines can be found in Appendix B.) On these pages, each system or area is identified in its own bordered "box" with the appropriate elements identified by bullets. All told, more than 60 different elements are listed, each providing a clue about what is currently happening in the patient's body. These clues help the clinician provide quality healthcare through an appropriate assessment of the patient's current body function and also help the clinician investigate for any signs of disease. All of these elements together provide a holistic snapshot of the patient's body at the time of the physical examination through documentation of specific findings.

An understanding of anatomy is one of the important keys to understanding the general multisystem physical examination requirements in the 1997 Documentation Guidelines. Although some of the elements identified by a bullet are anatomically separated into different locations of the human body, some elements are more closely localized in the patient's anatomy. The following example shows the difference between two systems/areas of the 1997 general multisystem physical examination: the ears, nose, throat, and mouth system, otherwise known as ENT/M, and the cardiovascular system.

evidentiary checklist the specifically identified clinical, pathological, and anatomic findings that are listed in the 1997 Documentation Guidelines for the general multisystem physical examination

otoscope examination instrument with magnifying lens and light that is used to examine the interior of the external surface of the ear as well as the interior tympanic membrane, interior tissues, and structures of the inner ear

nasal mucosa the layer of moist tissue that covers the inside of the nasal cavity

septum the natural barrier that divides one body cavity into different sections, as, for example, the nasal septum divides the nasal cavity into separate sections

turbinates three bony projections within each side of the nasal cavity; covered in mucosa; assist in filtering, warming, and humidifying the air inhaled through the nose

aorta the large artery leading away from the heart to the lower part of the human body; includes five sections—ascending aorta, arch of the aorta, and descending aorta, which divides into the thoracic aorta and the abdominal aorta

femoral arteries the large arteries found in the upper thigh, or femur

pedal pulse the area in the ankle where the physician can identify the peripheral pulse

> ### Examples of the 1997 General Multi-System Physical Examination of ENT/M and CV Organ Systems
>
> The ENT/M is located in the head and the far back of the mouth and the top of the throat. Therefore, while examining the health of the ears, nose, throat, and mouth of the patient, a clinician may do the following:
>
> - Visually inspect the outer appearance, shape, and continuity of the outer ear and nose
> - Use an **otoscope** to visually assess the interior of the ear (eardrum, ear canal, etc.)
> - Assess the patient's hearing using tuning fork, rubbing fingers beside the ear, whispering
> - Inspect the **nasal mucosa**, **septum**, **turbinates**
> - Inspect the patient's lips (outside and inside), gums, and teeth
> - Examine the oropharynx (back of the throat including the tonsils), the pharynx (the very back of the throat), oral mucosa, salivary glands, hard and soft palates, tongue (surface, underside), etc.
>
> However, the cardiovascular system extends from the head to the foot, through the entire human body. Therefore, during an examination of the patient's cardiovascular system, the clinician may do the following:
>
> - Identify the pulse and feel of the carotid artery in the neck
> - Listen to the heart
> - Determine the size of the heart by palpating the chest
> - Determine the size of the abdominal **aorta**
> - Assess the **femoral arteries** of the groin or thigh
> - Measure the **pedal pulse** of the ankle
> - Note any edema and or varicose veins in the extremities

Notice that the clinical language used to describe the individual physical examination findings suggests that a strong understanding of anatomy is helpful when reviewing the documentation of the physical examination while referencing the 1997 Documentation Guidelines.

There are 14 different systems/areas identified in the general multisystem physical examination of the 1997 Documentation Guidelines. Each of the systems/areas defined provides a different perspective into the general multisystem physical examination. ■ FIGURES 7.2 through 7.15 provide illustrations intended to visually support an understanding of the 14 areas/systems.

Constitutional	• Measurement of any 3 of the following 7 vital signs: (1) sitting or standing blood pressure, (2) supine blood pressure, (3) pulse rate and regularity, (4) respiration, (5) temperature, (6) height, (7) weight (May be measured and recorded by ancillary staff: nurse, medical assistant, etc.) • General appearance of patient (e.g., development, nutrition, body habitus, deformities, attention to grooming)

Figure 7.2 ■ General multisystem physical examination: constitutional.

Eyes	• Inspection of conjunctivae (inner membrane of eyelid & exposed white surface of eyeball) and eyelids • Examination of pupils and irises (e.g., reaction to light and accommodation, size, and symmetry) • Ophthalmoscopic examination of optic discs (e.g., size, C/D ratio, appearance) and posterior segments (e.g., vessel changes, exudates, hemorrhages)

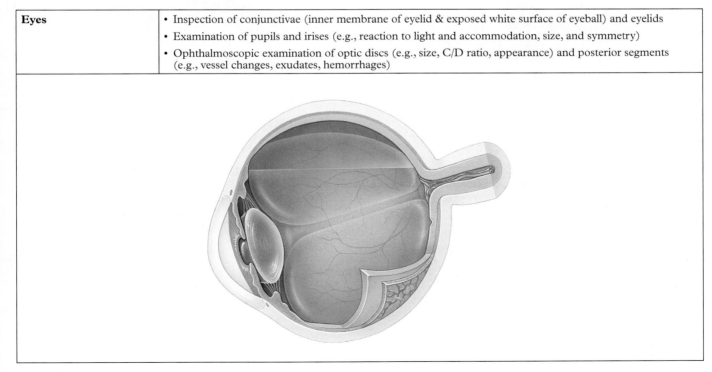

Figure 7.3 ■ General multisystem physical examination: eyes.

Ears, Nose, Throat, and Mouth	• External inspection of ears and nose (e.g., overall appearance, scars, lesions, masses)
	• Otoscopic examination of external auditory canals and tympanic membranes
	• Assessment of hearing (e.g., whispered voice, finger rub, tuning fork)
	• Inspection of nasal mucosa, septum. and turbinates
	• Inspection of lips, teeth, and gums
	• Examination of oropharynx: oral mucosa, salivary glands, hard and soft palates, tongue, tonsils. and posterior pharynx

Figure 7.4 ■ General multisystem physical examination: ears, nose, throat, and mouth.

Neck	• Examination of neck (e.g., masses, overall appearance, symmetry, tracheal position, crepitus)
	• Examination of thyroid (e.g., enlargement, tenderness, mass)

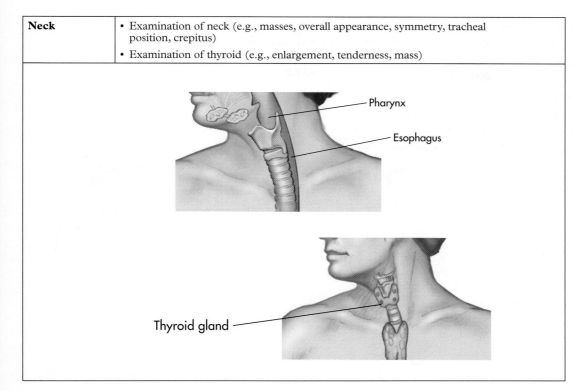

Figure 7.5 ■ General multisystem physical examination: neck.

Respiratory	• Assessment of respiratory effort (e.g., intercostal retractions, use of accessory muscles, diaphragmatic movement)
	• Percussion of chest (e.g., dullness, flatness, hyperresonance)
	• Palpation of chest (e.g., tactile fremitus)
	• Auscultation of lungs (e.g., breath sounds, adventitious sounds, rubs)

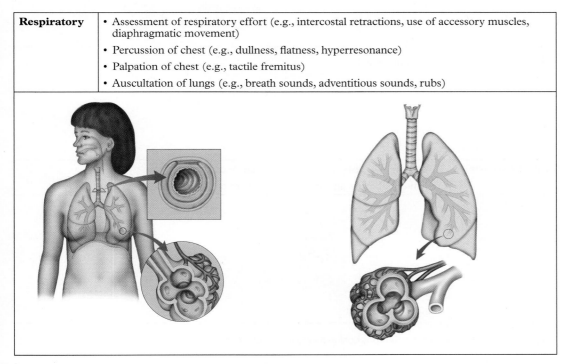

Figure 7.6 ■ General multisystem physical examination: respiratory.

Cardiovascular	• Palpation of heart (e.g., location, size, thrills) • Auscultation of heart with notation of abnormal sounds and murmurs Examination of • carotid arteries (e.g., pulse, bruits) • abdominal aorta (e.g., size, bruits) • femoral arteries (e.g., pulse amplitude, bruits) • pedal pulses (e.g., pulse amplitude) • extremities for edema and/or varicosities

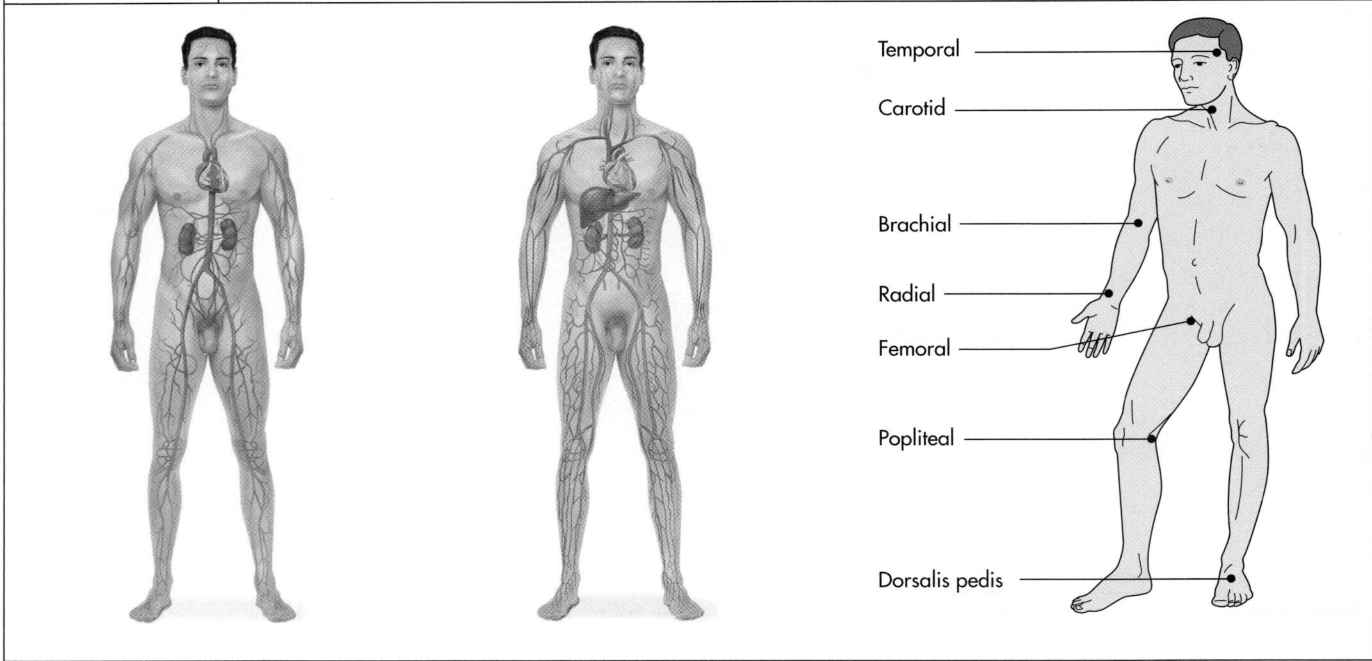

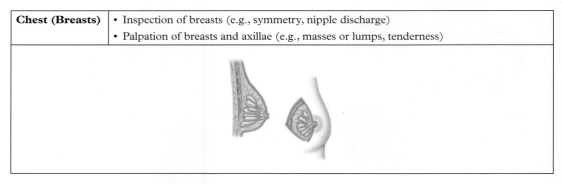

Figure 7.7 ■ General multisystem physical examination: cardiovascular.

Chest (Breasts)	• Inspection of breasts (e.g., symmetry, nipple discharge) • Palpation of breasts and axillae (e.g., masses or lumps, tenderness)

Figure 7.8 ■ General multisystem physical examination: chest (breasts).

Gastrointestinal	• Examination of abdomen with notation of presence of masses or tenderness
	• Examination of liver and spleen
	• Examination for presence or absence of hernia
	• Examination (when indicated) of anus, perineum and rectum, including sphincter tone, presence of hemorrhoids, rectal masses
	• Obtain stool sample for occult blood test when indicated

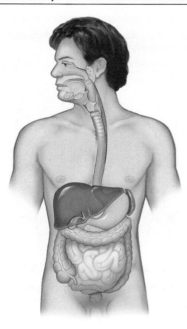

Figure 7.9 ■ General multisystem physical examination: gastrointestinal (abdomen).

Genitourinary: Male	• Examination of the scrotal contents (e.g., hydrocele, spermatocele, tenderness of cord, testicular mass)
	• Examination of the penis
	• Digital rectal examination of prostate gland (e.g., size, symmetry, nodularity, tenderness)

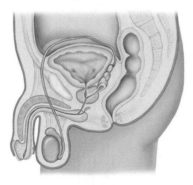

Figure 7.10a ■ General multisystem physical examination: genitourinary (male).

Genitourinary: Female	Pelvic examination (with or without specimen collection for smears and cultures) • Examination of external genitalia (e.g., general appearance, hair distribution, lesions) and vagina (e.g., general appearance, estrogen effect, discharge, lesions, pelvic support, cystocele, rectocele) • Examination of urethra (e.g., masses, tenderness, scarring) • Examination of bladder (e.g., fullness, masses, tenderness) • Cervix (e.g., general appearance, lesions, discharge) • Uterus (e.g., size, contour, position, mobility, tenderness, consistency, descent, or support) • Adnexa/parametria (e.g., masses, tenderness, organomegaly, nodularity)
	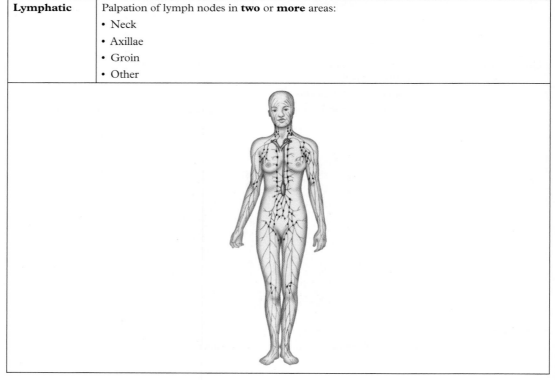

Figure 7.10b ▪ General multisystem physical examination: genitourinary (female).

Lymphatic	Palpation of lymph nodes in **two** or **more** areas: • Neck • Axillae • Groin • Other

Figure 7.11 ▪ General multisystem physical examination: lymphatic.

Musculoskeletal	• Examination of gait and station
	• Inspection and/or palpation of digits and nails (e.g., clubbing, cyanosis, inflammatory conditions, petechiae, ischemia, infections, nodes)
	Examination of **joints, bones, and muscles of one or more** of these six areas:(1) head and neck; (2) spine, ribs, and pelvis; (3) right upper extremity; (4) left upper extremity; (5) right lower extremity; and (6) left lower extremity-to include the following:
	• Inspection and/or palpation with notation of presence of any misalignment, asymmetry, crepitation, defects, tenderness, masses, effusions
	• Assessment of range of motion with notation of any pain, crepitation, or contracture
	• Assessment of stability with notation of any dislocation (luxation), subluxation, or laxity
	• Assessment of muscle strength and tone (e.g., flaccid, cog wheel, spastic) with notation of any atrophy or abnormal movements

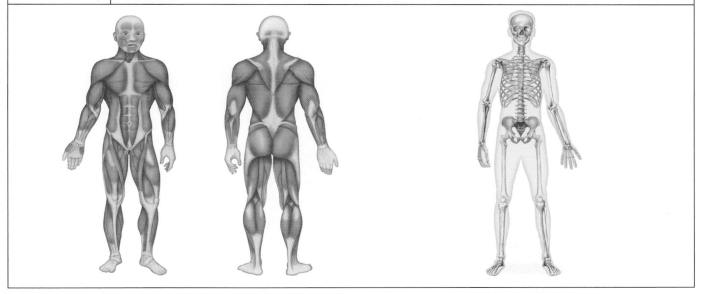

Figure 7.12 ■ General multisystem physical examination: musculoskeletal.

Skin (Integumentary)	• Inspection of skin and subcutaneous tissue (e.g., rashes, lesions, ulcers)
	• Palpation of skin and subcutaneous tissue (e.g., induration, subcutaneous nodules, tightening)

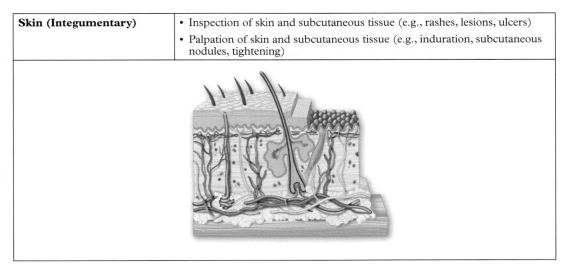

Figure 7.13 ■ General multisystem physical examination: skin.

Neurologic	• Test of cranial nerves with notation of any deficits
	• Examination of deep tendon reflexes with notation of pathological reflexes (e.g., Babinski reflex)
	• Examination of sensation (e.g., by touch, pin, vibration, proprioception)

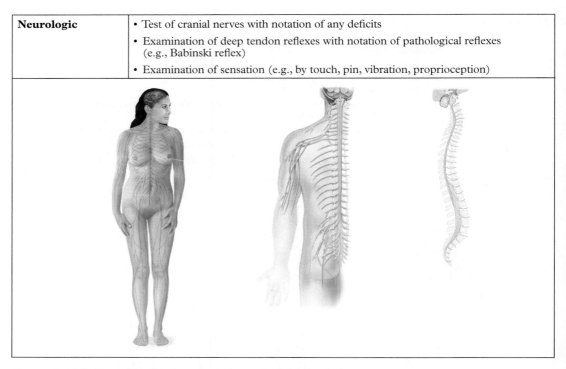

Figure 7.14 ■ General multisystem physical examination: neurologic.

Psychiatric	• Description of patient's judgment and insight
	Brief assessment of mental status:
	• Orientation to time, place, and person
	• Recent and remote memory
	• Mood and affect (e.g., depression, anxiety, agitation)

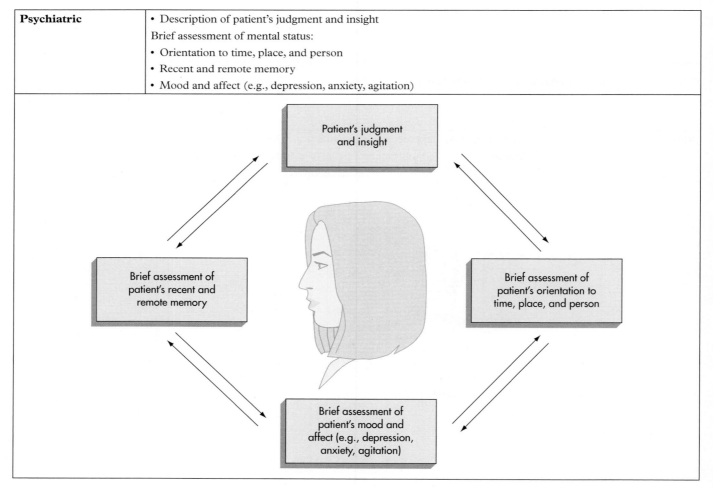

Figure 7.15   General multisystem physical examination: psychiatric.

Exercise 7.1   Patient's Sinus Pressure and Cough

Review the following medical documentation. Using the 1997 Documentation Guidelines for the general multisystem physical examination, identify the systems/body areas examined and each of the examination elements identified by a bullet.

History: Patient has presented for sinus pressure and cough. Patient's face hurts so much on the right cheek beneath eye that she feels she cannot open her eyes all the way due to the stabbing pain. She complains of a ringing in her right ear, and the right side of her throat hurts when she swallows. She has no appetite, complains of heartburn but no nausea. Nighttime has been interrupted by frequent urination without pain but very smelly urine. Patient denies joint pain other than a sore neck. Patient complains of heavy chest pressure and pain upon coughing. Patient states she can feel her heartbeat in her head as a throbbing but denies any heart palpitations. Patient is dizzy upon standing and reports she has spent 3 days lying down because of the discomfort. No report of sick contact at work, but her husband had the flu last month. Neither patient nor her husband smokes tobacco.

Exam: Patient is pale and appears very tired; she appears well groomed. Conjunctivae clear without swelling. Nasal passages quite congested and very swollen. Fluid noted within inner ear bilaterally; however, tympanic membrane does not appear significantly pressured. Throat mottled with yellow and white patches, and tonsils significantly red and swollen. Palpation of neck and behind ears reveals very tender, swollen lymph nodes. Patient expresses extreme discomfort when swallowing.

System/body area: _____
Elements identified by bullet: _____

System/body area: _____
Elements identified by bullet: _____

System/body area: _____
Elements identified by bullet: _____

System/body area: _____
Elements identified by bullet: _____

System/body area: _____
Elements identified by bullet: _____

System/body area: _____
Elements identified by bullet: _____

Exercise 7.2   Timmy's Abdominal Pain and Diarrhea

Review the following medical documentation. Using the 1997 Documentation Guidelines for the general multisystem physical examination, identify the systems/body areas examined and each of the examination elements identified by a bullet.

Timmy is an established patient and presents for abdominal pain and diarrhea.

PE: Timmy appears pale and slightly lethargic but responsive to questions. T, 98.7F; pulse, 130; resp, 20. Eyes clear with no **jaundice**. Pupils are reactive to light within normal limits. Lungs clear to auscultation and percussion. Auscultation of heart reveals normal but rapid heartbeat without murmur. Timmy complains of pain during palpation of **costovertebral angle** with painful **rebound**; however, bladder full upon palpation, although Timmy provided urinary specimen and claims he emptied his bladder. **Urinary meatus** appears red and inflamed. Testicles slightly retracted, but warm without tenderness.

System/body area: _____
Elements identified by bullet: _____

System/body area: _____
Elements identified by bullet: _____

System/body area: _____
Elements identified by bullet: _____

System/body area: _____
Elements identified by bullet: _____

System/body area: _____
Elements identified by bullet: _____

System/body area: _____
Elements identified by bullet: _____

System/body area: _____
Elements identified by bullet: _____

System/body area: _____
Elements identified by bullet: _____

System/body area: _____
Elements identified by bullet: _____

System/body area: _____
Elements identified by bullet: _____

Exercise 7.3 | **Joan's Lower Back Pain**

Review the following medical documentation. Using the 1997 Documentation Guidelines for the general multisystem physical examination, identify the systems/body areas examined and each of the examination elements identified by a bullet.

Joan is an established patient who presents for lower back pain. Her lower back hurts, down by beltline, and pain is sometimes very severe. The pain is sporadic, mostly when standing up after sitting in one place for an extended period. Ibuprofen used to help, but now it does not help back pain anymore. At its worst, low back pain is sharp and throbbing. Joan has had occasional back pain for about 20 years, since first in the service, but she first noticed this particular low back pain shortly after playing touch football with adult children this past Thanksgiving. Patient denies any other joint pain than low back pain. Patient denies double vision or dizziness, and no chest pain or shortness of breath. Patient denies tobacco or alcohol use. Pain has not affected her work as a fifth-grade teacher.

Exam: Back is soft to the touch and palpation and revealed no obvious lumps or masses. Percussion of back reveals tenderness in lower back, but no costovertebral tenderness. Patient performs **side-to-side flexion** to 30 degrees with minimal pain; however, she finds **forward flexion** at 50 degrees with pain localized to her lower back that does not radiate down legs or up her back. **Deep tendon reflexes** within normal limits: **ankle jerk reflex**, **patellar reflex**, **plantar reflexes** tested. Patient's range of motion is stable, within normal limits, and without pain.

System/body area: _____
Elements identified by bullet: _____

System/body area: _____
Elements identified by bullet: _____

System/body area: _____
Elements identified by bullet: _____

jaundice yellowing of skin, mucus membranes, and the whites of the eyes caused by an excess of bile in the tissues

costovertebral angle the angular space of the back between the lowest rib and the vertebrae, which is most commonly located over the kidneys

rebound a sudden tightening of muscles caused by an autonomic reflex, such as tightening of abdominal muscles because of disease, illness, or injury

urinary meatus the external opening of the urinary system, which allows urine to leave the body

side-to-side flexion bending from side to side

forward flexion bending forward

deep tendon reflexes one of many neurologic tests that provide indication of the integrity of the central nervous system and the peripheral nervous system; include Babinski test, ankle jerk reflex, and the knee jerk reflex

1997 GENERAL MULTISYSTEM PHYSICAL EXAMINATION REQUIREMENTS

The "1997 Documentation Guidelines for Evaluation and Management Services" states that any physician, regardless of the physician's specialty, may perform the general multisystem physical examination. The type of physical examination is determined by the physician's clinical judgment, the patient's history, and the nature of the presenting problem. Since the medical documentation is the record of all healthcare services performed during an E/M visit, the documented physical examination becomes the record of the physical examination that was performed by the physician during the E/M service visit.

Even as the "1995 Documentation Guidelines for Evaluation and Management Services" defines specific documentation requirements for the 1995 physical examination, the "1997 Documentation Guidelines for Evaluation and Management Services" defines specific documentation guidelines for the general multisystem physical examination. Like the 1995 guidelines, the 1997 guidelines call for documenting any findings considered to be abnormal, unexpected, or normal/negative during the performance of the physical examination. However, the language of the 1997 guidelines goes further than that of the 1995 guidelines in identifying the expectations of the general multisystem physical examination performed by the physician. In addition, the documentation guidelines for each of the four types of physical examination diverge widely from those of 1995.

FOUR TYPES OF GENERAL MULTISYSTEM PHYSICAL EXAMINATION

The purpose of identifying the four different types of physical examination remains the same in 1995 and 1997: consistency in documenting the physical examination provides continuity across the country and ensures accountability within the medical field, given the understanding that the documented physical examination reflects the physical examination that was performed by the physician during the E/M service. The four types of general multisystem physical examination defined by the 1997 Documentation Guidelines are problem-focused, expanded problem-focused, detailed, and comprehensive. Each of these four types reflects a different level of examination in relation to the affected body area or organ system, and to any inclusion of other symptomatic or related organ systems, as shown in ■ TABLE 7.1.

■ TABLE 7.1   **FOUR TYPES OF GENERAL MULTISYSTEM PHYSICAL EXAMINATIONS**

Problem-focused—The physician performing this type of general multisystem physical examination should assess one or more organ systems or body areas and should document one to five elements identified by a bullet (•) for the examined organ system(s) or body area(s).

Expanded problem-focused—The physician performing this type of general multisystem physical examination should assess one or more organ systems and/or body areas and should document at least six elements identified by a bullet (•) for the examined organ system(s) or body area(s).

Detailed—The physician performing this type of general multisystem physical examination should assess at least six organ systems or body areas and should document at least two elements identified by a bullet (•) for each of the six systems or areas examined OR, alternatively, should document at least 12 elements identified by a bullet (•) for two or more organ systems or body areas examined.

Comprehensive—The physician performing this type of general multisystem physical examination should assess at least nine organ systems or body areas (unless specific directions limit the content of the examination) and should document at least two elements identified by a bullet (•) for each examined system or area.

Source: Centers for Medicare and Medicaid Services, "1997 Documentation Guidelines for Evaluation and Management Services," pp. 11–12, www.cms.gov/Outreach-and-Education/Medicare-Learning-Network-MLN/MLNEdWebGuide/Downloads/97Docguidelines.pdf.

■ FIGURE 7.16 summarizes these four types of general multisystem physical examination in a chart format.

Notice that every level of the exam includes both body areas, such as the body area of the neck, and organ systems, such as the cardiovascular organ system. By including both body areas and organ systems in the 1997 general multisystem physical examination, not only is a quantifiable guideline listed for each individual type of exam, but also a higher level of clinical and anatomic specificity can be achieved for each type. This specificity is dependent upon the physician's documentation of the performed physical examination.

Example: Documentation of Problem-Focused General Multisystem Exam

Documentation of between one and five elements identified by a bullet in each of the examined organ system(s) and/or body area(s). There is a requirement that the physician will examine at least one organ system and/or body area.

Johnny's Irritating Cough

Auricle of left ear is bright red as Johnny has been pulling at it. Upon examination, **serous fluid** is apparent behind tympanic membrane. **Finger rub test** resulted in normal hearing, despite Johnny's sense of hearing loss. Johnny is uncomfortably congested and unable to inhale through either nostril. Significant mucus production noted via nares bilaterally. Patient's cough produces thick, white phlegm upon **expectoration**, and solid, white **exudates** apparent on tonsils and along back of pharynx.

Five separate elements identified by a bullet are documented:

Ears, Nose, Throat, and Mouth

- External inspection of ears and nose (red auricle due to Johnny pulling at his earlobe)
- Otoscopic examination of external auditory canals and tympanic membranes (otoscopic identification of serous fluid behind tympanic membrane)
- Assessment of hearing (could hear the sound of the physician's fingertips rubbing together near Johnny's ears)
- Inspection of nasal mucosa, septum, and turbinates (unable to inhale through his nostrils, and significant mucus production noted in both nostrils)
- Examination of oropharynx: oral mucosa, salivary glands, hard and soft palates, tongue, tonsils, and **posterior** pharynx (solid white exudates, or discharge, along the tonsils and the back of the pharynx visible to the physician's naked eye)

ankle jerk reflex also known as "Achilles reflex"; reveals the rate of contraction of the calf muscles and tendons when the Achilles tendon is struck; tests the neurologic reflexes that occur when the Achilles tendon is sharply struck by a physician during a physical examination

patellar reflex also known as "knee jerk test," which reveals the rate of contraction of the tendons that run along the front of the shinbone when the patellar, or kneecap, tendon is sharply struck

plantar reflexes another phrase for the Babinski test, when irritation of the sole of the foot causes contraction of toes and feet

auricle external surface of the ear that can be easily visualized, most commonly referred to as the external ear, earlobe

serous fluid bodily fluids that may include lymphatic fluid, or fluid that may include white blood cells, plasma proteins, platelets, or red blood cells, or other fluids

finger rub test an auditory test that identifies how well the patient can hear the sound of a finger and thumb being rubbed together beside the patient's ear

expectoration spitting up, coughing up, or clearing one's throat by coughing and spitting out collected mucus

exudates the collection of fluid that is secreted from inflamed, infected, or swollen cells or tissues; can include pus

posterior any area of the body located toward the back, or opposite of the front

Physical Examination	Problem-Focused	Expanded Problem-Focused	Detailed	Comprehensive
1995 PE	A limited examination of affected body area or organ system (1 body area/organ system)	A limited examination of the affected body area or organ system and other symptomatic or related organ systems (2–4 body areas/organ systems)	An extended examination of the affected body area(s) or organ system(s) and other symptomatic or related body areas or organ systems (5–7 body areas/organ systems)	A general multisystem examination or complete examination of a single organ system and other symptomatic or related body areas or organ systems; should include 8 or more of the 12 organ systems (8+ body systems OR organ systems, but they cannot be mixed)
1997 General Multisystem	1–5 elements identified by a bullet	At least 6 elements identified by a bullet	At least 2 elements identified by a bullet from each of 6 areas/systems OR at least 12 elements identified by a bullet in 2 or more areas/systems	Performance of all elements identified by a bullet in at least 9 organ systems or body areas and documentation of at least 2 elements identified by a bullet in each of the examined areas/systems

Figure 7.16 ■ Content of service element: 1997 general multisystem physical examination highlighted.

When more than five elements identified by a bullet need to be examined and documented, an expanded problem-focused general multisystem physical examination may be more appropriate.

Example: Documentation of Expanded Problem-Focused General Multisystem Exam

Documentation of at least six elements identified by a bullet in one or more examined organ system(s) and/or body area(s). There is a requirement that the physician will examine at least one organ system and/or body area.

Johnny's Irritating Cough

Patient is alert, however clearly uncomfortable. Vital signs: T, 99.32F; pulse, 120; BP 100/65. Eyes: conjunctivae inflamed, but clear. ENT/M: auricle of left ear is bright red as Johnny has been pulling at the auricle of his ear. Finger rub test resulted in normal hearing, despite Johnny's sense of hearing loss. Johnny is uncomfortably congested and unable to inhale through either nostril. Significant mucus production noted via nares bilaterally. Patient's cough produces thick, white phlegm upon expectoration, and solid, white exudates apparent on tonsils and along back of pharynx.

Eight separate elements identified by a bullet are documented:

Constitutional

- Measurement of *any three of the following seven* vital signs: (1) sitting or standing blood pressure, (2) supine blood pressure, (3) pulse rate and regularity, (4) respiration, (5) temperature, (6) height, (7) weight (three vital signs documented: temperature, pulse, and blood pressure)
- General appearance of patient (clearly uncomfortable)

Eyes

- Inspection of conjunctivae (inflamed but clear)

Ears, Nose, Throat, and Mouth

- External inspection of ears and nose (red auricle due to Johnny pulling at his earlobe)
- Otoscopic examination of external auditory canals and tympanic membranes (otoscopic identification of serous fluid behind tympanic membrane)
- Assessment of hearing (could hear the sound of the physician's fingertips rubbing together near Johnny's ears)
- Inspection of nasal mucosa, septum, and turbinates (unable to inhale through his nostrils, and significant mucus production noted in both nostrils)
- Examination of oropharynx: oral mucosa, salivary glands, hard and soft palates, tongue, tonsils, and posterior pharynx (solid white exudates, or discharge, along the tonsils and the back of the pharynx visible to the physician's naked eye)

As a physical examination becomes more complex, a detailed general multisystem physical examination may be more appropriate.

Example: Documentation of Detailed General Multisystem Exam

Documentation of at least two elements identified by a bullet from each of (at least) six of the examined organ systems or body areas OR documentation of at least 12 elements identified by a bullet in two or more of the examined organ systems or body areas. There is a requirement that the physician will examine at least two organ systems and/or body areas.

Johnny's Irritating Cough (and Stomachache)

Patient is clearly uncomfortable, but alert, in no distress, and curious about his surroundings. Vital signs: T, 99.32F; pulse, 120; BP, 100/65. Eyes: conjunctivae inflamed, but clear. ENT/M: auricle of left ear is bright red as Johnny has been pulling at it. Finger rub test resulted in normal hearing, despite Johnny's sense of hearing loss. Johnny is uncomfortably congested and unable to inhale through either nostril. Significant mucus production noted via nares bilaterally. Patient's cough produces thick, white phlegm upon expectoration, and solid, white exudates apparent on tonsils and along back of pharynx. Neck is soft without masses; no thyromegaly. No sign of respiratory distress, lungs clear without crackles, wheezes. **Regular rate and rhythm (RRR)**, without **gallop**, **murmur**, or **rub**. Abdomen: soft with mild tenderness noted in left lower quadrant with palpable stool. Patient states he has not passed stool for 3 days; no **hepatosplenomegaly** noted; however, patient reports pain upon palpation of left upper quadrant.

Fifteen separate elements identified by a bullet from two or more systems/body areas are documented:

Constitutional

* Measurement of *any three of the following seven* vital signs: (1) sitting or standing blood pressure, (2) supine blood pressure, (3) pulse rate and regularity, (4) respiration, (5) temperature, (6) height, (7) weight (three vital signs documented: temperature, pulse, and blood pressure)
* General appearance of patient (clearly uncomfortable)

Eyes

* Inspection of conjunctivae (inflamed but clear)

Ears, Nose, Throat, and Mouth

* External inspection of ears and nose (red auricle due to Johnny pulling at his earlobe)
* Otoscopic examination of external auditory canals and tympanic membranes (otoscopic identification of serous fluid behind tympanic membrane)
* Assessment of hearing (could hear the sound of the physician's fingertips rubbing together near Johnny's ears)
* Inspection of nasal mucosa, septum, and turbinates (unable to inhale through his nostrils, and significant mucus production noted in both nostrils)
* Examination of oropharynx: oral mucosa, salivary glands, hard and soft palates, tongue, tonsils, and posterior pharynx (solid white exudates, or discharge, along the tonsils and the back of the pharynx visible to the physician's naked eye)

Neck

* Examination of neck (soft without masses)
* Examination of thyroid (no thyromegaly)

Respiratory

* Assessment of respiratory effort (no sign of respiratory distress)
* Auscultation of lungs (clear without crackles, wheezes)

Cardiovascular

* Auscultation of heart with notation of abnormal sounds and murmurs (RRR, without gallop, murmur, or rub)

---

regular rate and rhythm (RRR) refers to a heartbeat with regular rate and rhythm and without any abnormal findings

gallop abnormal third or fourth beat that makes the heartbeat sound like a galloping horse

murmur an abnormal heart sound

rub the abnormal sound of friction caused by inflamed tissues rubbing together; can be caused by respiratory tissues rubbing together or cardiac tissues rubbing together

hepatosplenomegaly enlargement of the liver and spleen

Gastrointestinal (or Abdomen)

- Examination of abdomen with notation of presence of masses or tenderness (soft abdomen, mild tenderness noted in left lower quadrant with palpable stool; has not passed stool for 3 days)
- Examination of liver and spleen (no hepatosplenomegaly noted; pain noted upon palpation of left upper quadrant)

It is important to note that two different requirements are listed for a detailed general multisystem physical examination, and the documentation must meet one of the two. For this example, two or more elements identified by a bullet are documented in only five different systems/body areas. Therefore, the documentation must meet the alternative requirement of at least 12 elements identified by a bullet in two or more systems/body areas.

Example: Documentation of Comprehensive General Multisystem Exam

Documentation of at least two elements identified by a bullet in each of the examined organ systems and/or body areas. There is a requirement that the physician will examine at least nine organ systems and/or body areas.

Johnny's Irritating Cough (and Stomachache after a Bad Fall)

Patient is clearly uncomfortable because of his cold, but alert, in no distress, and curious about his surroundings. He correctly reports the day and place, correctly identifying this examiner by name, showing good judgment and insight for the questions. Johnny remembers everything about his fall but shows no anxiety about getting on the examination table. Vital signs: T, 99.32F; pulse, 120; BP, 100/65. Eyes: conjunctivae inflamed, but clear. **Pupils equal, round, reactive to light (and accommodation) (PERRL[A])**. No **hemorrhages** noted in posterior segments of eye or indication of lasting injury after fall. **Normal visual field test** with normal **extra-ocular movements**. ENT/M: auricle of left ear is bright red as Johnny has been pulling at it. Finger rub test resulted in normal hearing, despite Johnny's sense of hearing loss. Johnny is uncomfortably congested and unable to inhale through either nostril. Significant mucus production noted via nares bilaterally. Patient's cough produces thick, white phlegm upon expectoration. Gums are red and slightly inflamed. Solid, white exudates apparent on tonsils and along back of pharynx. Neck is soft without masses; no thyromegaly. No sign of respiratory distress, lungs clear without crackles, wheezes. No **fremitus** upon palpation. Percussion reveals resonant lung sounds. RRR, without gallop, murmur, or rub. Abdomen: soft with mild tenderness noted in left lower quadrant with palpable stool. Patient states he has not passed stool for 3 days; no hepatosplenomegaly noted; however, patient reports pain upon palpation of left upper quadrant. Bladder palpated with minimal pain; testicles descended, warm, and nontender to palpation. Extremities: a total of four healing abrasions are noted on knees, lower legs, and forearms where the patient landed after falling onto driveway. The **abrasions** are healing without tenderness, redness, swelling, or signs of infection. No **indurations** noted in surrounding tissues, and Johnny can move his fingers without pain. Good grip strength of forefinger and thumb. Patient is able to move all joints without pain. Patient displayed normal **proprioception** responses upon request. **Babinski test** reveals appropriate **plantar flexion** response and laughter from patient. No swelling or pain noted in both patient's knee and wrist joints upon palpation. No **crepitation** noted when patient asked to demonstrate appropriate range of motion; Johnny seemed happy to move freely and skipped back and forth across exam room with excellent balance and with no pain.

Thirty-six separate elements identified by a bullet are documented:

Psychiatric (4/4 elements identified by a bullet are documented)

- Description of patient's judgment and insight (shows good judgment and insight for the questions)

---

pupils equal, round, reactive to light (and accommodation) (PERRL[A]) an ocular and neurologic test to identify the dilation of the pupils and the neuromuscular and ocular response when a bright light is shined into the patient's eyes

hemorrhage excessive bleeding

normal visual field test an assessment of the scope of the patient's visual field

extra-ocular movements an indication of the coordinated function of the seven muscles that control the movement of the eye; typically occur during a physical examination when a patient is instructed to look up, to the side, or down or to track a moving finger; considered "intact" when the movements are within normal limits

fremitus vibrations that can be felt externally when breathing or speaking; if respiratory, indicates excessive secretions that vibrate when air flows through the lungs

Brief assessment of mental status:

- **Orientation to time, place, and person** (correctly reports day and place, as well as correctly identifying examiner by name)
- Recent and remote memory (remembers everything about his fall)
- Mood and affect (shows no anxiety about getting on the examination table)

Constitutional (2/2 elements identified by a bullet are documented)

- Measurement of *any three of the following seven* vital signs: (1) sitting or standing blood pressure, (2) supine blood pressure, (3) pulse rate and regularity, (4) respiration, (5) temperature, (6) height, (7) weight (three vital signs documented: temperature, pulse, and blood pressure)
- General appearance of patient (clearly uncomfortable)

Eyes (3/3 elements identified by a bullet are documented)

- Inspection of conjunctivae (inflamed but clear)
- Examination of pupils and irises (PERRL[A])
- Ophthalmoscopic examination of optic discs (no indication of injury after fall) and posterior segments (no hemorrhages)

Ears, Nose, Throat, and Mouth (6/6 elements identified by a bullet are documented)

- External inspection of ears and nose (red auricle due to Johnny pulling at his earlobe)
- Otoscopic examination of external auditory canals and tympanic membranes (otoscopic identification of serous fluid behind tympanic membrane)
- Assessment of hearing (could hear the sound of the physician's fingertips rubbing together near Johnny's ears)
- Inspection of nasal mucosa, septum, and turbinates (unable to inhale through his nostrils, and significant mucus production noted in both nostrils)
- Inspection of lips, teeth, and gums (gums red and inflamed)
- Examination of oropharynx: oral mucosa, salivary glands, hard and soft palates, tongue, tonsils, and posterior pharynx (solid white exudates, or discharge, along the tonsils and the back of the pharynx visible to the physician's naked eye)

Neck (2/2 elements identified by a bullet are documented)

- Examination of neck (soft without masses)
- Examination of thyroid (no thyromegaly)

Respiratory (4/4 elements identified by a bullet are documented)

- Assessment of respiratory effort (no sign of respiratory distress)
- Percussion of chest (reveals resonant sounds)
- Palpation of chest (no fremitus)
- Auscultation of lungs (clear without crackles, wheezes)

Cardiovascular (1/7 of the elements identified by a bullet are documented)

- Auscultation of heart with notation of abnormal sounds and murmurs (RRR, without gallop, murmur, or rub)

Gastrointestinal (or Abdomen) (2/5 of the elements identified by a bullet are documented)

- Examination of abdomen with notation of presence of masses or tenderness (soft abdomen, mild tenderness noted in left lower quadrant with palpable stool; has not passed stool for 3 days)
- Examination of liver and spleen (no hepatosplenomegaly noted; however, pain noted upon palpation of left upper quadrant)

Genitourinary: Male (1/3 elements identified by a bullet are documented)

- Examination of the scrotal contents (testicles descended, warm, and nontender to palpation)

---

abrasion a minor wound of the skin that is most commonly identified as a scrape; caused by friction

induration abnormal hardening of tissues

proprioception subconscious awareness (with eyes closed) of one's body and extremities, including posture and position of arms, legs, hands, and feet; identified in a patient's verbal responses to a physician's queries

Babinski test checks the neurologic reaction of the toes and soles of the feet when the bottoms of the feet are stroked; provides a neurologic indication for the physician, depending on where the soles of the feet are stroked, which causes the toes and feet to curl in different manners

plantar flexion the motion of pointing toes downward while the patient is standing upright

crepitation a crackling or grating sound; in the lungs, associated with lung disease; also occurs when two ends of a broken bone rub together

orientation to time appropriate identification of the date, month, year

examination of gait a physician's examination of the patient's natural method, form, and process of movement; provides indicators about neuromuscular function, as well as balance, sense of space, and other indicators

effusion the abnormal collection of fluid in a body cavity or organ

contracture an abnormal tightening or shortening of muscles, usually in the extremities, that permanently limits the movement of the body part

dislocation the displacement of a joint, bone, organ, or structure from its normal position

luxation the act of dislocating a bone, organ, or joint out of alignment

subluxation a partial dislocation or misalignment of a joint, an organ, or tissues

laxity the condition of abnormal loosening of tissues, as in a loss of firmness in skin

flaccid loose, flabby, weak

cog wheel a specific form of muscular rigidity caused by tension in the muscles

spastic referring to abnormal spasms of muscles

atrophy the decrease of mass in a muscle, organ, or other tissue, most often caused by changes in nutrition or disease

cranial nerves the 12 nerves that connect the brain to 12 various sensory and motor sections of the head, or cranium

Skin (2/2 elements identified by a bullet are documented)

* Inspection of skin and subcutaneous tissue (abrasions healing well)
* Palpation of skin and subcutaneous tissue (no tenderness, redness, swelling, signs of infection, or indurations)

Musculoskeletal (6/6 elements identified by a bullet are documented)

* **Examination of gait and station** (skipped back and forth across the room)
* Inspection and/or palpation of digits and nails (can move fingers without pain)

  Examination of joints, bones, and muscles of one or more of these—(1) right upper extremity, (2) left upper extremity, (3) right lower extremity, and (4) left lower extremity— to include the following:
* Inspection and/or palpation with notation of presence of any misalignment, asymmetry, crepitation, defects, tenderness, masses, **effusions** (no swelling or pain noted in patient's knees or wrist joints upon palpation)
* Assessment of range of motion with notation of any pain, crepitation, or **contracture** (demonstrates appropriate range of motion)
* Assessment of stability with notation of any **dislocation** (**luxation**), **subluxation**, or **laxity** (skipped across the room without pain)
* Assessment of muscle strength and tone (e.g., **flaccid**, **cog wheel**, **spastic**) with notation of any **atrophy** or abnormal movements (good grip strength of forefinger and thumb)

Neurologic (3/3 elements identified by a bullet are documented)

* Test of **cranial nerves** with notation of any deficits (normal visual field test with normal extra-ocular movement)
* Examination of deep tendon reflexes with notation of pathological reflexes (appropriate plantar flexion response to Babinski test and laughter from patient)
* Examination of sensation (normal proprioception responses upon request)

One of the requirements for a comprehensive general multisystem physical examination states that all of the elements identified by a bullet in at least nine systems/body areas must be performed. In addition, at least two elements identified by a bullet in each of the nine systems/body areas are required to be documented. For the purposes of this example, a total of 36 elements identified by a bullet are documented, 32 of which account for the first half of the requirements plus four elements identified by a bullet in three other systems/body areas.

Even though something unique differentiates every human being as a distinctive individual, human anatomy remains consistent across the global experience. The beauty of the general multisystem physical examination guidelines lies in the compilation of the elements identified by bullets listed within the 14 different organ systems and body areas. Each of these elements offers another facet of the physical examination performed during the E/M service visit. When the 1995 guidelines do not provide enough anatomic detail to properly reflect the extent of the performing physician's specificity, effort, and focus during the physical examination, the general multisystem physical examination affords a more inclusive reflection of the physical examination actually performed by the physician.

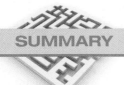

SUMMARY

* The "1997 Documentation Guidelines for Evaluation and Management Services" lists the general multisystem physical examination documentation requirements, which reflect a more exhaustive documentation. The documentation requirements reflect the status of the patient's health at the time of the E/M visit through the identification of specific clinical elements during an examination of multiple organ systems and/or body areas.

* These clinical elements are listed in an evidentiary checklist within the 1997 Documentation Guidelines; it is divided into 14 different anatomical categories known as systems/body areas. Within each system/body area, a separate bullet

identifies each individual clinical element. The elements identified by a bullet should be findings revealed by the physician's physical, visual, and auditory interaction with the patient.

- The 1997 Documentation Guidelines state that any physician, regardless of specialty, may perform the general multisystem physical examination. The type of examination is determined by the physician's clinical judgment, the patient's history, and the nature of the presenting problem. The clinical specificity of the elements identified by bullets provides guidance for those reading the documented physical examination.

- The four types of general multisystem physical examination defined by the 1997 Documentation Guidelines are problem-focused, expanded problem-focused, detailed, and comprehensive. The documentation that supports a problem-focused examination should include between one and five elements identified by a bullet. The documentation that supports an expanded problem-focused examination should include at least six elements identified by a bullet. The documentation that supports a detailed examination should include at least two elements identified by a bullet in each of six systems/body areas OR at least 12 elements identified by a bullet in two or more systems/body areas. The documentation that supports a comprehensive examination should include performance of all elements identified by a bullet in at least nine areas/systems AND documentation of at least two elements identified by a bullet in each of the nine areas/systems.

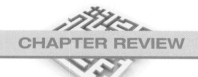

CHAPTER REVIEW

Multiple Choice

Choose the letter that best answers each question or completes each statement.

1. Which of the following best defines the nature of the presenting problem?

   a. The physician's collection of the patient's description of the chief complaint

   b. The physician's holistic view of the patient's illness, symptom, chief complaint, disease process, or other reason for care before the definition of a diagnosis

   c. The physician's documentation of the physical examination findings

   d. The physician's documented clinical findings according to the general multisystem physical examination requirements

2. In the medical documentation of the E/M service visit, the physical examination reflects which of the following?

   a. The past medical history, family medical history, and day-to-day activities of the patient

   b. An inventory of the patient's status of health prior to the E/M service visit

   c. Descriptions provided by the patient, which provide a personalized illustration of the symptom the patient is currently experiencing

   d. A snapshot of the patient's health at the time of the E/M service visit, including the functions, performance, structure, and health of the patient's body

3. How are the documentation requirements for the general multisystem physical examination presented in the "1997 Documentation Guidelines for Evaluation and Management"?

   a. The documentation requirements are presented in the form of specific clinical elements, which are each identified by a bullet.

   b. The documentation requirements are presented in the form of organ systems and body areas.

   c. The documentation requirements are presented in the form of the physician's documentation of the physical examination.

   d. The documentation requirements are presented in the form of the preprinted questionnaire completed by the patient.

4. How many types of general multisystem physical examination are listed in the 1997 Documentation Guidelines?

   a. Two

   b. Three

   c. Four

   d. Five

5. Which of the following choices represents the problem-focused type of physical examination?

   a. The documentation of at least six elements identified by a bullet

   b. The documentation of between one and five elements identified by a bullet

   c. The performance of all elements identified by a bullet in at least nine areas/systems AND documentation of at least two elements identified by a bullet in each of the nine areas/systems

   d. The documentation of at least two elements identified by a bullet in each of six systems/body areas OR at least 12 elements identified by a bullet in two or more systems/body areas

6. Which of the following choices represents an expanded problem-focused type of physical examination?

   a. The performance of all elements identified by a bullet in at least nine areas/systems AND documentation of at least two elements identified by a bullet in each of the nine areas/systems

   b. The documentation of at least six elements identified by a bullet

   c. The documentation of between one and five elements identified by a bullet

d. The documentation of at least two elements identified by a bullet in each of six systems/body areas OR at least 12 elements identified by a bullet in two or more systems/body areas

7. Which of the following choices represents a detailed type of physical examination?

   a. The documentation of at least two elements identified by a bullet in each of six systems/body areas OR at least 12 elements identified by a bullet in two or more systems/body areas

   b. The performance of all elements identified by a bullet in at least nine areas/systems AND documentation of at least two elements identified by a bullet in each of the nine areas/systems

   c. The documentation of at least six elements identified by a bullet

   d. The documentation of between one and five elements identified by a bullet

8. Which of the following choices represents a comprehensive type of physical examination?

   a. The documentation of at least six elements identified by a bullet

   b. The documentation of at least two elements identified by a bullet in each of six systems/body areas OR at least 12 elements identified by a bullet in two or more systems/body areas

   c. The documentation of between one and five elements identified by a bullet

   d. The performance of all elements identified by a bullet in at least nine areas/systems AND documentation of at least two elements identified by a bullet in each of the nine areas/systems

9. In order to perform the physical examination, the physician must do which of the following?

   a. Be sure to use the otoscope and the ophthalmoscope

   b. Perform the examination according to the order of the 1997 general multisystem physical examination evidentiary checklist

   c. Physically interact with the patient, such as touching or palpating, listening to or auscultation, looking at or inspecting different parts of the patient's body

   d. Obtain the patient's verbal permission before beginning the physical examination

10. How many different systems/body areas are listed in the general multisystem physical examination guidelines?

   a. Four

   b. Ten

   c. Fourteen

   d. Fifty-nine

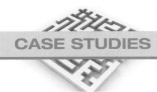

CASE STUDIES

Case Study 7-1

Read the following documentation, and then answer questions 1–10 by identifying the most appropriate element identified by a bullet that is referenced in the case study documentation. Be sure to follow the 1997 general multisystem physical examination guidelines. Directions for accessing the guidelines can be found in Appendix B.

Exam: Light head contusion along lateral hairline with no pain upon examination. Neck is soft without masses. No thyromegaly. Palpation and percussion reveal no cervical spine tenderness, no thoracic spine tenderness, and no lumbar spine tenderness. Patient does have a dark, category 3 contusion along entire URQ, and expresses significant pain upon any palpation. Lower abdomen tense with no rebound, patient "holding breath against pain." Patient expressed nausea upon palpation and vomited immediately after abdominal exam; face flushed with temperature of 101.2. Pulse rapid, respiration shallow. Patient calmed after a few moments' interruption, pulse slowed, and respiration became more regular. Inguinal hernia incision site is well healed with no redness, pain, or other s/s of infection or dehiscence. Fever remained stable at 101.1.

1. Which element identified by a bullet is documented in the words "light head contusion along lateral hairline with no pain upon examination"?

   a. Cardiovascular: auscultation of heart with notation of abnormal sounds and murmurs

   b. Skin: inspection of skin and subcutaneous tissue (e.g., rashes, lesions, ulcers)

   c. Psychiatric: description of patient's judgment and insight

   d. Constitutional: general appearance of patient (e.g., development, nutrition, body habitus, deformities, attention to grooming)

2. Which element identified by a bullet is documented in the words "neck is soft without masses"?

   a. Cardiovascular: auscultation of heart with notation of abnormal sounds and murmurs

   b. Neck: examination of neck (e.g., masses, overall appearance, symmetry, tracheal position, crepitus)

   c. Respiratory: palpation of chest (e.g., tactile fremitus)

   d. Lymphatic: palpation of lymph nodes in neck

3. Which element identified by a bullet is documented in the words "palpation and percussion reveal no cervical spine tenderness, no thoracic spine tenderness, and no lumbar spine tenderness"?

   a. Skin: palpation of skin and subcutaneous tissue (e.g., induration, subcutaneous nodules, tightening)

b. Neurologic: test of cranial nerves with notation of any deficits

c. Constitutional: general appearance of patient (e.g., development, nutrition, body habitus, deformities, attention to grooming)

d. Musculoskeletal: inspection and/or palpation with notation of presence of any misalignment, asymmetry, crepitation, defects, tenderness, masses, effusions

4. Which element identified by a bullet is documented in the words "face flushed with temperature of 101.2," "pulse rapid, respiration shallow," "fever remained stable at 101.1"?

   a. Constitutional: measurement of *any three of the following seven* vital signs: (1) sitting or standing blood pressure, (2) supine blood pressure, (3) pulse rate and regularity, (4) respiration, (5) temperature, (6) height, (7) weight

   b. Respiratory: assessment of respiratory effort (e.g., intercostal retractions, use of accessory muscles, diaphragmatic movement)

   c. Cardiovascular: auscultation of heart with notation of abnormal sounds and murmurs

   d. Skin: inspection of skin and subcutaneous tissue (e.g., rashes, lesions, ulcers)

5. Which element identified by a bullet is documented in the phrase "no thyromegaly"?

   a. Neck: examination of thyroid (e.g., enlargement, tenderness, mass

   b. Lymphatic: palpation of lymph nodes in *two* or *more* areas (neck, axillae, groin, other)

   c. Neurologic: examination of sensation (e.g., by touch, pin, vibration, proprioception)

   d. Ears, Nose, Throat, and Mouth: examination of oropharynx: oral mucosa, salivary glands, hard and soft palates, tongue, tonsils, and posterior pharynx

6. Which element identified by a bullet is documented in the words "patient does have a dark, category 3 contusion along entire URQ, and expresses significant pain upon any palpation. Lower abdomen tense with no rebound, patient 'holding breath against pain.' Patient expressed nausea upon palpation and vomited immediately after abdominal exam"?

   a. Cardiovascular: examination of abdominal aorta (e.g., size, bruits)

   b. Psychiatric: brief assessment of mental status, including mood and affect (e.g., depression, anxiety, agitation)

   c. Neurologic: examination of sensation (e.g., by touch, pin, vibration, proprioception)

   d. Gastrointestinal: examination of abdomen with notation of presence of masses or tenderness

7. Which element identified by a bullet is documented in the words "inguinal hernia incision site is well healed with no redness, pain, or other s/s of infection or dehiscence"?

   a. Lymphatic: palpation of lymph nodes in *two* or *more* areas (neck, axillae, groin, other)

   b. Psychiatric: brief assessment of mental status, including orientation to time, place, and person

   c. Skin: palpation of skin and subcutaneous tissue (e.g., induration, subcutaneous nodules, tightening)

   d. Genitourinary: examination of the scrotal contents (e.g., hydrocele, spermatocele, tenderness of cord, testicular mass)

8. Which element identified by a bullet is documented in the words "patient calmed after a few moments' interruption"?

   a. Constitutional: measurement of *any three of the following seven* vital signs: (1) sitting or standing blood pressure, (2) supine blood pressure, (3) pulse rate and regularity, (4) respiration, (5) temperature, (6) height, (7) weight

   b. Psychiatric: brief assessment of mental status, including mood and affect (e.g., depression, anxiety, agitation)

   c. Cardiovascular: auscultation of heart with notation of abnormal sounds and murmurs

   d. Neurologic: examination of sensation (e.g., by touch, pin, vibration, proprioception)

9. How many elements identified by a bullet have been documented in this medical documentation?

   a. Between one and five

   b. More than six

   c. Two elements identified by a bullet from each of six systems/body areas OR at least 12 elements identified by a bullet in two or more systems/body areas

   d. All elements identified by a bullet in at least nine areas/systems AND documentation of at least two elements identified by a bullet in each of the nine areas/systems

10. What type of general multisystem physical examination best reflects the documented physical examination?

    a. Problem-focused

    b. Expanded problem-focused

    c. Detailed

    d. Comprehensive

Case Study 7-2

Read the following documentation, and then identify the documented levels of history *as well as* the documented elements and type of general multisystem physical examination described.

Complaint: Frank is well-known to me and presents for sharp left flank pain and dark-orange-colored urine after a fall resulting in blunt abdominal trauma on Saturday afternoon, 2 days ago. He tripped on his dog and fell against the patio railing, striking his upper left abdomen against the decorative wrought iron. Patient reports experiencing immediate stabbing pain across his upper abdomen and down his left flank, which subsided quickly without recurrence. Upon rising on Sunday morning, Frank noticed sharp stabbing pain across ULQ abdomen accompanied by dark, painful bruising in the area of his URQ where he was struck by the decorative railing. The pain is most severe when he breathes deeply, rating pain at 8/10, and Frank cannot bend his torso without significant pain. Frank reports his urine sample to be very dark and **odorous** but denies painful urination. He denies any chest pain or racing heartbeat. No reports of tingling of extremities, dizziness, nausea, bloody stool. All other reviews of systems pertinent to this problem are negative. No report of ill contact at work or family, although Frank reports a higher stress level than usual, as budget cuts at work have caused many layoffs, and he is anxious about his employment status at work. There is no history of gastrointestinal disease in family or past medical history.

Physical Exam: T, 97.8; BP, 106/88; P, 68. Eyes clear without jaundice. Head is atraumatic without tenderness, nodules, or swelling. Neck: no thyromegaly. Auscultation of lungs is clear without wheezes or rub. No tactile fremitus noted upon palpation of chest. Auscultation of heart reveals regular rate and rhythm with no abnormal sounds noted. No cervical spine tenderness. No thoracic spine tenderness and no lumbar spine tenderness; however, costovertebral tenderness noted upon palpation. No referred pain in left shoulder. Palpation of lower abdomen reveals soft, nontender abdomen, and no hepatomegaly or tenderness upon upper right quadrant palpation or percussion. Upper left abdomen mildly inflamed with dark circular bruise where patient identifies blow to abdomen. Very tender upper left quadrant upon palpation, and patient's pain precludes deep palpation of spleen. No dullness noted upon percussion of left or right flank. Stool sample collected for occult blood test.

Laboratory: CBC reveals white blood count normal; hemoglobin and hematocrit are normal. A FAST scan abdominal CT scan was reviewed with radiologist. Review of KUB revealed significant stool within sigmoid and rectum. Occult blood test negative.

Assessment: It is quite probable that at least one of the lower left ribs has been fractured, although the patient's pain makes specific rib identification impossible. A splenic injury should be ruled out through CT scan. In my opinion, it would be prudent to begin oral Augmentin treatment at 875 mg twice a day for 7 days and increase fluid intake. Follow-up in 10 days for recheck.

1. Identify the appropriate level of the documented HPI:

   _____

2. Identify the appropriate level of the documented ROS:

   _____

3. Identify the appropriate level of the documented PFSH:

   _____

odorous foul smelling

4. Circle the level of overall history:

   Problem-focused

   Expanded problem-focused

   Detailed

   Comprehensive

5. Using the 1997 Documentation Guidelines for the general multisystem physical examination, identify each system/body area examined and each of the general multisystem physical examination elements identified by a bullet:

   System/body area: _____
   Elements identified by bullet:_____

   System/body area: _____
   Elements identified by bullet:_____

   System/body area: _____
   Elements identified by bullet:_____

   System/body area: _____
   Elements identified by bullet:_____

   System/body area: _____
   Elements identified by bullet:_____

   System/body area: _____
   Elements identified by bullet:_____

   System/body area: _____
   Elements identified by bullet:_____

   System/body area: _____
   Elements identified by bullet:_____

   System/body area: _____
   Elements identified by bullet:_____

   System/body area: _____
   Elements identified by bullet:_____

6. What type of general multisystem physical examination is documented?_____

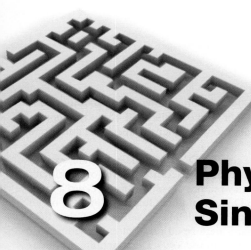

8 Physical Examination—Single Organ

Learning Objectives

After completing this chapter, you should be able to do the following:

- Spell and define the key terms and abbreviations presented in this chapter
- Define the single organ–system physical examination
- Distinguish the difference between the general multisystem physical examination and the single organ–system physical examination
- Identify the guidelines for the 10 different single organ–system physical examinations listed in the "1997 Documentation Guidelines for Evaluation and Management"
- List and define the four types of single organ–system physical examination documentation according to the 1997 Documentation Guidelines

Key Terms

adenoids

atraumatic

cervical

choanae

clinical speech reception thresholds

crackles

epiglottis

eustacian tube

false vocal cords

larynx

nares

pharyngeal walls

pneumo-otoscopy

pyriform sinuses

salivary glands

shaded border

single organ–system physical examination

solid white exudates

supine

thyromegaly

true vocal cords

unshaded border

INTRODUCTION

During the course of a student's entire education, the student's foundation of knowledge becomes stronger, and he or she may choose to specialize in a particular area of study. As the field of study becomes more specialized, the examinations encountered change according to the student's experience and scope of knowledge.

Physicians devote years of study and hard work to earn the title "MD." This education, skill, experience, and professional knowledge allow the performing physician to discern the level of specificity required for a physical examination. Certain E/M service visits may require the physician to record a more general physical examination. In those circumstances, the 1995 Documentation Guidelines and the organ system/body area physical examination may be the most appropriate guidelines to reference. Other E/M service visits demand more anatomic specificity in the physician's performed physical examination. For these circumstances, the general multisystem physical examination in the 1997 Documentation Guidelines provides the more appropriate reference. However, certain E/M service visits demand an even higher degree of anatomic specificity in the physical examination. For these circumstances, the single organ–system physical examination in the 1997 Documentation Guidelines may be the most appropriate reference. This chapter focuses on that single organ–system physical examination.

SINGLE ORGAN–SYSTEM PHYSICAL EXAMINATION

single organ–system physical examination a physical examination that narrows its focus to the elements supporting one single organ system, according to the requirements listed in the 1997 Documentation Guidelines

Whereas the evidentiary checklist for the general multisystem physical examination presents a holistic view of the human anatomy, the **single organ–system physical examination** narrows the focus to the elements supporting one single organ system. For instance, respiratory function is directly related to the cardiovascular system. Therefore, respiratory effort provides important evidence about the status of the patient's cardiovascular health; if the patient is struggling to breathe, the physician is informed about factors influencing the condition of the patient's cardiovascular health. Thus, certain clinical elements become crucial indicators for identifying the status of a specific single organ system.

The "1997 Documentation Guidelines for Evaluation and Management Services" lists separate documentation guidelines for 10 different single organ systems. Each of the separate guidelines enumerates clinical elements identified by a bullet that lead to particular clinical findings and evidence regarding that specific single organ system. The 10 different single organ systems are these:

- Cardiovascular
- Ears, Nose, and Throat
- Eyes
- Genitourinary
- Hematologic/Lymphatic/Immunologic
- Musculoskeletal
- Neurological
- Psychiatric
- Respiratory
- Skin

SINGLE ORGAN SYSTEM VS. GENERAL MULTISYSTEM

The guidelines for the general multisystem physical examination give an evidentiary checklist that includes elements identified by a bullet for each of the 14 different systems/body areas. This evidentiary checklist is provided in the form of a chart, or table, that lists all 14 of the systems/body areas and the corresponding elements identified by bullets. ■ FIGURE 8.1 shows the first three systems/body areas listed in the general multisystem evidentiary checklist.

Each of the separate single organ–system guidelines contains an individualized evidentiary checklist. Since different systems/body areas support different single organ systems, each of the evidentiary checklists looks a little different. Certain borders on the evidentiary checklist are shaded, indicating specific elements of particular importance for this single organ system. ■ FIGURE 8.2 shows the first three systems/body areas listed in the cardiovascular single organ–system evidentiary checklist.

Name of System/ Body Area	The elements that may be examined during the general multisystem physical exam (each individual element identified by an individual bullet): • Anatomic location of specific clinical finding
Constitutional	• Measurement of any three of the following seven vital signs: (1) sitting or standing blood pressure, (2) supine blood pressure, (3) pulse rate and regularity, (4) respiration, (5) temperature, (6) height, (7) weight • General appearance of patient
Eyes	• Inspection of conjunctivae and lids • Examination of pupils and irises • Ophthalmoscopic examination of optic discs and posterior segments
Ears, Nose, Throat, and Mouth	• External inspection of ears and nose • Otoscopic examination of external auditory canals and tympanic membranes • Assessment of hearing • Inspection of nasal mucosa, septum, and turbinates • Inspection of lips, teeth, and gums • Examination of oropharynx

Figure 8.1 ■ An example from the general multisystem physical examination evidentiary checklist.

Name of System/ Body Area	**Cardiovascular** Single Organ–System Physical Exam (each individual element identified by an individual bullet):
Constitutional	• Measurement of any three of the following seven vital signs: (1) sitting or standing blood pressure, (2) supine blood pressure, (3) pulse rate and regularity, (4) respiration, (5) temperature, (6) height, (7) weight • General appearance of patient
Head and Face	
Eyes	• Inspection of conjunctivae and lids

Figure 8.2 ■ An example from the cardiovascular single organ–system evidentiary checklist.

In Figure 8.2, a dark border surrounds the constitutional system/body area, indicating that those elements identified by bullets reveal very important clinical evidence about the health of the cardiovascular system. The 1997 Documentation Guidelines refer to this dark border as a **shaded border**.

The eye system/body area listed in Figure 8.2 shows a different, thinner outline than the shaded border surrounding the constitutional system/body area. This thinner outline indicates that this particular element is not a critical piece of clinical evidence about the health of the cardiovascular single organ system; a lighter outline indicates that the findings within those specific systems/body areas are relevant to the single organ system but do not carry the same weight and importance as the shaded systems/body areas. The 1997 Documentation Guidelines refer to this thinner outline as an **unshaded border**.

The second system/body area listed in Figure 8.2, the head and face system/body area, lists no elements identified by a bullet since any clinical findings concerning the head and face provide little information or evidence regarding the health of the cardiovascular system. These "empty" systems/body areas are anatomically involved in the single organ system, but any findings are not relevant to the health of the single organ system being examined.

In this way, the evidentiary checklists for the 10 single organ systems contain shaded and unshaded borders that indicate the relationship between the single organ system examined by the physician and the individually listed systems/body areas and their corresponding elements. Instructions for accessing the complete requirements for each single organ–system physical examination in the "1997 Documentation Guidelines for Evaluation and Management Services" are provided in Appendix B.

shaded border a dark border outlining a specific system/body area in the 1997 Documentation Guidelines that bears considerable importance to the examination of a single organ system

unshaded border a light line outlining a system/ body area in the 1997 Documentation Guidelines that bears a lower significance to the examination of a single organ system

| Exercise 8.1 | Patient's Sinus Pressure and Cough |

After reading the following medical documentations, identify which systems/body areas have a shaded border and which have an unshaded border. Be sure to reference the 1997 single organ–system physical examination by following the instructions provided in Appendix B.

1. **History:** Patient has presented for sinus pressure and cough. Patient's face hurts so much on the right cheek beneath eye that she feels she cannot open her eyes all the way due to the stabbing pain. She complains of a ringing in her right ear, and the right side of her throat hurts when she swallows. She has no appetite, complains of heartburn but no nausea. Nighttime has been interrupted by frequent urination without pain but very smelly urine. Patient denies joint pain other than a sore neck. Patient complains of heavy chest pressure and pain upon coughing. Patient states she can feel her heartbeat in her head as a throbbing but denies any heart palpitations. Patient is dizzy upon standing and reports she has spent 3 days lying down because of the discomfort. No report of sick contact at work; however, her husband had the flu last month. Neither patient nor her husband smokes tobacco.

Exam: Patient is pale and appears very tired; she appears well groomed. Conjunctivae clear without swelling. Nasal passages quite congested and very swollen. Fluid noted within inner ear bilaterally; however, tympanic membrane does not appear significantly pressured. Throat mottled with yellow and white patches, and tonsils significantly red and swollen. Palpation of neck and behind ears reveals very tender, swollen lymph nodes. Patient expresses extreme discomfort when swallowing.

Respiratory single organ system

System/body area with shaded border: _____

System/body area with shaded border: _____

System/body area with shaded border: _____

System/body area with unshaded border: _____

| Exercise 8.2 | Timmy's Abdominal Pain and Diarrhea |

After reading the following medical documentation, identify which systems/body areas have a shaded border and which have an unshaded border. Be sure to reference the 1997 single organ–system physical examination by following the instructions provided in Appendix B.

Timmy is an established patient and presents for abdominal pain and diarrhea. Timmy says his stomach hurts, down low on the right side, and that it hurts really, really badly, but not all the time. Timmy's father reports his son complains most about the pain in the morning after getting up, and Timmy describes that pain as an 8 on pain scale. Per father's report, Timmy feels better after eating breakfast, but the pain became bad last week. Per father's report, Timmy had stomach flu last month with no vomiting but explosive diarrhea. Timmy's father denies bloody stools but states that Timmy's urine is dark and odorous, but that Timmy denies painful urination. Upon query, Timmy complains of some pain in his back during the last week, placing his hands on his midback. Timmy states he felt dizzy during the past week after walking upstairs at school and home. Patient is second grader at Hardy Oaks Elementary and active in peewee soccer as a goalie where, per father, Timmy was recently involved in a goal-side tackle with resultant sharp abdominal pain. Timmy reported domestic incident between his parents at practice; father corroborates Timmy's report. Patient's primary residence is with father, with joint custody with mother, and Timmy states visitation with mother is occasional with stressful transitions. Timmy's father denies use of tobacco or alcohol.

PE: Timmy appears pale and slightly lethargic but responsive to questions. T, 98.7F; pulse, 130; resp., 20. Eyes clear with no jaundice. Pupils are reactive to light within normal limits. Lungs clear to auscultation and percussion. Auscultation of heart reveals normal but rapid heartbeat without murmur. Timmy complains of pain during palpation of costovertebral angle. Abdomen firm with rebound; however, bladder full upon palpation, although Timmy provided urinary specimen and claims he emptied his bladder. Urinary meatus appears red and inflamed. Testicles are slightly retracted, but warm and without tenderness.

Hematologic, lymphatic, immunologic single organ system

System/body area with shaded border: _____

System/body area with shaded border: _____

System/body area with shaded border: _____

System/body area with shaded border: _____

System/body area with unshaded border: _____

System/body area with unshaded border: _____

System/body area with unshaded border: _____

Joan's Lower Back Pain

After reading the following medical documentation, identify which systems/body areas have a shaded border and which have an unshaded border. Be sure to reference the 1997 single organ–system physical examination by following the instructions provided in Appendix B.

Joan is an established patient who presents for lower back pain. Her lower back hurts, down by beltline, and pain is sometimes very severe. The pain is sporadic, mostly when standing up after sitting in one place for an extended period. Ibuprofen used to help, but now it does not help back pain anymore. At its worst, low back pain is sharp and throbbing. Joan has had occasional back pain for about 20 years, since first in the service, but she first noticed this particular low back pain shortly after playing touch football with adult children this past Thanksgiving. Patient denies any other joint pain than this low back pain. Patient denies double vision or dizziness, and no chest pain or shortness of breath. Patient denies tobacco or alcohol use. Pain has not affected her work as a fifth-grade teacher.

Exam: Back is soft to the touch and palpation and revealed no obvious lumps or masses. Percussion of back reveals tenderness in lower back, but no costovertebral tenderness. Patient performs side-to-side flexion to 30 degrees with minimal pain; however, she finds forward flexion at 50 degrees with pain localized to her lower back that does not radiate down legs or up her back. Deep tendon reflexes within normal limits: ankle jerk reflex, patellar reflex, plantar reflexes tested. Patient's range of motion is stable, within normal limits, and without pain.

Musculoskeletal single organ system

System/body area with shaded border: _____

System/body area with shaded border: _____

1997 SINGLE ORGAN–SYSTEM PHYSICAL EXAMINATION REQUIREMENTS

The "1997 Documentation Guidelines for Evaluation and Management Services" states that any physician, regardless of specialty, may perform the single organ–system physical examination. The type of physical examination is determined by the physician's clinical judgment, the patient's history, and the nature of the presenting problem. Remember that whereas the chief complaint is the patient's description of the specific health issue, complaint, or disease for which the patient sought care, the nature of the presenting problem is the physician's holistic view of the patient's illness, symptom, chief complaint, disease process, or other reason for care before the definition of a diagnosis.

The 1997 Documentation Guidelines clearly define specific requirements for the documentation of abnormal, unexpected, and normal, or negative, physical examination findings. These documentation requirements remain as true for the single organ–system physical examination as for the 1995 physical examination and the general multisystem physical examination.

FOUR TYPES OF 1997 SINGLE ORGAN–SYSTEM PHYSICAL EXAMINATION

Four different types of examination are defined for the single organ–system physical examination. The four types remain the same as for the 1995 organ system/body area exam and the 1997 general multisystem exam, thus providing consistency of documentation across the spectrum of E/M service visits (see ■ FIGURE 8.3).

The four types of single organ–system physical examination, as defined by the 1997 Documentation Guidelines, are problem-focused, expanded problem-focused, detailed, and comprehensive. The amount of clinical and anatomic specificity provided in each of these four types differs in relation to the affected body area or organ system and to any inclusion of other symptomatic or related organ systems (see ■ TABLE 8.1).

By including both body areas and organ systems in the single organ–system physical examination, a quantifiable guideline is identified for each of the four types. This clinical specificity is dependent upon the physician's documentation of the performed physical examination, as shown in the following example.

> ### Example: Documentation of Problem-Focused Single Organ–System Exam
>
> Documentation of one to five elements identified by a bullet (•), whether in a shaded or an unshaded border, is required for this type of exam.
>
> #### Johnny's Irritating Cough
>
> Auricle of left ear is bright red as Johnny has been pulling at it. Upon examination, serous fluid is apparent behind tympanic membrane. Finger rub test resulted in normal hearing, despite Johnny's sense of hearing loss. Johnny is uncomfortably congested

pneumo-otoscopy the use of an otoscope to identify and diagnose otitis media (an infection of the middle ear); utilizes a puff of air to determine how much pressure is behind the eardrum and to assess the mobility of the eardrum

clinical speech reception thresholds determination of a patient's ability to hear, retain, and repeat two-syllable words prompted by the physician

nares nostrils

solid white exudates secretions covering the back of the throat that might suggest an infection

and unable to inhale through either nostril. Significant mucus production noted via nares bilaterally. Patient's cough produces thick, white phlegm upon expectoration, and solid, white exudates apparent on tonsils and along back of pharynx.

Five separate elements identified by a bullet are documented:

Ears, Nose, Throat, and Mouth

- External inspection of ears and nose (red auricle due to Johnny pulling at his earlobe)
- Otoscopic examination of external auditory canals and tympanic membranes, including **pneumo-otoscopy** with notation of mobility of membranes (otoscopic identification of serous fluid behind tympanic membrane)
- Assessment of hearing with tuning forks and **clinical speech reception thresholds** (could hear the sound of the physician's fingertips rubbing together near Johnny's ears)
- Inspection of nasal mucosa, septum, and turbinates (unable to inhale through his nostrils, and significant mucus production noted via **nares** bilaterally)
- Examination of oropharynx: oral mucosa, hard and soft palates, tongue, tonsils, and posterior pharynx (**solid white exudates,** or discharge, along the tonsils and the back of the pharynx visible to the physician's naked eye)

Physical Examination	Problem-Focused	Expanded Problem-Focused	Detailed	Comprehensive
1995 PE	A limited examination of affected body area or organ system (1 body area/organ system)	A limited examination of the affected body area or organ system and other symptomatic or related organ systems (2–4 body areas/organ systems)	An extended examination of the affected body area(s) or organ system(s) and other symptomatic or related body areas or organ systems (5–7 body areas/organ systems)	A general multisystem examination or complete examination of a single organ system and other symptomatic or related body areas or organ systems; should include 8 or more of the 12 organ systems (8+ body systems OR organ systems, but they cannot be mixed)
1997 General Multisystem	1–5 elements identified by a bullet	At least 6 elements identified by a bullet	At least 2 elements identified by a bullet from each of 6 areas/systems OR at least 12 elements identified by a bullet in 2 or more areas/systems	Performance of all elements identified by a bullet in at least 9 organ systems or body areas and documentation of at least 2 elements identified by a bullet in each of 9 areas/systems
1997 Single Organ System	1–5 elements identified by a bullet, whether in a shaded or unshaded border	At least 6 elements identified by a bullet, whether in a shaded or unshaded border	At least 12 elements identified by a bullet, whether within a shaded or unshaded border (Eye & psychiatric: at least 9 elements identified by a bullet, whether within a shaded or unshaded border)	All elements identified by a bullet within each shaded border and at least 1 element identified by a bullet within each unshaded border

Figure 8.3 ■ Content of service element: 1997 single organ–system physical examination.

■ **TABLE 8.1   THE FOUR TYPES OF SINGLE ORGAN–SYSTEM PHYSICAL EXAMINATIONS**

Problem-Focused—performance and documentation of one to five elements identified by a bullet (•), whether in a shaded or an unshaded border

Expanded Problem-Focused—performance and documentation of at least six elements identified by a bullet (•), whether in a shaded or an unshaded border

Detailed for the following single organ systems: cardiovascular; ears, nose, throat, and mouth; genitourinary; hematologic, lymphatic, immunologic; musculoskeletal; neurologic; respiratory; skin—documentation of at least 12 elements identified by a bullet (•), whether in a shaded or an unshaded border

Detailed for the following single organ systems: eyes, psychiatric—documentation of at least nine elements identified by a bullet (•), whether in a shaded or an unshaded border

Comprehensive—documentation of every element identified by a bullet (•) within a shaded border and at least one element within each unshaded border

Source: Centers for Medicare and Medicaid Services, "1997 Documentation Guidelines for Evaluation and Management Services," pp. 12–13, www.cms.gov/Outreach-and-Education/Medicare-Learning-Network-MLN/MLNEdWebGuide/Downloads/97Docguidelines.pdf.

As the documentation reflects the complexity of the performed physical examination, the level of the single organ–system physical examination changes depending on the documented elements identified by a bullet, as seen in the following example.

Example: Documentation of Expanded Problem-Focused Single Organ–System Exam

Documentation of at least six elements identified by a bullet (•), whether in a shaded or an unshaded border, is required for this type of exam.

Johnny's Irritating Cough

Patient is alert, however clearly uncomfortable. Vital signs: T, 99.32F; pulse, 120; BP 100/65. Eyes: conjunctivae inflamed, but clear. ENT/M: auricle of left ear is bright red as Johnny has been pulling at it. Finger rub test resulted in normal hearing, despite Johnny's sense of hearing loss. Johnny is uncomfortably congested and unable to inhale through either nostril. Significant mucus production noted via nares bilaterally. Patient's cough produces thick, white phlegm upon expectoration, and solid, white exudates apparent on tonsils and along back of pharynx.

Seven separate elements identified by a bullet are documented:

Constitutional

- Measurement of <u>any three of the following seven</u> vital signs: (1) sitting or standing blood pressure, (2) **supine** blood pressure, (3) pulse rate and regularity, (4) respiration, (5) temperature, (6) height, (7) weight (three vital signs documented: temperature, pulse, and blood pressure)
- General appearance of patient (clearly uncomfortable)

Ears, Nose, Throat, and Mouth

- External inspection of ears and nose (red auricle due to Johnny pulling at his earlobe)
- Otoscopic examination of external auditory canals and tympanic membranes, including pneumo-otoscopy with notation of mobility of membranes (otoscopic identification of serous fluid behind tympanic membrane)
- Assessment of hearing with tuning forks and clinical speech reception thresholds (could hear the sound of the physician's fingertips rubbing together near Johnny's ears)
- Inspection of nasal mucosa, septum, and turbinates (unable to inhale through his nostrils, and significant mucus production noted in both nostrils)
- Examination of oropharynx: oral mucosa, hard and soft palates, tongue, tonsils, and posterior pharynx (solid white exudates, or discharge, along the tonsils and the back of the pharynx visible to the physician's naked eye)

supine lying on the back; refers to blood pressure that is taken when the patient is lying down

---

Within the 1997 single organ–system physical examination, the elements found within unshaded borders are important for the single organ system, even though they may not be essential to the physician's examination of that single organ system. This distinction between unshaded and shaded border elements can be seen in the following example, which illustrates a detailed physical examination of the ear, nose, and throat single organ system.

Example: Documentation of Detailed Single Organ–System Exam

Documentation of at least 12 elements identified by a bullet (•), whether in a shaded or an unshaded border, is required for this type of exam.

Johnny's Irritating Cough (and Stomachache)

Patient is clearly uncomfortable, but alert, in no distress, and curious about his surroundings. Vital signs: T, 99.3F; pulse, 120; BP, 100/65. Eyes: conjunctivae inflamed, but clear. ENT/M: auricle of left ear is bright red as Johnny has been pulling at it. Finger rub test resulted in normal hearing, despite Johnny's sense of hearing loss. Johnny is uncomfortably congested and unable to inhale through either nostril. Significant mucus production noted via nares bilaterally. Patient's cough produces thick, white phlegm upon expectoration, and solid, white exudates apparent on tonsils and along back of pharynx. Neck is soft without masses; no thyromegaly. No sign of respiratory distress, lungs clear without crackles, wheezes. RRR, without gallop, murmur, or rub. Abdomen: soft with mild tenderness noted in left lower quadrant with palpable stool. Patient states he has not passed stool for 3 days; no hepatosplenomegaly noted; however, patient reports pain upon palpation of left upper quadrant.

Twelve separate elements identified by a bullet are documented:

Constitutional

- Measurement of <u>any three of the following seven</u> vital signs: (1) sitting or standing blood pressure, (2) supine blood pressure, (3) pulse rate and regularity, (4) respiration, (5) temperature, (6) height, (7) weight (three vital signs documented: temperature, pulse, and blood pressure)
- General appearance of patient (clearly uncomfortable)

Ears, Nose, Throat, and Mouth

- External inspection of ears and nose (red auricle due to Johnny pulling at his earlobe)
- Otoscopic examination of external auditory canals and tympanic membranes (otoscopic identification of serous fluid behind tympanic membrane)
- Assessment of hearing (could hear the sound of the physician's fingertips rubbing together near Johnny's ears)
- Inspection of nasal mucosa, septum, and turbinates (unable to inhale through his nostrils, and significant mucus production noted in both nostrils)
- Examination of oropharynx: oral mucosa, **salivary glands**, hard and soft palates, tongue, tonsils, and posterior pharynx (solid white exudates, or discharge, along the tonsils and the back of the pharynx visible to the physician's naked eye)

Neck

- Examination of neck (soft without masses)
- Examination of thyroid (no **thyromegaly**)

Respiratory

- Assessment of respiratory effort (no sign of respiratory distress)
- Auscultation of lungs (clear without **crackles**, wheezes)

Cardiovascular

- Auscultation of heart with notation of abnormal sounds and murmurs (RRR, without gallop, murmur, or rub)

salivary glands glands located in the mouth and beneath the tongue that secrete saliva

thyromegaly enlargement of the thyroid gland

crackles abnormal, sharp sounds that can be heard during auscultation of the lungs

Note that the 1997 Documentation Guidelines include different requirements for a detailed physical examination of the eye or psychiatric single organ system: just nine separate elements identified by a bullet.

Example: Documentation of Comprehensive Single Organ–System Exam

Documentation of every element identified by a bullet within a shaded border as well as at least one element identified by a bullet within each unshaded border, is required for this type of exam.

Johnny's Irritating Cough (and Stomachache after a Bad Fall)

Patient is clearly uncomfortable because of his cold, but alert, in no distress, and curious about his surroundings. His voice is hoarse, but clear and understandable. He correctly reports the day and place, correctly identifying this examiner by name, showing good judgment and insight for the questions. Johnny remembers everything about his fall but shows no anxiety about getting on the examination table. Vital signs: T, 99.32F; pulse, 120; BP, 100/65. Eyes: conjunctivae inflamed, but clear. PERRL. No hemorrhages noted in posterior segments of eye or indication of lasting injury after fall. Normal visual field test with normal extra-ocular movements. ENT/M: auricle of left ear is

continued

bright red as Johnny has been pulling at it. Finger rub test resulted in normal hearing, despite Johnny's sense of hearing loss. Johnny is uncomfortably congested and unable to inhale through either nostril. Significant mucus production noted via nares bilaterally. Patient's cough produces thick, white phlegm upon expectoration. Gums are red and slightly inflamed with adequate salivary production. Solid white exudates apparent on tonsils and along back of pharynx. No lesions noted along **pharyngeal walls**. **Larynx** swollen but within normal limits. Although larynx was not directly viewed, **epiglottis** is red and inflamed. **Adenoids** swollen per direct visualization. Patient's gag reflex prevented further direct visualization with mirror. Head **atraumatic** and face without lesions. Exquisite tenderness upon palpation of sinuses, and facial muscles reaction bilaterally accurate and within normal limits. **Cervical** lymph nodes swollen and tender upon palpation. Neck is soft without masses; no thyromegaly. No sign of respiratory distress, lungs clear without crackles, wheezes. No fremitus upon palpation. Percussion reveals resonant lung sounds. RRR, without gallop, murmur, or rub.

Each of the elements identified by a bullet within the shaded borders is documented, as well as at least one element identified by a bullet within each of the unshaded borders:

Constitutional (shaded)

* Measurement of <u>any three of the following seven</u> vital signs: (1) sitting or standing blood pressure, (2) supine blood pressure, (3) pulse rate and regularity, (4) respiration, (5) temperature, (6) height, (7) weight (three vital signs documented: temperature, pulse, and blood pressure)
* General appearance of patient (clearly uncomfortable)
* Assessment of ability to communicate and quality of voice (voice is hoarse but clear)

Head (shaded)

* Inspection of head and face (head atraumatic and face without lesions)
* Palpation and/or percussion of face with notation of presence or absence of sinus tenderness (exquisite tenderness upon palpation of sinuses)
* Examination of salivary glands (adequate salivary production)
* Assessment of facial strength (facial muscles reaction bilaterally accurate and within normal limits)

Ears, Nose, Throat, and Mouth (shaded)

* Otoscopic examination of external auditory canals and tympanic membranes (otoscopic identification of serous fluid behind tympanic membrane)
* Assessment of hearing with tuning forks and clinical speech reception (could hear the sound of the physician's fingertips rubbing together near Johnny's ears)
* External inspection of ears and nose (red auricle due to Johnny pulling at his earlobe)
* Inspection of nasal mucosa, septum, and turbinates (unable to inhale through his nostrils, and significant mucus production noted in both nostrils)
* Inspection of lips, teeth, and gums (gums red and inflamed)
* Examination of oropharynx: oral mucosa, salivary glands, hard and soft palates, tongue, tonsils, and posterior pharynx (solid white exudates, or discharge, along the tonsils and the back of the pharynx visible to the physician's naked eye)
* Inspection of pharyngeal walls and **pyriform sinuses** (no lesions noted along pharyngeal walls)
* Examination by mirror of larynx, including the condition of the epiglottis, **false vocal cords**, **true vocal cords**, and mobility of larynx; use of mirror not required in children (larynx swollen but within normal limits; epiglottis red and inflamed)
* Examination by mirror of nasopharynx, including appearance of the mucosa, adenoids, posterior **choanae**, and **eustacian tubes**; use of mirror not required in children (adenoids swollen per direct visualization, gag reflex preventing further direct visualization with mirror)

Neck (shaded)

* Examination of neck (soft without masses)
* Examination of thyroid (no thyromegaly)

pharyngeal walls the mucosal tissues covering the surface of the throat, extending from the mouth and nasal cavities down to the tracheoesophageal junction; the sides of the pharynx, through which food passes to the esophagus and air passes to the lungs

larynx the section of the throat that contains the voice box

epiglottis the flap of tissue that covers and protects the larynx during the act of swallowing

adenoids lymphatic tissue located behind the nose, in the roof of the nasopharynx

atraumatic without sign or indication of trauma or injury

cervical referring to lymph nodes located in the neck

pyriform sinuses a pear-shaped recess near the larynx, which is a common location where food may be caught

false vocal cords the mucus membrane that covers the true vocal cords

true vocal cords the vocal folds responsible for the production of sounds

choanae the funnel-shaped channels that form large openings through which air leaves the nose; also referred to as *posterior nares*

eustacian tube a tube or passage linking the middle ear to the throat, which helps to regulate internal air pressure and drain mucus

Respiratory (unshaded)

- Assessment of chest, including symmetry, expansion, and/or assessment of respiratory effort (no sign of respiratory distress)
- Auscultation of lungs (clear without crackles, wheezes)

Cardiovascular (unshaded)

- Auscultation of heart with notation of abnormal sounds and murmurs (RRR, without gallop, murmur, or rub)

Lymphatic (unshaded)

- Palpation of lymph nodes in neck, axillae, groin, and/or other location (cervical lymph nodes swollen and tender upon palpation)

Neurologic/Psychiatric (unshaded)

Brief assessment of mental status:

- Orientation to time, place, and person (correctly reports day and place, as well as correctly identifying examiner by name)
- Recent and remote memory (remembers everything about his fall)
- Mood and affect (shows no anxiety about getting on the examination table)

It is important to remember that each of the different single organ systems would reveal very different findings in the documentation, with different elements identified by bullets. The importance of logic and reason remains paramount for medical documentation and is most apparent with single organ–system physical examinations.

When Should the Single Organ–System Physical Examination Be Referenced?

Unlike the other two types of physical examination, the 1995 organ system/body area and the general multisystem, the single organ–system physical examination requires a much higher level of anatomic specificity. Although this specificity may seem daunting, these distinctive guidelines become tremendously helpful in a specialist's setting. For example, a cardiologist's documentation may contain more specific clinical findings than may be supported by the documentation requirements for the organ system/body area or even the general multisystem exams. For the performing physician, the medical documentation stands as the testament to the effort, skill, and expertise he or she has devoted to the completion of the physical examination.

However, in reviewing the medical documentation of an E/M service visit, how does the reviewer know which of the three physical examinations to reference? The answer can be simplified to one simple criterion: it is recommended for the reviewer to determine which of the three physical examinations best reflects the physician's documented physical examination for the patient encounter—the organ system/body area exam of the 1995 Documentation Guidelines or the general multisystem or single organ–system exams of the 1997 Documentation Guidelines.

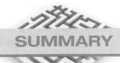

SUMMARY

- The single organ–system physical examination reflects the status of the patient's health at the time of the E/M visit through the documentation of specific clinical elements identified during an examination of one specific organ system. The "1997 Documentation Guidelines for Evaluation and Management Services" lists the single organ–system physical examination documentation requirements, which provide individual guide-

lines for the 10 different organ systems: cardiovascular; ear, nose, throat, and mouth; eyes; genitourinary; hematologic, lymphatic, immunologic; musculoskeletal; neurologic; psychiatric; respiratory; and skin.

- Each of the 10 single organ systems contains a specific evidentiary checklist that identifies the systems/body areas most pertinent to its examination and the unique elements identified by a bullet. These elements represent findings to be identified by the physician's physical, visual, and auditory interaction with the patient.

- According to the 1997 Documentation Guidelines, any physician, regardless of specialty, may perform the general multisystem physical examination. The inclusion of the physician's specialty highlights the importance of the single organ–system physical examination. The physician's clinical judgment, the patient's history, and the nature of the presenting problem inform the physician's decision regarding not only the type of physical examination, but also its specificity.

- There are four types of single organ–system physical examination: problem-focused, expanded problem-focused, detailed, and comprehensive. The requirements for problem-focused, expanded problem-focused, and comprehensive types of single organ–system exams are consistent across all 10 of the single organ systems. Documentation supporting the problem-focused type should include one to five elements identified by a bullet (•), whether in a shaded or an unshaded border. Documentation supporting the expanded problem-focused type should include at least six elements identified by a bullet (•), whether in a shaded or an unshaded border. Documentation supporting the comprehensive type should include documentation of all elements identified by a bullet (•) within a shaded border as well as at least one element within each unshaded border. The detailed type of single organ–system exam is unique because two different requirements are listed: For the eye and psychiatric single organ systems, the documentation should include at least nine elements identified by a bullet (•), whether in a shaded or an unshaded border. However, for the other eight single organ systems, documentation should include at least 12 elements identified by a bullet (•), whether in a shaded or an unshaded border.

CHAPTER REVIEW

Multiple Choice

Choose the letter that best answers each question or completes each statement.

1. Which of the following best defines the nature of the presenting problem?
   a. The documentation of the physical examination findings
   b. The physician's documented clinical findings according to the single organ–system physical examination findings
   c. The medical documentation of the patient's description of the chief complaint
   d. The physician's holistic view of the patient's illness, symptom, chief complaint, disease process, or other reason for care before the definition of a diagnosis

2. In the medical documentation of the E/M service visit, the physical examination reflects which of the following?
   a. An inventory of the patient's status of health prior to the E/M service visit
   b. A snapshot of the patient's health at the time of the E/M service visit, including the functions, performance, structure, and health of the patient's body
   c. Documented findings of the previous medical history of the patient and patient's family
   d. Descriptions provided by the patient that provide a personalized illustration of the symptom the patient is currently experiencing

3. How are the documentation requirements for the single organ–system physical examination presented in the "1997 Documentation Guidelines for Evaluation and Management Services"?
   a. The documentation requirements for the single organ–system physical examination are presented in the form of specific clinical elements, which are each identified by a bullet.

b. The documentation requirements for the single organ–system physical examination are presented in the form of organ systems and body areas.
   c. The documentation requirements for the single organ–system physical examination are presented in the form of the physician's documentation of the physical examination.
   d. The documentation requirements for the single organ–system physical examination are presented in the form of the preprinted questionnaire completed by the patient.

4. How many different single organ–system physical examinations are listed in the 1997 Documentation Guidelines?
   a. Four
   b. Five
   c. Eight
   d. Ten

5. How many types of single organ–system physical examination are listed in the 1997 Documentation Guidelines?
   a. Two
   b. Three
   c. Four
   d. Five

6. Which of the following choices represents the problem-focused type of single organ–system physical examination?
   a. The documentation should include at least six elements identified by a bullet (•) whether in a shaded border or an unshaded border.
   b. The documentation should include one to five elements identified by a bullet (•) whether in a shaded border or an unshaded border.
   c. The documentation should include at least 12 elements identified by a bullet (•) whether in a shaded border or an unshaded border.

d. The documentation should include all elements identified by a bullet (•) within a shaded border as well as at least one element within each unshaded border.

7. Which of the following choices represents an expanded problem-focused type of physical examination?

   a. The documentation should include all elements identified by a bullet (•) within a shaded border as well as at least one element in every unshaded border.

   b. The documentation should include at least six elements identified by a bullet (•) whether in a shaded border or an unshaded border.

   c. The documentation should include at least 12 elements identified by a bullet (•) whether in a shaded border or an unshaded border.

   d. The documentation should include one to five elements identified by a bullet (•) whether in a shaded border or an unshaded border.

8. Which of the following choices represents a detailed type of single organ–system physical examination for the eye system/body area?

   a. The documentation should include between five and seven organ systems and/or body areas that have been examined by the clinician.

   b. The documentation should include at least two elements identified by a bullet (•) from each of six systems/body areas OR at least 12 elements identified by a bullet (•) in two or more systems/body areas.

   c. The documentation should include at least nine elements identified by a bullet (•) whether in a shaded border or an unshaded border.

   d. The documentation should include at least 12 elements identified by a bullet (•) whether in a shaded border or an unshaded border.

9. Which of the following choices represents a comprehensive type of single organ–system physical examination?

   a. The documentation should include all elements identified by a bullet (•) within a shaded border, as well as at least one element in each unshaded border.

   b. The documentation should include at least two elements identified by a bullet (•) from each of six systems/body areas OR at least 12 elements identified by a bullet (•) in two or more systems/body areas.

   c. The documentation should include performance of all elements identified by a bullet (•) in at least nine areas/systems AND documentation of at least two elements identified by a bullet (•) in each of the nine areas/systems.

   d. The documentation of eight or more organ systems OR body areas that have been examined.

10. Which of the following choices represents a detailed type of single organ–system physical examination for the cardiovascular system?

    a. The documentation should include at least two elements identified by a bullet (•) from each of six systems/body areas OR at least 12 elements identified by a bullet (•) in two or more systems/body areas.

    b. The documentation should include between five and seven organ systems and/or body areas that have been examined by the clinician.

    c. The documentation should include at least 12 elements identified by a bullet (•) whether in a shaded border or an unshaded border.

    d. The documentation should include at least nine elements identified by a bullet (•) whether in a shaded border or an unshaded border.

11. In order to perform the physical examination, the physician must do which of the following?

    a. Obtain the patient's verbal permission before beginning the physical examination

    b. Perform the examination according to the order of the 1997 single organ–system physical examination evidentiary checklist

    c. Be sure to use the appropriate tools such as an otoscope and an ophthalmoscope

    d. Physically interact with the patient, such as by touching or palpating, listening to or auscultation, looking at or inspecting different parts of the patient's body

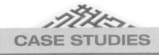

CASE STUDIES

Case Study 8-1

Read the following documentation, and then answer questions 1–9 by identifying the most appropriate element identified by a bullet referenced in the case study. Be sure to reference the single organ systems of the "1997 Documentation Guidelines for Evaluation and Management Services" found in Appendix B.

Light head contusion along lateral hairline with no pain upon examination. Neck is soft without masses. No thyromegaly. Palpation and percussion reveal no cervical spine tenderness, no thoracic spine tenderness, and no lumbar spine tenderness. Patient does have a dark, category 3 contusion along entire URQ, and patient expresses significant pain upon any palpation. Lower abdomen tense with no rebound, patient "holding breath against pain." Patient expressed nausea upon palpation and vomited immediately after abdominal exam; face flushed with temperature of 101.2. Pulse rapid, respiration shallow. Patient calmed after a few moments' interruption, pulse slowed, and respiration became more regular. Inguinal hernia incision site is well healed with no redness, pain, or other s/s of infection or dehiscence. Fever remained stable at 101.1°F.

1. Which element identified by a bullet is documented in the phrase "light head contusion along lateral hairline with no pain upon examination"?

   a. Constitutional (shaded)—general appearance of patient

   b. Skin (unshaded)—inspection of skin and/or palpation of skin and/or subcutaneous tissue

c. Musculoskeletal (unshaded)—examination of back with notation of kyphosis or scoliosis

d. Cardiovascular (shaded)—extremities for peripheral edema and/or varicosities

2. Which element identified by a bullet is documented in the words "neck is soft without masses … no thyromegaly"?

   a. Cardiovascular (shaded)—examination of carotid artery

   b. Neck (unshaded)—examination of thyroid

   c. Skin (unshaded)—inspection and/or palpation of skin and subcutaneous tissue

   d. Respiratory (shaded)—assessment of respiratory effort

3. Which element identified by a bullet is documented in the words "palpation and percussion reveal no cervical spine tenderness, no thoracic spine tenderness, and no lumbar spine tenderness"?

   a. Constitutional (shaded)—general appearance of patient

   b. Respiratory (shaded)—assessment of respiratory effort

   c. Gastrointestinal (shaded)—examination of abdomen with notation of presence of tenderness or masses

   d. Musculoskeletal (unshaded)—examination of back with notation of kyphosis or scoliosis

4. Which element identified by a bullet is documented in the words "face flushed with temperature of 101.2, pulse rapid, respiration shallow . . . fever remained stable at 101.1"?

   a. Cardiovascular (shaded)—examination of carotid arteries

   b. ENT (unshaded)—inspection of oral mucosa with notation of presence of pallor of cyanosis

   c. Respiratory (shaded)—assessment of respiratory effort

   d. Constitutional (shaded)—measurement of any three of seven listed vital signs

5. Which element identified by a bullet is documented in these words: "Patient does have a dark, category 3 contusion along entire URQ, and patient expresses significant pain upon any palpation. Lower abdomen tense with no rebound, patient 'holding breath against pain.' Patient expressed nausea upon palpation and vomited immediately after abdominal exam"?

   a. Skin (unshaded)—inspection and/or palpation of skin and subcutaneous tissue

   b. Constitutional (shaded)—general appearance of patient

   c. Gastrointestinal (shaded)—examination of abdomen with notation of presence of tenderness or masses

   d. Cardiovascular (shaded)—examination of abdominal aorta

6. Which element identified by a bullet is documented in the words "inguinal hernia incision site is well healed with no redness, pain, or other s/s of infection or dehiscence"?

   a. Skin (unshaded)—inspection and/or palpation of skin and subcutaneous tissue

   b. Gastrointestinal (shaded)—examination of abdomen with notation of presence of tenderness or masses

   c. Respiratory (shaded)—assessment of respiratory effort

   d. Eyes (unshaded)—inspection of conjunctivae and lids

7. Which element identified by a bullet is documented in the phrase "patient calmed after a few moments' interruption"?

   a. Constitutional (shaded)—general appearance of patient

   b. Neurologic/Psychiatric (shaded)—brief assessment of mental status, including mood and affect

   c. Respiratory (shaded)—assessment of respiratory effort

   d. Eyes (unshaded)—inspection of conjunctivae and lids

8. How many elements identified by a bullet have been included in this medical documentation?

   a. Four

   b. Six

   c. Eight

   d. Twenty

9. What type of cardiovascular single organ–system physical examination best reflects this documented physical examination?

   a. Problem-focused

   b. Expanded problem-focused

   c. Detailed

   d. Comprehensive

Case Study 8-2

Read the following documentation, and then answer the questions that follow.

Complaint: Frank is well-known to me and presents for sharp left flank pain and dark-orange-colored urine after a fall resulting in blunt abdominal trauma on Saturday afternoon, 2 days ago. He tripped on his dog and fell against the patio railing, striking his upper left abdomen against the decorative wrought iron. Patient reports experiencing immediate stabbing pain across his upper abdomen and down his left flank, which subsided quickly without recurrence. Upon rising on Sunday morning, Frank noticed sharp stabbing pain across ULQ abdomen accompanied by dark, painful bruising in the area of his URQ where he was struck by the decorative railing. The pain is most severe when he breathes deeply, rating pain at 8/10, and Frank cannot bend his torso without significant pain. Frank reports his urine sample to be very dark and odorous but denies painful urination. He denies any chest pain or racing heartbeat. No reports of tingling of extremities, dizziness, nausea, bloody stool. All other reviews of systems pertinent to this problem are negative. No report of ill contact at work or family, although Frank reports a higher stress level than usual, as budget cuts at work have caused many layoffs, and he is anxious about his employment status at work. There is no history of gastrointestinal disease in family or past medical history.

Physical Exam: T, 97.8; BP, 106/88; P, 68. Eyes clear without jaundice. Head is atraumatic without tenderness, nodules, or swelling. Neck: no thyromegaly. Auscultation of lungs clear without wheezes or rub. No tactile fremitus noted upon palpation of chest. Auscultation of heart reveals regular rate and rhythm with no abnormal sounds noted. No cervical spine tenderness. No thoracic spine tenderness and no lumbar spine tenderness; however, costovertebral tenderness noted upon palpation. No referred pain in left shoulder. Palpation of lower abdomen reveals soft, nontender abdomen, and no hepatomegaly or tenderness upon upper right quadrant palpation or percussion. Upper left abdomen mildly inflamed with dark circular bruise where patient identifies blow to abdomen. Very tender upper left quadrant upon palpation; patient's pain precludes deep palpation of spleen. No dullness noted upon percussion of left or right flank. Stool sample collected for occult blood test.

Laboratory: CBC reveals white blood count normal; hemoglobin and hematocrit are normal. A FAST scan abdominal CT scan was reviewed with radiologist. Review of KUB revealed significant stool within sigmoid and rectum. Occult blood test negative.

Assessment: It is quite probable that at least one of the lower left ribs has been fractured, although the patient's pain makes specific rib identification impossible. A splenic injury should be ruled out through CT scan. In my opinion, it would be prudent to begin oral Augmentin treatment at 875 mg twice a day for 7 days and increase fluid intake. Follow-up in 10 days for recheck.

History Utilizing prior knowledge, identify each documented level of HPI, ROS, and PFSH, and identify the documented level of overall history.

1. Identify the appropriate level of the documented HPI:

   _____

2. Identify the appropriate level of the documented ROS:

   _____

3. Identify the appropriate level of the documented PFSH:

   _____

4. Circle the level of overall history:
   Problem-focused
   Expanded problem-focused
   Detailed
   Comprehensive

Single Organ–System Physical Examination

Referencing *one* of these single organ–system guidelines—cardiovascular, musculoskeletal, or hematologic/lymphatic/immunologic—identify the type of single organ–system physical examination that has been documented, including which documented systems/body areas have a shaded border and which have an unshaded border.

Referenced single organ–system physical examination guidelines:

_____

System/body area with shaded border: _____

System/body area with shaded border: _____

System/body area with shaded border: _____

System/body area with shaded border: _____

System/body area with unshaded border: _____

System/body area with unshaded border: _____

System/body area with unshaded border: _____

System/body area with shaded border: _____

System/body area with shaded border: _____

System/body area with unshaded border: _____

System/body area with unshaded border: _____

System/body area with unshaded border: _____

Type of single organ–system physical examination:_____

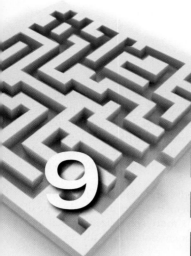

9 Medical Decision Making: Number of Diagnoses and/or Management Options

Learning Objectives

After completing this chapter, you should be able to do the following:

- Spell and define the key terms and abbreviations presented in this chapter
- Distinguish medical decision making in the medical documentation
- Identify medical decision making in the medical documentation
- Identify the management options and/or number of diagnoses
- Distinguish the number of diagnoses, specifically the new problem and established problem
- Identify the documentation requirements for the number of diagnoses and management options

Key Terms

azithromycin

diagnostic results

established problem

established problem, stable or improving

established problem, worsening

hemodynamically

laboratory

management option

new problem

new problem with diagnostic workup

number of diagnoses

otitis media

pathology

pharyngitis

possible diagnosis

probable diagnosis

radiology

rapid antigen test

rule-out diagnosis

suppurative

workup

Abbreviation

NSAID nonsteroidal anti-inflammatory drug; an analgesic used to treat inflammation or pain, sometimes available only by prescription but sometimes available over-the-counter, such as aspirin, ibuprofen, and naproxen

INTRODUCTION

Medical documentation tells the story of a patient's health from the context of the E/M service visit: what was, what is now, and what is yet to occur. The documentation of the history reflects what has happened before the patient arrived at the E/M service visit. The documentation of the physical examination reflects the status of the patient's health at the time of the E/M service visit. Knowing the patient's history and physical examination findings provides the foundation for looking into the future of the patient's health. This component of E/M documentation, medical decision making, reflects the physician's decision-making process.

Making a decision requires the collection of information, both subjective and objective, for deliberation. Depending on the nature of the decision to be made, this deliberation may require a limited scope of knowledge and expertise, or perhaps a physician with experience that is more specialized in skill and training. During an E/M service visit, the medical decision-making component documents the process by which the physician identifies the diagnosis for the patient's condition.

Medical decision making involves the chief complaint, the nature of the presenting problem, any possible diagnostic tests, and any available management options, as well as the state of the patient's health at the time of the visit. Regardless of the complexity of the medical decision making, the 1995 and 1997 Documentation Guidelines provide clear and specific direction for the documentation of the decision making, as well as the review of this documentation.

As with each of the other key components of an E/M service, medical decision making is composed of different parts: the number of diagnoses and management options, the amount or complexity of data to be reviewed, and the risk of complications, morbidity, or mortality. This chapter focuses specifically on the first element of medical decision making, the **number of diagnoses** and **management options**.

MEDICAL DECISION MAKING IN THE MEDICAL DOCUMENTATION

The documentation of each E/M service has an inherent structure. Within that structure, a pattern emerges: the past, present, and expected future of the patient's health regarding the presenting problem. Since the history commonly documents what *has* happened in the patient's health, the language can generally be identified as past tense. Correspondingly, the physical examination documents the physician's clinical identification of the patient's health during the E/M service visit, and the documented physical examination findings generally tend to be more clinical in nature, since they reflect the current anatomical and physiological status of the patient's health. In the same way, documented medical decision making reflects specific clinical and pathological changes occurring within the patient's body as determined by the physician's clinical expertise and professional knowledge, as well as by the physician's review of the patient's **pathology** or **laboratory** results, radiological scans, or other diagnostic tests. Because of the quantifiable nature of the medical decision-making findings, the language used in the documentation of medical decision making tends to be much more scientific in nature.

Understanding the language used to document the medical decision-making findings can help the reader more easily identify these findings. However, language alone cannot ensure correct identification of the elements of a documented E/M service visit. Even as the three components—history, physical examination, and medical decision making—could be characterized as the past, present, and future of an E/M service visit, each of these components can be identified in specific locations of the E/M service visit documentation. In most cases, the documentation supporting the history tends to be found in the beginning of the medical documentation, and the documentation supporting the physical examination can be identified in the middle of the medical documentation. The documentation supporting the medical decision making is most likely to be found near the end of the medical documentation.

However, not every piece of medical documentation follows one specific pattern. Even as every patient is a distinct individual experiencing unique circumstances, each E/M service visit takes place in a different setting with different factors and distinctive participants. Therefore, in order to identify the medical decision-making findings within the medical documentation, it is important to understand the foundation of those findings. The quantifiable medical decision-making findings reflect clinical findings that cannot ordinarily be identified with the eyes, ears, or sense of touch of the performing physician or the patient, but instead are identified with laboratory or pathology results, **radiology** images or films, or other **diagnostic results**.

Nevertheless, not every element of medical decision making requires specific clinicopathological or radiology results. The first element of medical decision making does not require laboratory, pathology,

number of diagnoses the documentation that reflects the physician's familiarity or unfamiliarity with the patient's presenting problem

management option documentation of any existing or initiated method of treatment, care, or management of the presenting problem; could range from something as simple as getting a little rest, to having an invasive medical procedure

pathology a scientific study of tissues to determine the nature of a disease and its causes, processes, development, and potential consequences

laboratory a facility that provides scientific study of clinical specimens such as blood, fluids, or other tissues for the purpose of identifying information about the health of the patient, specifically in relation to diagnosis

radiology a scientific study obtaining images of the body with the use of imaging technologies such as X-ray, ultrasound, computed tomography

diagnostic results the results of any laboratory, pathology, radiology, medical, or other diagnostic testing to determine a final diagnosis; may be presented in a variety of forms, including, but not limited to, a report, itemized results, images, scans, or compiled records

radiology, or diagnostic results. Instead, the first element of medical decision making is the physician's documentation of his or her medical decision-making process in diagnosing the presenting problem and any management options.

NUMBER OF DIAGNOSES AND/OR MANAGEMENT OPTIONS

Ultimately, it is the goal of every medical professional to promote and maintain the health of the patient. However, ill health, disease, or sickness still occur and, thankfully, trained physicians and medical professionals dedicate themselves to identify, or diagnose, the ill health, disease, or sickness. If the disease has been diagnosed, the physician can create a plan of care, or an option for managing the diagnosed condition.

The documentation requirements for this first element of medical decision making—identifying the number of diagnoses and management options—require that the performing physician document his or her familiarity with the patient's presenting problem and any potential or current management options for this presenting problem. Both of the concepts—"number of diagnoses" and "management options"— work together in concert to identify the patient's presenting problem and provide treatment in order to manage the patient's presenting problem.

Although the 1995 and 1997 DGs refer to these elements in this order—number of diagnoses and management options—this chapter reviews these concepts in a reverse order, which provides the greatest understanding of how these two concepts work together to clearly document the care provided during the E/M service visit.

Management Options

The word *management* conjures up a variety of meanings and situations. An elementary school teacher manages a classroom filled with young students. An agent manages the career of a movie star. A banker manages financial transactions. A physician manages the maintenance of a patient's health and any treatment of disease. A person manages his or her own health through healthy choices.

Management options vary in complexity and content. A management option documents any existing or initiated method of treatment, care, or management of the presenting problem and could range from something as simple as getting a little rest, to having an invasive medical procedure. Consider a woman who presents to her family physician because she suffers from frequent headaches. During the course of the E/M service visit, the physician's understanding about possible management options is informed by the history of the patient, as well as the status of the patient's current health. The management option for treating the headache depends on the nature of the headache, as well as the cause of the headache.

Identification of the diagnosis, or diagnoses—regardless of whether the diagnosis is a **possible diagnosis**, a **probable diagnosis**, or a **rule-out diagnosis**—provides some guidance for possible management options for the physician. However, the diagnosis does not provide this guidance without the necessary information about the patient's history and the physical examination. The physician utilizes the data about the patient's past health and the findings regarding the patient's current state of health to determine the potential management options.

Consider the person suffering from a headache. Several management options exist for her. If she is a preschool teacher and the students were particularly boisterous and gregarious that day, the management option for the headache may be some quiet, relaxing time in a darkened space. This meditative rest is a simple management option and requires no diagnostic testing.

However, if a person is suffering from a headache 2 days after being struck on the head by a baseball during practice, at which time a loss of consciousness occurred, this headache could simply be related to the blow to the head. However, it could also be related to a concussion. Further, this headache could be related to a cardiovascular issue that was exacerbated by the blow to the head. Any management option for this headache may require further clinical interaction between the physician and the patient, laboratory or diagnostic testing, or perhaps radiological testing. Regardless of whether the physician changes an existing management option or initiates a new management option, the 1995 and 1997 DGs require that the management option be recorded in the medical documentation. The management option includes treatment with prescription medication, specific therapies, and instructions for the clinical or nursing staff.

Management options may not only be a form of clinical treatment or therapy. They may even extend to specific instructions for the patient given by the performing physician. At times, the performing physician may request a consultation, or may seek advice, from another physician or specialist about the presenting problem. Regardless of what the management option may be—whether it involves

possible diagnosis considered to be an uncertain likelihood, but one that could be the final diagnosis

probable diagnosis a diagnosis that is considered to be very plausible by the physician because of the findings, data, and information gathered about the presenting problem and the patient

rule-out diagnosis a diagnosis intended to do one of two things: either prove that a specific diagnosis is the definitive diagnosis through diagnostic testing, data, and findings, or dismiss it from any future consideration as the final diagnosis of the presenting problem

therapeutic treatment, a request for professional advice or consultation, or additional diagnostic testing—the medical documentation should clearly indicate each part of this important part of the physician's medical decision making.

Number of Diagnoses

In a way, the determination of the management options remains dependent upon the diagnosis of the presenting problem and any required diagnostic, laboratory, or pathological testing. Ultimately, the management option cannot be discerned until the diagnosis or diagnoses have been determined. The number of diagnoses deals with the physician's familiarity with the presenting problem. Every clinical encounter between physician and patient creates another layer of experience and clinical understanding between them. The number of diagnoses specifically identifies the documentation necessary to reflect the physician's familiarity with the patient's presenting problem. That familiarity is reflected in three different documentation classifications of the number of diagnoses: an **established presenting problem that is stable or improving**, an **established presenting problem that is worsening**, and a **new problem**.

Established Presenting Problem: Stable or Improving

An **established problem** is any presenting problem that has already been diagnosed by the performing physician. Once the presenting problem has been diagnosed, it can be treated or managed, at which point it may stabilize or improve. If the patient returns to the physician for follow-up care of this specific presenting problem, the performing physician should document this improvement or stabilization of the presenting problem clearly. Generally, when the diagnosed problem has stabilized or improved, the medical decision making becomes more streamlined.

established problem, stable or improving a patient's presenting problem that has already been diagnosed by the performing physician and that has remained stable or shows improvement

established problem, worsening a patient's presenting problem that has already been diagnosed by the performing physician and that has become worse

new problem a patient's presenting problem that is new or unfamiliar to the performing physician

established problem any patient's presenting problem that has already been diagnosed by the performing physician

pharyngitis inflammation of the throat

> ### Example: Documentation of Established Presenting Problem: Stable or Improving
>
> #### Johnny's Irritating Cough (Improving)
>
> Johnny is an established patient who presents for follow-up for acute **pharyngitis**. Patient's sore throat has greatly improved. The cough lingers, but Johnny denies any chest pain or dizziness when he coughs, and his cough produces thin clear mucus. Johnny's ocular discomfort has lessened, and he uses Visine with positive results. Johnny's live-in girlfriend has quit smoking. His employer changed the smoking policy at Johnny's workplace, Smoky's Sports Bar, and patrons are no longer allowed to smoke in the bar, which has made a big, positive change in Johnny's condition.
>
> > **Physical Exam:** Patient is alert and comfortable. Vital signs: T, 97.6°F; pulse, 65; BP, 98/62. Eyes: clear. ENT/M: serous fluid apparent behind left tympanic membrane; however, right tympanic membrane clear. Patient's cough easily produces thin, clear mucus; oropharynx is slightly red, but benign.
> >
> > **Assessment:** Slight irritation to throat due to secondhand smoke inhalation
> >
> > **Plan:** Return if needed.

Notice in the previous example that, although the documentation of the improving presenting problem can be found scattered throughout the entire medical documentation, the documented management option is simply stated at the end of the medical documentation: "Return if needed." In this way, the number of diagnoses and management options work together to reflect not only the relationship between the performing physician and the patient, but the patient's story of health.

Established Presenting Problem: Worsening

When the physician has diagnosed the presenting problem and developed a plan of treatment to manage the patient's presenting problem, this initiates the care of the patient's health. However, if the patient's presenting problem does not improve, but actually worsens, then the next time the patient presents to the physician's office, the patient's presenting problem is considered an established, worsening presenting problem.

> **Example: Documentation of Established Presenting Problem: Worsening**
>
> **Johnny's Irritating Cough**
>
> Johnny is an established patient who presents for follow-up for a red, painful throat and barking cough. Patient appears haggard and weak, and Johnny states that his nasal drainage has turned green and thick. His cough has become much worse since his last visit, and he now states that he has a severe burning sensation in his chest and back when he coughs. Johnny's live-in girlfriend has quit smoking entirely since his cough has gotten worse at night and has interfered with his sleep. His employer changed the smoking policy at Johnny's workplace, Smoky's Sports Bar, and patrons are no longer allowed to smoke in the bar. Although Johnny feels confident this will help when he is better, he states that his cough now "rules his life."
>
> > **Physical Exam:** Patient is alert, however clearly uncomfortable. Vital signs: T, 99.32°F; pulse, 120; BP, 100/65. Eyes: conjunctivae red and inflamed bilaterally. ENT/M: serous fluid apparent behind right tympanic membrane, but **suppurative** serous fluid apparent behind left tympanic membrane with significant pressure. Patient is uncomfortably congested with significant green mucus production via nares. Patient's cough produces green chunks of phlegm upon expectoration, and solid, white exudates apparent on tonsils and along back of pharynx.
> >
> > **Laboratory:** Throat swab negative
> >
> > **Assessment:** Left **otitis media**. Acute pharyngitis exacerbated by secondhand smoke inhalation
> >
> > **Plan:** Single dose **azithromycin** prescribed for the otitis media and OTC nonsteroidal anti-inflammatory drug (**NSAID**) recommended for painful throat.

suppurative pus-producing or puslike

otitis media an infection of the middle ear

azithromycin an antibiotic, commonly known as Zithromax, often used to treat respiratory infections and other bacterial infections

The documentation supporting the established, worsening problem is scattered throughout the medical documentation but is most significantly in the documented history, which reflects how the presenting problem has worsened in the patient's life. However, the documented physical examination reflects the physician's clinical identification of the worsening presenting problem. In addition, the worsening established problem is documented in the assessment of the pharyngitis, as well as the prescription of azithromycin for the otitis media.

New Problem

A new problem is any presenting problem that has neither been seen by nor been diagnosed by the performing physician. Whether the patient is a new patient or an established patient does not pertain to the new problem. The new problem is, by definition, unfamiliar to the performing physician, which means that the performing physician must discern the diagnosis.

It could be said that the primary reason for any patient's presence in an E/M service visit is the diagnosis. After all, when a person feels unwell, understanding the cause of the illness can be the first step toward health. Therefore, the 1995 and 1997 DGs make specific requirements for the documentation of the diagnosis: "The assessment or clinical impression may be stated in the form of differential diagnoses or as a 'possible,' 'probable,' or 'rule-out' diagnosis."[1] The process of determining the diagnosis requires the collection of necessary data, impressions, and findings about the presenting problem, in conjunction with the impressions, data, and findings about the patient. This requirement reveals that the final documented diagnosis should be possible, probable, rule-out, or differential.

Possible Diagnosis   A possible diagnosis is considered an uncertain likelihood, but it could be the final diagnosis. Even though a possible diagnosis could be feasible and logical, there may be other diagnoses that are more likely that have not yet been considered. For example, if the documentation states "possible appendicitis," this reflects the physician's medical decision-making process regarding the patient's sharp abdominal pain in the lower right quadrant. The word *possible* reflects that the phy-

---

[1]Centers for Medicare and Medicaid Services, "1995 Documentation Guidelines for Evaluation and Management Services," p. 11, www.cms.gov/Outreach-and-Education/Medicare-Learning-Network-MLN/MLNEdWebGuide/Downloads/95Docguidelines.pdf, and "1997 Documentation Guidelines for Evaluation and Management Services," p. 47, www.cms.gov/Outreach-and-Education/Medicare-Learning-Network-MLN/MLNEdWebGuide/Downloads/97Docguidelines.pdf.

sician may consider appendicitis as a possible diagnosis but has not identified appendicitis as a final diagnosis.

Probable Diagnosis A probable diagnosis is very plausible given the findings, data, and information gathered about the presenting problem and the patient. However, although the probable diagnosis is very likely the final diagnosis, it is not certain. For example, if the documentation states "probable appendicitis," this reflects the physician's medical decision-making process regarding the patient's high fever, nausea, and sharp abdominal pain in the lower right quadrant. The word *probable* reflects that the physician may consider appendicitis as a probable diagnosis but has not identified appendicitis as a final diagnosis.

To rule something out means to dismiss it from consideration. Therefore, a rule-out diagnosis is intended to do one of two things: either prove that it is the definitive diagnosis through diagnostic testing, data, and findings or dismiss the rule-out diagnosis from any future consideration as the final diagnosis of the presenting problem.

For example, if the documentation states "rule out appendicitis," this reflects the physician's medical decision-making process regarding the patient's high fever, nausea, sharp lower right abdominal pain, high white blood count, and abnormal findings on the abdominal X-ray. The phrase "rule out" reflects that the physician must either prove or disprove appendicitis as the final diagnosis, but that current findings, data, information, and results make appendicitis very likely, even though not yet the final diagnosis.

workup documentation of any ordered or requested diagnostic testing to identify the final diagnosis

Regardless of how the diagnosis is determined, this process requires the synthesis of the documented history, physical examination, and any laboratory, pathology, or diagnostic results that have been ordered by the performing physician for a diagnostic **workup**. When the performing physician orders the laboratory, pathology, or diagnostic tests, this process is commonly referred to as "working up the problem" to determine the diagnosis. This workup must be documented to properly reflect the performing physician's medical decision making; it illustrates what the performing physician ordered as well as how the workup helps the determination of the final diagnosis.

New Problem with Diagnostic Workup Sometimes the diagnosis of the presenting problem is difficult to identify because of the nature of the signs, symptoms, and possible causes of the presenting problem. At such times the performing physician may specifically request certain diagnostic testing to facilitate the systematic process of discriminating the final diagnosis from the possible or probable diagnoses. When a diagnostic workup is required to determine the diagnosis of the presenting problem, that situation is referred to as a **new problem with diagnostic workup**.

new problem with diagnostic workup an undiagnosed new presenting problem that requires specific laboratory, pathology, or other diagnostic tests to identify the differential diagnosis

---

Example: Documentation of New Problem with Diagnostic Workup

Working Up Johnny's Irritating Cough

Johnny is an established patient who presents with a very sore throat and barking cough. Patient has no complaints of nasal drainage. Cough lozenges and cough suppressants have not helped his throat or cough. Johnny recently moved in with his girlfriend, who smokes. Johnny also recently started work as a bartender at Smoky's Sports Bar, where the patrons are allowed to smoke in the bar. Grandfather died last year of lung cancer.

> **Physical Exam:** Serous fluid is apparent behind tympanic membrane. Patient is uncomfortably congested with significant mucus production via nares. Patient's cough produces thick, white phlegm upon expectoration, and solid, white exudates apparent on tonsils and along back of pharynx.
>
> **Laboratory:** Rapid antigen test negative; throat swab sent for culture.
>
> **Assessment:** Acute pharyngitis exacerbated by increased secondhand smoke inhalation
>
> **Plan:** NSAID recommended for painful throat

In the previous example, the results provided by the rapid antigen test and the pending results of the throat culture deliver laboratory information to the performing physician that can be identified only through diagnostic testing. This workup provides the physician the information needed to make a diagnosis based on the gathered findings of the patient's history, physical examination, and any diagnostic results.

New Problem without Diagnostic Workup   Diagnostic workup may not be required for determination of a diagnosis. When no workup is required, the medical decision making becomes uncomplicated; the documentation should reflect the straightforward determination of the diagnosis without any diagnostic testing ordered by the performing physician.

Example: Documentation of New Problem without Diagnostic Workup

Johnny's Irritating Cough

Johnny is an established patient who presents with a very sore throat and barking cough. Patient has no complaints of nasal drainage. Cough lozenges and cough suppressants have not helped his throat or cough. Johnny recently moved in with his girlfriend, who smokes. Johnny also recently started work as a bartender at Smoky's Sports Bar, where the patrons are allowed to smoke in the bar. Grandfather died last year of lung cancer.

Physical Exam: Serous fluid is apparent behind tympanic membrane. Patient is uncomfortably congested with significant mucus production via nares. Patient's cough produces clear, thin mucus upon expectoration. The oropharynx is red and inflamed without evidence of exudates or infection.

Assessment: Likely irritation of eyes, nose, throat due to increased secondhand smoke inhalation

Plan: OTC NSAID recommended for painful throat. Recommend that Johnny have an honest conversation with his employer regarding the secondhand smoke and encourage girlfriend to either quit smoking or smoke outside the home.

In this example, the physician required no workup to diagnose the presenting problem. The gathered findings of the patient's history and physical examination provided enough information for the physician to make a final diagnosis. In the event that the performing physician reviews diagnostic results that were ordered and performed by another physician, this review would not be considered additional workup because the performing physician has not ordered the diagnostic workup.

All of these individual elements can be compiled in an easy-to-read chart format that provides an easy reference (see ■ FIGURE 9.1).

rapid antigen test a quick laboratory test to determine whether the patient has strep throat

---

Exercise 9.1   **Patient's Sinus Pressure**

After reading the following medical documentation, identify the number of diagnoses and management options, specifically whether the presenting problem is new or established and any documented management option. If the presenting problem is established, identify whether the presenting problem is stable/improving or worsening.

History: Patient returns for worsening sinus pressure. The right side of the patient's head hurts so much that she feels she cannot hold her head up due to the throbbing pain. Patient states every part of her hurts now. Patient recognizes flu is likely but is concerned about strep throat.

Exam: Patient is very pale and appears very tired. Conjunctivae red, swollen, and inflamed. Exquisite pain upon palpation of face, particularly the forehead and maxillary sinuses. Copious production of thick, white/brown mucus per nares. Patient unable to open mouth due to pain. Palpation of neck and behind ears reveals exquisitely tender, swollen lymph nodes. Patient expresses extreme discomfort when swallowing. Auscultation of lungs reveals pleural rub. Heart: no murmur identified. **Laboratory: Rapid antigen test** negative; throat swab sent for culture. Influenza swab deferred per patient.

Assessment: Sinus infection, probable influenza.

Plan: Azithromycin, increased fluids, rest. Per patient's request, note written for employer indicating need for 3-day release from work for bed rest.

1. Is this problem new or established?

   _____

2. If this is an established problem, is it stable/improving or worsening?

   _____

3. Is a management option documented?

   _____

4. If a management option is documented, what is the management option?

   _____

Complexity of Medical Decision Making	Straightforward	Low	Moderate	High
Number of Diagnoses and/or Management Options	Established presenting problem, stable or improving	Established presenting problem, worsening	New presenting problem, without workup	New presenting problem, with workup

Figure 9.1 ■ Content of service element: medical decision making, number of diagnoses and management options.

Exercise 9.2   Timmy's Recurrent Abdominal Pain

Read the following medical documentation, then identify the number of diagnoses and management options, specifically whether the presenting problem is new or established and any documented management option. If the presenting problem is established, identify whether the presenting problem is stable/improving or worsening.

Timmy is a 12-year-old established patient and presents for recurrent abdominal pain. Timmy's pain is localized in the right lower quadrant. Since Timmy's previous visit, his abdominal pain has increased in severity and frequency, preventing him from attending school and requiring him to take pain relievers.

Review of systems: Diarrhea has subsided, and negative for bloody stools. Negative for dysuria, hematuria. Negative for fevers, sick contact, or trauma other than the goal-side tackle reported during Timmy's previous visit dated 09/23. All other ROS pertaining to this problem are negative.

PE: Timmy is not in distress, although he is very pale. T, 98.7°F; pulse, 130; resp., 20. Eyes clear with no jaundice. Pupils are reactive to light within normal limits. Lungs clear to auscultation and percussion. Auscultation of heart reveals normal but rapid heartbeat without murmur. Timmy complains of mild discomfort pain during palpation of lower right quadrant. No hepatosplenomegaly. No peritoneal signs noted and no evidence of abdominal or inguinal hernias. No edema noted in extremities.

Assessment: The severity of the pain makes it prudent to rule out appendiceal abscess.

Plan: Recommend abdominal CT scan, KUB, complete blood panel, and urinalysis. Timmy will return tomorrow morning to provide urine and blood samples for workup. Radiology scheduled for tomorrow afternoon. Return for recheck in 2 days after receipt of radiology scans.

1. Is this problem new or established?

   _____

2. If this is an established problem, is it stable/improving or worsening?

   _____

3. Is a management option documented?

   _____

4. If a management option is documented, what is the management option? _____

Exercise 9.3   Joan's Lower Back Pain

Read the following medical documentation, then identify the number of diagnoses and management options, specifically whether the presenting problem is new or established and any documented management option. If the presenting problem is established, identify whether the presenting problem is stable/improving or worsening.

Joan is an established patient who presents for lower back pain. Her lower back hurts, down by beltline, and pain is sometimes very severe. The pain is sporadic, mostly when standing up after sitting in one place for an extended period. Ibuprofen used to help, but now it does not help back pain anymore. At its worst, low back pain is sharp and throbbing. Joan has had occasional back pain for about 20 years, since first in the service, but she first noticed this particular low back pain shortly after playing touch football with adult children this past Thanksgiving. Patient denies any other joint pain than this low back pain. Patient denies double vision or dizziness, and no chest pain or shortness of breath. Patient denies tobacco or alcohol use. Pain has not affected her work as a fifth-grade teacher.

Exam: Back is soft to the touch and palpation and revealed no obvious lumps or masses. Percussion of back reveals tenderness in lower back but no costovertebral tenderness. Patient performs side-to-side flexion to 30 degrees with minimal pain; however, she finds forward flexion at 50 degrees with pain localized to her lower back that does not radiate down legs or up her back. Deep tendon reflexes within normal limits: ankle jerk reflex, patellar reflex, plantar reflexes tested. Patient's range of motion is stable, within normal limits, and without pain.

Plan: Recommend physical therapy, NSAID as needed for inflammation. Follow-up in 6 weeks.

1. Is this problem new or established?

   _____

2. If this is an established problem, is it stable/improving or worsening?

   _____

3. Is a management option documented?

   _____

4. If a management option is documented, what is the management option?

   _____

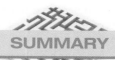

SUMMARY

- The first element of medical decision making is the number of diagnoses and management options, both of which address the documentation required to illustrate the physician's medical decision-making process regarding the patient's presenting problem.

- The management options include any existing or initiated method of treatment, care, or management of the presenting problem. The physician's identification of any existing or potential management options is informed by the history of the patient, the current health of the patient, and the diagnosis, or diagnoses. Management options can vary widely and could be as simple as getting a little rest or as complex as an invasive medical procedure. Regardless of how many management options are involved or whether the management option involves therapeutic treatment, a request for professional advice or consultation, or additional diagnostic testing, this important part of the physician's medical decision making is dependent upon the diagnosis, or the diagnoses, identified by the physician.

- The number of diagnoses identifies the documentation necessary to reflect the physician's familiarity with the patient's presenting problem. That familiarity is described as either a new problem or an established problem for the physician. If the presenting problem is an established problem, the number of diagnoses identifies whether the problem is improving or stable or whether the problem has worsened since the patient's most recent visit. If the presenting problem is a new problem, the number of diagnoses identifies whether or not the problem requires additional workup to diagnose it. If a definite diagnosis can be made, the number of diagnoses records the identification of the possible diagnoses, probable diagnoses, rule-out diagnoses, or differential, or comparative, diagnoses.

- The documentation guidelines for the number of diagnoses and management options work in concert to show whether diagnostic workup is required to help the performing physician identify the final diagnosis, or diagnoses. These documentation guidelines include the clear documentation of whether the presenting problem is a new diagnosis or an established diagnosis for the performing physician. The diagnosis should be formed through the physician's clinical impression, collection of data and findings, and any necessary workup; it can be stated in the form of a differential, or comparative, diagnosis or a possible, probable, or rule-out diagnosis.

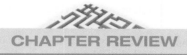

CHAPTER REVIEW

Multiple Choice

Choose the letter that best answers each question or completes each statement.

1. Which of the following best defines "number of diagnoses"?
   a. Documentation that reflects the physician's familiarity or unfamiliarity with the patient's presenting problem
   b. Documentation of any existing or initiated method of treatment, care, or management of the presenting problem; could range from getting a little rest, to having an invasive medical procedure
   c. Documentation that reflects the physician's specific findings during the E/M service visit with the patient
   d. Documentation of any ordered or requested diagnostic testing to identify the final diagnosis

2. Which of the following best defines "management options"?
   a. Documentation that reflects the physician's familiarity or unfamiliarity with the patient's presenting problem
   b. Documentation of any existing or initiated method of treatment, care, or management of the presenting problem; could range from getting a little rest, to having an invasive medical procedure

   c. Documentation of any ordered or requested diagnostic testing to identify the final diagnosis
   d. Documentation of the clinical tools used during the physical examination

3. Which of the following best defines "workup"?
   a. Documentation of any ordered or requested diagnostic testing to identify the final diagnosis
   b. Documentation that reflects the physician's familiarity or unfamiliarity with the patient's presenting problem
   c. Documentation of any existing or initiated method of treatment, care, or management of the presenting problem; could range from getting a little rest, to having an invasive medical procedure
   d. Documentation of the patient's willingness or reluctance to participate in the E/M service visit

4. Which of the following best defines an established problem?
   a. A patient's presenting problem that has already been diagnosed by the performing physician and has become worse
   b. When the performing physician orders specific laboratory, pathology, or diagnostic tests for the purpose of identifying the differential diagnosis of the undiagnosed new presenting problem

c. A patient's presenting problem that has already been diagnosed by the performing physician and has remained stable or shows improvement

d. A patient's presenting problem that has already been diagnosed by the performing physician

5. Which of the following best defines a new problem with a diagnostic work up?

a. A patient's presenting problem that has already been diagnosed by the performing physician and has become worse

b. A patient's presenting problem that has already been diagnosed by the performing physician

c. When the performing physician orders specific laboratory, pathology, or diagnostic tests for the purpose of identifying the differential diagnosis of the undiagnosed new presenting problem

d. A patient's presenting problem that has already been diagnosed by the performing physician and has remained stable or shows improvement

6. Which of the following best defines an established problem, worsening?

a. When the performing physician orders specific laboratory, pathology, or diagnostic tests for the purpose of identifying the differential diagnosis of the undiagnosed new presenting problem

b. A patient's presenting problem that has already been diagnosed by the performing physician and has become worse

c. A patient's presenting problem that has already been diagnosed by the performing physician and has remained stable or shows improvement

d. A patient's presenting problem that has already been diagnosed by the performing physician

7. Which of the following options best completes this sentence: "An established problem is stable or improving when . . . "?

a. the performing physician orders specific laboratory, pathology, or diagnostic tests for the purpose of identifying the differential diagnosis of the undiagnosed new presenting problem.

b. the patient's presenting problem that has already been diagnosed by the performing physician has become worse.

c. the patient's presenting problem that has already been diagnosed by the performing physician has remained stable or shows improvement.

d. the patient's presenting problem has already been diagnosed by the performing physician.

8. Which of the following statements best reflects a possible diagnosis?

a. It is considered to be very plausible by the physician because of the findings, data, and information gathered about the presenting problem and the patient.

b. It is considered to be an uncertain likelihood, but one that could be the final diagnosis.

c. It is intended to either prove that a specific diagnosis is the definitive diagnosis through diagnostic testing, data, and findings, or dismiss it from any future consideration as the final diagnosis of the presenting problem.

d. It is the final diagnosis identified through careful consideration, discernment, and clinical judgment.

9. Which of the following statements best reflects a probable diagnosis?

a. It is the final diagnosis identified through careful consideration, discernment, and clinical judgment.

b. It is considered to be an uncertain likelihood, but one that could be the final diagnosis.

c. It is a preliminary diagnosis subject to careful consideration, discernment, and clinical judgment.

d. It is considered to be very plausible by the physician because of the findings, data, and information gathered about the presenting problem and the patient.

10. Which of the following statements best reflects a rule-out diagnosis?

a. It is the final diagnosis identified through careful consideration, discernment, and clinical judgment.

b. It is considered to be an uncertain likelihood, but one that could be the final diagnosis.

c. It is intended to either prove that a specific diagnosis is the definitive diagnosis through diagnostic testing, data, and findings, or dismiss that specific diagnosis from any future consideration as the final diagnosis of the presenting problem.

d. It is considered to be very plausible by the physician because of the findings, data, and information gathered about the presenting problem and the patient.

CASE STUDIES

Case Study 9-1

Read the following documentation, and then answer questions 1–3 by identifying the phrase that best supports the number of diagnoses and/or management options.

Complaint: I have been asked to consult on James Roberts's abdominal trauma. James Roberts is a 45-year-old new patient who suffered a fall in his home office. Mr. Roberts tripped on the computer cords in his home office and fell onto his office chair, striking his upper abdomen on the armrest of the chair and striking his forehead on the edge of his desk. Patient reports experiencing immediate URQ pain that he reported as 5/10 at time of fall, but has increased in severity to 7/10. Per patient, there was no LOC. Since that time, he has experienced occasional dizziness and three nosebleeds, each lasting at least 20 minutes. Patient has vomited twice and has noted significant midback pain during each emesis, which he rates at a 7–8/10.

Laboratory: Hemoglobin, 13.5; WBC, 18,000. An abdominal CT scan was reviewed with radiologist; scan showed a small amount of free fluid in ULQ with grade 3 laceration of spleen. Evidence of significant amount of stool within sigmoid and rectum.

Assessment: Hemodynamically stable patient with grade 3 splenic laceration. No immediate correlation between splenic trauma and previous hernia repair is being considered at this time, although Mr. Robert's history of alcoholism could affect treatment of splenic trauma. Contacted patient's primary physician in Charleston, Texas, by phone to discuss Pt's previous hernia surgery, complications, alcohol-related conditions, and healthcare management related to long history of alcohol use. Pertinent records to be reviewed upon receipt by fax.

Plan: Patient admitted for overnight observation, IV antibiotics with rehydration. Gastroenterology consultation requested for splenic trauma.

1. Which of the following best reflects the number of diagnoses for this medical documentation?

   a. Established problem, stable or improving

   b. Established problem, worsening

   c. New problem without diagnostic workup

   d. New problem with diagnostic workup

2. Which of the following best reflects the documented excerpt titled "Assessment"?

   a. A possible diagnosis because the performing physician is not sure how the patient's history of alcoholism has impacted the patient's health

   b. A probable diagnosis because the performing physician is requesting records from the previous physician in Texas

   c. A definite diagnosis because the performing physician documents the splenic laceration by specific grade based on the radiologic findings

   d. A rule-out diagnosis because the performing physician has not definitively diagnosed the presenting problem

3. Which of the following excerpts best documents a management option in this medical documentation?

   a. Contacted patient's primary physician in Charleston, Texas, by phone to discuss pt's previous hernia surgery, complications, alcohol-related conditions, and healthcare management related to long history of alcohol use

   b. Patient admitted for overnight observation, IV antibiotics with rehydration

   c. Gastroenterology consultation requested for splenic trauma

   d. All of the above

Case Study 9-2

Read the following documentation, and then answer the questions that follow.

Complaint: Frank is well-known to me and presents for sharp left flank pain and dark-orange-colored urine after a fall resulting in blunt abdominal trauma on Saturday afternoon, 2 days ago. He tripped on his dog and fell against the patio railing, striking his upper left abdomen against the decorative wrought iron. Patient reports experiencing immediate stabbing pain across his upper abdomen and down his left flank, which subsided quickly without recurrence. Upon rising on Sunday morning, Frank noticed sharp stabbing pain across ULQ abdomen accompanied by dark, painful bruising in the area of his ULQ where he was struck by the decorative railing. The pain is most severe when he breathes deeply, rating pain at 8/10, and Frank cannot bend his torso without significant pain. Frank reports his urine sample to be very dark and odorous but denies painful urination. He denies any chest pain or racing heartbeat. No reports of tingling of extremities, dizziness, nausea, bloody stool. All other reviews of systems pertinent to this problem are negative. No report of ill contact at work or family, although Frank reports a higher stress level than usual, as budget cuts at work have caused many layoffs, and he is anxious about his employment status at work. There is no history of gastrointestinal disease in family or past medical history.

Physical Exam: T, 97.8; BP, 106/88; P, 68. Eyes clear without jaundice. Head is atraumatic without tenderness, nodules, or swelling. Neck: no thyromegaly. Auscultation of lungs clear without wheezes or rub. No tactile fremitus noted upon palpation of chest. Auscultation of heart reveals regular rate and rhythm with no abnormal sounds noted. No cervical, thoracic, or lumbar spine tenderness; however, costovertebral tenderness noted upon palpation. No referred pain in left shoulder. Palpation of lower abdomen reveals soft, nontender abdomen, and no hepatomegaly or tenderness upon upper right quadrant palpation or percussion. Upper left abdomen mildly inflamed with dark circular bruise where patient identifies blow to abdomen. Very tender upper left quadrant upon palpation, and patient's pain precludes deep palpation of spleen. No dullness noted upon percussion of left or right flank. Stool sample collected for occult blood test.

Laboratory: CBC reveals white blood count normal; hemoglobin and hematocrit are normal. A FAST scan abdominal CT scan was reviewed with radiologist. Review of KUB revealed significant stool within sigmoid and rectum. Occult blood test negative.

Assessment: It is quite probable that at least one of the lower left ribs has been fractured, although the patient's pain makes specific rib identification impossible. A splenic injury should be ruled out through CT scan. In my opinion, it would be prudent to begin oral Augmentin treatment at 875 mg twice a day for 7 days and increase fluid intake. Follow-up in 10 days for recheck.

   Identify the documented elements of history, referencing the following portion of the content of service worksheet. Circle each individual history element as well as the overall level of history on this worksheet.

History (chief complaint included)	Problem-Focused	Expanded Problem-Focused	Detailed	Comprehensive
History of Present Illness Location, severity, timing, mod fact, quality, duration, context, assoc s/s	Brief (1)	Brief (2–3)	Ext. (4+, or 3 chronic problems)	Ext. (4+, or 3 chronic problems)
Review of Systems Constitutional, ENT/M, respiratory, GU, skin/breast, endocrine, all/imm, eyes, CV, GI, musculoskeletal, psychiatric, neurologic, hem/lymph	None	Pert. (1 system)	Extended (2–9 systems)	Complete (10+ systems)
Past, Family, and Social History New/initial/consults	Pertinent (1–2 elements)	Pertinent (1–2 elements)	Pertinent (1–2 elements)	Complete (3 elements)
Past, Family, and Social History Established patient/subsequent hospital	Pertinent (1 element)	Pertinent (1 element)	Pertinent (1 element)	Complete (2–3 elements)

Identify the type of physical examination by referencing this next portion of the content of service worksheet. Circle the following on this worksheet: the physical examination guidelines referenced—body area/organ system; general multisystem; or single organ system, identifying the single organ system referenced—as well as the specific type of physical examination (problem-focused, expanded problem-focused, detailed, or comprehensive).

Physical Examination	Problem-Focused	Expanded Problem-Focused	Detailed	Comprehensive
1995 PE	A limited examination of affected body area or organ system (1 body area/organ system)	A limited examination of the affected body area or organ system and other symptomatic or related organ systems (2–4 body areas/organ systems)	An extended examination of the affected body area(s) or organ system(s) and other symptomatic or related body areas or organ systems (5–7 body areas/organ systems)	A general multisystem examination or complete examination of a single organ system and other symptomatic or related body areas or organ systems; should include 8 or more of the 12 organ systems (8+ body systems or organ systems, but they cannot be mixed)
1997 General Multisystem	1–5 elements identified by a bullet	At least 6 elements identified by a bullet	At least 2 elements identified by a bullet from each of 6 areas/systems OR at least 12 elements identified by a bullet in 2 or more areas/systems	Performance of all elements identified by a bullet in at least 9 organ systems or body areas and documentation of at least 2 elements identified by a bullet in each of the examined areas/systems
1997 Single Organ System	1–5 elements identified by a bullet, whether in a shaded or unshaded border	At least 6 elements identified by a bullet, whether in a shaded or unshaded border	At least 12 elements identified by a bullet, whether in a shaded or unshaded border (Eyes & psychiatric: at least 9 elements identified by a bullet, whether in a shaded or unshaded border)	All elements identified by a bullet within each shaded border and at least 1 element identified by a bullet within each unshaded border

Identify the number of diagnoses and/or management options.

1. Is the diagnosis (or diagnoses) a possible, probable, rule-out, or final diagnosis (or diagnoses)? Include the rationale for your answer.

_____

_____

_____

2. Is the diagnosis (or diagnoses) an established problem or a new problem? Include the status of the presenting problem—stable or improving, worsening, or requiring workup—and include the rationale for your answer.

_____

_____

_____

3. What management options have been documented in this case study?

_____

_____

_____

hemodynamically
regarding the movement of blood through the patient's body

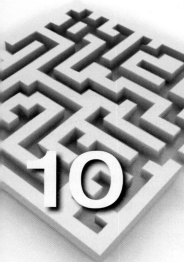

10 Medical Decision Making: Amount and/or Complexity of Data to Be Reviewed

Learning Objectives

After completing this chapter, you should be able to do the following:

- Spell and define the key terms and abbreviations presented in this chapter
- Define the amount and/or complexity of data to be reviewed
- Recognize each of the six documentation guidelines for the amount and/or complexity of data to be reviewed

Key Terms

abdominal CT scan

amount of data

AVantage A/H5N1 Flu test

bronchoscopy

Cefotaxime

complexity of data

computed tomography (CT) scan

data

diagnostic data

diagnostic results

diagnostic testing

echoencephalography

expectoration

hydrocodone cough suppressant

indomethacin

sputum gram stain

Streptococcus pneumonia

Abbreviations

CBC complete blood count, a laboratory test requiring a small amount of blood to determine the components within the patient's blood; can indicate the state of health or pathology the patient is currently experiencing

KUB an abdominal X-ray used to identify the structure and status of the kidney, ureters, and bladder

S. pneumonia the abbreviation that identifies Streptococcus pneumonia

INTRODUCTION

In general, the collection of history findings requires verbal interchange between the performing physician and the patient, whereas the collection of physical examination findings requires physical interaction between the physician and the patient through a variety of examination techniques, including palpation, auscultation, and visual inspection. In a similar vein, the collection of medical decision-making findings generally involves the gathering of **data** and information to assist the performing physician in diagnostic deliberation. The first element of medical decision making, number of diagnoses and management options, addresses the physician's familiarity with the presenting problem and any need for **diagnostic testing** to discern the possible, probable, rule-out, or final diagnosis, or diagnoses. The second element of medical decision making specifically addresses the amount and/or **complexity of data** to be reviewed during the collection of any clinical, laboratory, pathology, or radiology results. This chapter focuses on the documentation guidelines for the performing physician's review of diagnostic findings during the E/M service visit.

DATA TO BE REVIEWED

The 1995 and 1997 Documentation Guidelines recognize that a broad scope of **diagnostic data** could be reviewed during an E/M service visit, including results of laboratory, pathology, or medical tests; radiology reports; review of old medical records; and the independent review of the radiology image by the performing physician. For the second element of medical decision making—the amount and/or complexity of data to be reviewed—different documentation guidelines reflect the performing physician's review of these **diagnostic results** during the process of medical decision making. The 1995 and 1997 DGs recognize that the scope of data to be reviewed may be quite broad and provide six different guidelines for the data to be reviewed. These guidelines simultaneously address the performing physician's documentation of the **amount of data** to be reviewed and the complexity of data to be reviewed during the E/M service visit.

Amount of Data

The data to be reviewed can best be identified by the type of data. The word *data* refers to steps taken by the performing physician to obtain information that could help facilitate the diagnosis of the presenting problem. This information could be obtained through ordering diagnostic testing or reviewing the results of diagnostic testing. It could be obtained through acquiring and reviewing the patient's old medical records, which could inform the physician about the nature of the presenting problem. It could also be obtained through collecting additional history from the patient's family or caretaker or from a supplemental source.

Ultimately, the nature of the data to be reviewed could be referred to as any clues identified and used by the performing physician for the discernment of diagnosing the presenting problem. Only the performing physician can ensure the complete documentation of any identified clues, thus underlining the importance of the physician's thorough documentation of the E/M service visit. In order to clearly define the expected parameters for the amount and/or complexity of data to be reviewed, the 1995 and 1997 Documentation Guidelines list six distinct guidelines for the required documentation of the data. Since the clarity of documentation is of paramount importance and the 1995 and 1997 DGs provide such clear guidelines, if any confusion about the data to be reviewed exists on the part of the medical coder, the performing physician should be queried to ensure clarity of documentation.

Complexity of Data

Certain types of data may be simple to review, such as laboratory diagnostic tests (e.g., white blood count or urinalysis). Other types of data to be reviewed may be more complex, such as old patient medical records or a patient's **computed tomography (CT) scan**. The documentation of this complexity not only clearly reflects the effort, expertise, and clinical skill of the performing physician, but also details the complexity of the diagnosing process.

When a radiology test is performed, an actual image or scan is produced, which is then reviewed and interpreted, or read, by a specially trained physician or qualified healthcare professional. After the scan or image is read, the findings are dictated into the patient's record as a radiology report. It is reasonable

---

data information that could help facilitate the diagnosis of the presenting problem; includes the results of diagnostic testing, the patient's old medical records, and additional history from the patient's family or caretaker

diagnostic testing a specific test used to determine the internal function, status, structure, and/or pathology occurring within the patient; includes laboratory tests, radiology rests, or even endoscopies

complexity of data identification of how multifaceted, difficult, or intricate the presented data are, as well as the level of difficulty the data present to the physician performing the E/M service

diagnostic data information obtained by the physician that identifies the internal structure, status, physiology, or pathology within the patient's body through tests that facilitate identification and diagnosis of the presenting problem

diagnostic results the results of any laboratory, pathology, radiology, medical, or other diagnostic testing to determine a final diagnosis; may be presented in a variety of forms, including, but not limited to, a report, itemized results, images, scans, or compiled records

amount of data the quantity of data that has been reviewed and interpreted by the physician performing the E/M service

computed tomography (CT) scan known as computed tomography, or CT; a specific radiological diagnostic test that creates a three-dimensional image of the inside of the human body or cavity

Complexity of Medical Decision Making	Straightforward	Low	Moderate	High
Number of Diagnoses and/or Management Options	Established presenting problem, stable or improving	Established presenting problem, worsening	New presenting problem, without workup	New presenting problem, with workup
Amount and/or Complexity of Data to Be Reviewed	Ordering or reviewing diagnostic data	Obtaining old records or additional history from someone other than patient	Discussion of diagnostic results with physician who performed diagnostic testing	Independent visualization of image, tracing, or scan by physician performing the E/M service

Figure 10.1 ■ Content of service element: amount and/or complexity of data to be reviewed, highlighted.

that actually reviewing and interpreting the **abdominal CT scan** requires a different set of skills and is more complex than reading the radiologist's report of the same CT abdominal scan. Although it is not necessary for the performing physician to document that "this is a complex set of data to review," common sense should prevail when reading the documentation of the complexity of data. In other words, when the physician performing the E/M service documents that he or she "personally reviewed the chest X-ray," this indicates a higher level of complexity. Similarly, an undiagnosed presenting problem may require the collection of more information, which increases the complexity of the data to be reviewed. Even though the specific, individual pieces of collected information and data may not be complex, the compilation of numerous sources of diagnostic information may increase the complexity of the data to be reviewed.

Interestingly, the 1995 and 1997 Documentation Guidelines identify no quantifiable levels associated with the amount and/or complexity of data to be reviewed. Rather, this element of medical decision making recognizes the various types of data to be reviewed and the various diagnostic tools available for physicians performing E/M service visits. ■ FIGURE 10.1 summarizes what the 1995 and 1997 Documentation Guidelines endorse for the amount and/or complexity of data, specifically the objective categorization of the data that could be reviewed during an E/M service visit.

abdominal CT scan the CT scan used to identify structure, anatomy, and pathologies within the patient's abdominal cavity

THE SIX DOCUMENTATION GUIDELINES FOR AMOUNT AND/OR COMPLEXITY OF DATA

During an E/M service, a wide range of data may be identified and collected—including, but not limited to, laboratory pathology tests such as blood tests, sputum cultures, or urinalysis, and radiology tests such as chest X-rays, CT scans, or ultrasounds. However the data are collected, the 1995 and 1997 DGs identify six different guidelines for documenting the amount and complexity of the data to be reviewed: ordering diagnostic data, reviewing diagnostic data, obtaining additional history or old medical records, discussion of diagnostic results, and independent visualization of the image, scan, or specimen by the physician performing the E/M service. Since each of these different guidelines identifies the correct documentation of the complexity and/or amount of data to be reviewed, these guidelines provide clear parameters for anyone reviewing the documentation of the E/M service.

Ordering Diagnostic Data

In order for a patient to undergo diagnostic testing, the diagnostic test must be identified as a recommended workup for diagnosing the patient's presenting problem. Diagnostic testing may be in the form of a laboratory test, such as a white blood count; a pathology test, such as determining the nature of a growth; or even a diagnostic procedure, such as an **echoencephalography**, which uses ultrasound to study the brain. In order to achieve the diagnostic benefit of these tests, the diagnostic test must first be ordered, planned, and scheduled, or it may even be performed in the E/M service visit. The documentation should include the type of diagnostic service that has been ordered, planned, scheduled, or performed—for instance, an occult blood test in the laboratory, a pathology test to determine the nature of an abscess, or a chest X-ray to provide diagnostic information about the patient's lungs.

echoencephalography a diagnostic scan that utilizes ultrasound waves to study the brain

> **Example: Documentation of Ordering Diagnostic Testing**
>
> Johnny is an established patient who presents with a sore throat and cough. Patient has no complaints of nasal drainage. Nothing has helped his cough. Grandfather died last year of lung cancer.
>
> **Physical Exam:** Serous fluid is apparent behind tympanic membrane. Patient is uncomfortably congested with significant mucus production via nares. Patient's cough produces thick, white phlegm upon **expectoration**, and solid, white exudates apparent on tonsils and along back of pharynx.
>
> **Laboratory:** Throat culture ordered.

expectoration spitting up, coughing up, or clearing one's throat by coughing and spitting out collected mucus

---

Exercise 10.1 Sinus Pressure

For the following medical documentation, identify the data to be reviewed and the complexity of the data to be reviewed.

History: Patient returns for worsening sinus pressure. The right side of the patient's head hurts so much that she feels she cannot hold her head up due to the throbbing pain. Patient states every part of her hurts now. Patient recognizes flu is likely but is concerned about strep throat.

Exam: Patient is very pale and appears very tired. Conjunctivae red, swollen, and inflamed. Exquisite pain upon palpation of face, particularly the forehead and maxillary sinuses. Copious production of thick, white/brown mucus per nares. Patient unable to open mouth due to pain. Palpation of neck and behind ears reveals exquisitely tender, swollen lymph nodes. Patient expresses extreme discomfort when swallowing. Auscultation of lungs reveals pleural rub. Heart: no murmur identified.

Laboratory: Rapid antigen test negative; throat swab sent for culture. Influenza swab deferred per patient.

Assessment: Sinus infection, probable influenza.

Plan: Azithromycin. Increased fluids, rest. Per patient's request, note written for employer indicating need for 3-day release from work for bed rest.

1. What is the documented data to be reviewed?

   _____

   _____

2. Identify the complexity of the data to be reviewed.

   _____

   _____

Review of Diagnostic Test Results

If, once the diagnostic test has been completed, the physician performing the E/M service visit reviews the laboratory report, radiologist report, or other diagnostic test results, this review should be included in the medical documentation of the E/M service visit. For instance, consider the physician who has ordered a CBC laboratory test to be performed. Once that physician receives the CBC lab results, he or she reviews the red blood cell count, the white blood cell count, hematocrit, and other results pertinent to the patient's presenting problem. Common sense suggests that this physician's review of the laboratory results should be documented in order to fully record the data pertinent to the diagnosis of the patient's problem. Again, there is a tremendous amount of effort, expertise, and clinical skill utilized by the performing physician during the review of these diagnostic results, and the documentation not only reflects and stands as a testament to that effort and skill, but also ensures that these recorded results can contribute to the continuation of the patient's healthcare. To ensure clear documentation of the data review by the performing physician, the 1995 and 1997 Documentation Guidelines state that the performing physician may document his or her review of the diagnostic test results by initialing and dating the diagnostic report.

Within the laboratory or pathology data that are reviewed, certain results may be completely normal or are not pertinent to the patient's presenting problem, such as a urinalysis that is completely normal. In these situations, clear, simple documentation such as "urinalysis normal" is acceptable. Similarly, identification of specific data used in the diagnosis of the presenting problem may be clear and simple as well, such as "white blood count elevated," which may suggest an infection.

However, radiology results are produced in two different forms: the actual radiologic image, tracing, scan, or film and the radiologist's report. When the physician performing the E/M service visit reviews the radiologist's report, he or she reviews the report that has been dictated by the radiologist who performed the diagnostic radiology test. Therefore, for example, when the performing physician documents that the patient's chest X-ray shows nothing abnormal, the note "chest X-ray unremarkable" acceptably documents the results. Regardless of the results, the 1995 and 1997 Documentation Guidelines stress that simple documentation is acceptable for the documentation of the review of diagnostic results, which requires careful reading of the medical documentation.

Example: Documentation of Review of Diagnostic Test Results

Date of Visit: 11-01-20XX

Johnny returns for follow-up for a red, painful throat and barking cough. Patient appears much more haggard and weak, with thick, green nasal drainage. Johnny's girlfriend accompanies him today, since Johnny is unable to speak either without pain or without coughing. His cough has become much worse since his last visit, and his girlfriend says Johnny cannot move when he coughs because he is in so much pain. Johnny motions that both his chest and back hurt when he coughs.

> **Physical Exam:** Patient is alert, however clearly uncomfortable. Vital signs: T, 99.32°F; pulse, 120; BP, 100/65. Eyes: conjunctivae red and inflamed bilaterally. ENT/M: serous fluid apparent behind right tympanic membrane; however, suppurative serous fluid apparent behind left tympanic membrane with significant pressure. Patient is uncomfortably congested with significant green mucus production via nares. Patient's cough produces green chunks of phlegm upon expectoration, and solid, white exudates apparent on tonsils and along back of pharynx.
>
> **Laboratory:** Throat culture results negative. **Sputum gram stain** and culture positive for **Streptococcus pneumonia**. Urinalysis positive for S. pneumonia antigen.
>
> **Assessment:** Streptococcus pneumonia.
>
> **Plan:** Prescribed **cefotaxime** antibiotic for streptococcus pneumonia. NSAID recommended for painful throat. Wrote note for work ordering 3-day bed rest.

Obtaining Old Records or Additional History

At times, the circumstances of the E/M service visit require the performing physician to gather more expansive information about the patient's past medical history than can be collected from the patient. This additional, expansive information about the patient's past medical history is collected by reviewing the patient's old medical records; this does not mean the review of the patient's medical records from a few weeks or months prior, but from several years ago or longer. If these older medical records are not easily available within the patient's chart, the physician performing the E/M service must make a specific request to obtain the old medical records. Regardless of whether the physician must obtain these old medical records from the healthcare facility in which he or she works or from an outside source, the review of these old medical records increases the complexity of the data to be reviewed.

Obtaining Old Records Perhaps the patient is not able to recall the clinical specifics of a previous health condition or the treatment received for it. Perhaps the information required by the performing physician is too clinical, too specific, and can be found only in the previous medical records. In these circumstances, the 1995 and 1997 Documentation Guidelines provide guidance for the documentation of this collection and review of old medical records, specifically that the performing physician should document the decision for obtaining these old medical records, as well as the review of these old medical records.

The results of this review should also be documented, specifically any pertinent findings that inform the performing physician regarding the diagnosis of the presenting problem. The documentation of any pertinent data not only reflects the medical decision-making process but also ensures continuity in the patient's medical record.

As with the review of diagnostic results, if the performing physician has gathered no relevant information or data, a simple, clear statement documenting "old records reviewed" reflects the performing physician's effort in obtaining and reviewing the old medical records. Contrarily, any reviewed data that inform the performing physician's medical decision making should be documented clearly, again to ensure the reflection of the effort, skill, and clinical expertise of the performing physician's medical decision making.

Obtaining Additional History The 1995 and 1997 Documentation Guidelines recognize that, sometimes, the performing physician must collect additional history. For instance, after gathering the history of present illness, review of systems, or past, family, and social history from the patient, the performing physician may need to collect additional history from the patient's caregiver, family member, or other source. Common sense would suggest that the reason for this additional collection of data should be included in the documentation, even though the 1995 and 1997 Documentation Guidelines do not explicitly state the need to document the rationale for additional history collection. Regardless, any pertinent data that inform the medical decision making of the performing physician should be

sputum gram stain a commonly used laboratory test that uses stains to determine specific bacterial infection

Streptococcus pneumonia a bacterial infection that causes pneumonia, sinusitis, ear infections, and many other pathologies

Cefotaxime a broad spectrum antibiotic used for infections of the skin, bones, respiratory tract, and urinary tract; septicemia; and other infections

documented, along with the source of the pertinent data, such as family member, caretaker, and so on. Any informing or pertinent data that provide no insight for the medical decision making can be documented with a simple, but clear "additional history obtained," along with identification of the source of the additional history.

Example: Documentation of Obtaining Additional History

Date of Visit: 11-01-20XX

Johnny returns for follow-up for a red, painful throat and barking cough. Patient appears much more haggard and weak, with thick, green nasal drainage. Johnny's girlfriend accompanies him today, since Johnny is unable to speak either without pain or without coughing. His cough has become much worse since his last visit, and his girlfriend says Johnny cannot move when he coughs because he is in so much pain. Johnny tries to motion that both his chest and back hurt when he coughs, but his cough prevents his movement. Per Johnny's girlfriend, Johnny had been camping with friends for the first good hunting weekend and two wild geese had been killed and dressed at the campsite. Johnny's girlfriend stated that Johnny helped in dressing the carcasses. Johnny's girlfriend expressed concern about bird flu.

> **Physical Exam:** Patient is alert, however clearly uncomfortable. Vital signs: T, 99.32°F; pulse, 120; BP, 100/65. Eyes: conjunctivae red and inflamed bilaterally. ENT/M: serous fluid apparent behind right tympanic membrane; however, suppurative serous fluid apparent behind left tympanic membrane with significant pressure. Patient is uncomfortably congested with significant green mucus production via nares. Patient's cough produces green chunks of phlegm upon expectoration, and solid, white exudates apparent on tonsils and along back of pharynx.
>
> **Laboratory:** Throat culture results negative. Sputum gram stain and culture positive for Streptococcus pneumonia. Urinalysis positive for S. pneumonia antigen. Ordered **AVantage A/H5N1 Flu test** per Johnny's written request.
>
> **Assessment:** Streptococcus pneumonia.
>
> **Plan:** Prescribed cefotaxime antibiotic for streptococcus pneumonia. NSAID recommended for painful throat. Wrote note for work ordering 3-day bed rest.

AVantage A/H5N1 Flu test a minimally invasive test involving a nasal or throat swab, used to quickly determine whether a person has been infected with the H5N1 avian flu

Discussion of Diagnostic Results

The performing physician may seek to discuss the results of a diagnostic test with the physician who actually performed the diagnostic test or interpreted the results of the test, regardless of whether the diagnostic test is a laboratory, radiology, or any other diagnostic test. The content of this discussion provides information and data for the performing physician, and the results of this discussion should be included in the medical documentation of the E/M service visit.

It is important to note that this documentation guideline regarding the discussion of diagnostic results is the shortest of all the documentation guidelines for the amount and/or complexity of data to be reviewed. Again, common sense dictates recognition of the effort and time required for the physician performing the E/M service visit to discuss the results and/or interpretation of the results with the individual physician who performed and/or interpreted the diagnostic test. The documentation of this discussion reflects the medical decision making of the physician performing the E/M service visit in relation to the laboratory, radiology, or other diagnostic results.

Example: Documentation of Discussion of Diagnostic Results

Date of Visit: 11-01-20XX

Johnny returns for follow-up for a red, painful throat and barking cough. Patient appears much more haggard and weak, with thick, green nasal drainage. Johnny's girlfriend accompanies him today, since Johnny is unable to speak either without pain or without coughing. His cough has become much worse since his last visit, and his girlfriend says Johnny cannot move when he coughs because he is in so much pain. Johnny tries to motion that both his chest and back hurt when he coughs, but his cough prevents his movement.

continued

Physical Exam: Patient is alert, however clearly uncomfortable. Vital signs: T, 99.32°F; pulse, 120; BP, 100/65. Eyes: conjunctivae red and inflamed bilaterally. ENT/M: serous fluid apparent behind right tympanic membrane; however, suppurative serous fluid apparent behind left tympanic membrane with significant pressure. Patient is uncomfortably congested with significant green mucus production via nares. Patient's cough produces green chunks of phlegm upon expectoration, and solid, white exudates apparent on tonsils and along back of pharynx.

Laboratory: Throat culture results negative. Sputum gram stain and culture negative for Streptococcus pneumonia. Urinalysis positive for S. pneumonia antigen. Ordered chest X-ray.

Assessment: Discussed laboratory results with laboratory pathologist, specifically regarding the conflicting results of the negative sputum gram stain and culture results and the positive S. pneumonia urinalysis results. Per pathology recommendation, repeat sputum gram stain with **bronchoscopy** ordered for probable streptococcus pneumonia.

Plan: Patient will be notified of bronchoscopy-assisted sputum gram stain test. Rx cefotaxime will be made available for Johnny if sputum gram stain is positive for streptococcus pneumonia. Patient should return to clinic if sputum gram stain is negative for S. pneumonia. NSAID recommended for painful throat. Wrote note for work ordering 3-day bed rest.

bronchoscopy the act of inserting a cylindrical fiber optic tube with a video function into the airway; allows direct visualization of the mucosal tissues of the airways for diagnostic purposes

---

Exercise 10.2 **Recurrent Abdominal Pain**

For the following medical documentation, identify the data to be reviewed and the complexity of the data to be reviewed.

Timmy is a 12-year-old established patient and presents for recurrent abdominal pain. Timmy's pain is localized in the right lower quadrant. Since Timmy's previous visit, his abdominal pain has increased in severity and frequency, preventing him from attending school and requiring him to take pain relievers.

Review of systems: Diarrhea has subsided, and negative for bloody stools. Negative for dysuria, hematuria. Negative for fevers, sick contact, or trauma other than the goal-side tackle reported during Timmy's previous visit dated 09/23. All other ROS pertaining to this problem are negative.

PE: Timmy is not in distress, although he is very pale. T, 98.7°F; pulse, 130; resp., 20. Eyes clear with no jaundice. Pupils are reactive to light within normal limits. Lungs clear to auscultation and percussion. Auscultation of heart reveals normal but rapid heartbeat without murmur. Timmy complains of mild discomfort pain during palpation of lower right quadrant. No hepatosplenomegaly. No peritoneal signs noted and no evidence of abdominal or inguinal hernias. No edema noted in extremities.

Assessment: The severity of the pain makes it prudent to rule out appendiceal abscess.

Plan: Recommend abdominal CT scan, KUB, complete blood panel, and urinalysis. Timmy will return tomorrow morning to provide urine and blood samples for workup. Radiology scheduled for tomorrow afternoon. Return for recheck in 2 days after receipt of radiology scans.

1. What is the documented data to be reviewed?

   _____
   _____

2. Identify the complexity of the data to be reviewed.

   _____
   _____

Independent Visualization of Image, Tracing, or Scan

As mentioned earlier, radiology results are produced in two different forms: the actual radiologic image, tracing, scan, or film and the radiologist's report. On the occasions when the physician performing the E/M service visit may need to personally view the radiology scan or image, this requires additional effort, skill, and expertise on that physician's part. The 1995 and 1997 Documentation Guidelines refer to this as "direct visualization" and "independent interpretation" of the radiology image, scan, film, or specimen. This direct visualization requires the physician performing the E/M service visit to personally invest his or her own clinical and diagnostic skills in the medical decision making and should be documented clearly, particularly identifying that the physician personally and independently visualized the radiology scan. This investment of effort on the part of the physician performing the E/M service visit is significant in the effort to better discern the diagnosis of the patient's presenting problem.

Although this specific guideline is most commonly associated with radiology results, the 1995 and 1997 Documentation Guidelines do not specifically state that it relates only to radiology. Therefore, the independent visualization and interpretation of an image, tracing, or specimen may apply to any diagnostic result. One of the most important aspects of this guideline is that this image, tracing, or specimen has been previously or subsequently reviewed or interpreted by another physician than the physician performing the E/M service visit.

Example: Documentation of Independent Visualization of Radiology Scan or Image

Date of Visit: 11-01-20XX

Johnny returns for follow-up for a red, painful throat and barking cough. Patient appears much more haggard and weak, with thick, green nasal drainage. Johnny's girlfriend accompanies him today, since Johnny is unable to speak either without pain or without coughing. His cough has become much worse since his last visit, and his girlfriend says Johnny cannot move when he coughs because he's in so much pain. Johnny tries to motion that both his chest and back hurt when he coughs, but his cough prevents his movement.

Physical Exam: Patient is alert, however clearly uncomfortable. Vital signs: T, 99.32°F; pulse, 120; BP, 100/65. Eyes: conjunctivae red and inflamed bilaterally. ENT/M: serous fluid apparent behind right tympanic membrane; however, suppurative serous fluid apparent behind left tympanic membrane with significant pressure. Patient is uncomfortably congested with significant green mucus production via nares. Patient's cough produces green chunks of phlegm upon expectoration, and solid, white exudates apparent on tonsils and along back of pharynx.

Assessment: Throat culture results negative. Sputum gram stain and culture positive for Streptococcus pneumonia. Urinalysis positive for S. pneumonia antigen. Independent visualization of chest X-ray reveals significant inflammation of pleural lining as well as the bronchi.

Diagnosis: Streptococcal pneumonia, pleurisy, and bronchitis.

Plan: Prescribed cefotaxime antibiotic for Streptococcus pneumonia. **Indomethacin** prescribed to reduce inflammation of pleural lining. **Hydrocodone cough suppressant** prescribed for reduction of cough. Wrote note for work ordering 3 days' bed rest.

---

indomethacin an NSAID used to reduce fever, pain, swelling, and stiffness; used in the treatment of various conditions, including rheumatoid arthritis and patent ductus arteriosus

hydrocodone cough suppressant a cough suppressant combined with a narcotic analgesic, or pain reliever

Ultimately, the documentation of the amount and/or complexity of the data to be reviewed is the culmination of the objective review of the data collected by the physician performing the E/M service visit.

Exercise 10.3 Lower Back Pain

For the following medical documentation, identify the data to be reviewed and the complexity of the data to be reviewed.

Joan is an established patient who presents for lower back pain. Her lower back hurts, down by beltline, and pain is sometimes very severe. The pain is sporadic, mostly when standing up after sitting in one place for an extended period. Ibuprofen used to help, but now it does not help back pain anymore. At its worst, low back pain is sharp and throbbing. Joan has had occasional back pain for about 20 years, since first in the service, but she first noticed this particular low back pain shortly after playing touch football with adult children this past Thanksgiving. Patient denies any other joint pain than this low back pain. Patient denies double vision or dizziness, and no chest pain or shortness of breath. Patient denies tobacco or alcohol use. Pain has not affected her work as a fifth-grade teacher.

Exam: Back is soft to the touch and palpation and revealed no obvious lumps or masses. Percussion of back reveals tenderness in lower back but no costovertebral tenderness. Patient performs side-to-side flexion to 30 degrees with minimal pain; however, she finds forward flexion at 50 degrees with pain localized to her lower back that does not radiate down legs or up her back. Deep tendon reflexes within normal limits: ankle jerk reflex, patellar reflex, plantar reflexes tested. Patient's range of motion is stable, within normal limits, and without pain.

Plan: Recommend physical therapy, NSAID as needed for inflammation. Follow-up in 6 weeks.

1. What is the documented data to be reviewed?

_____

_____

2. Identify the complexity of the data to be reviewed.

_____

_____

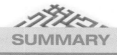

SUMMARY

- The 1995 and 1997 "Documentation Guidelines for Evaluation and Management Services" recognize that a broad scope of diagnostic information could be reviewed during an E/M service visit. This diagnostic information may include results of laboratory, pathology, or medical tests; radiology reports; review of old medical records; and the independent review of a radiology image by the physician performing the E/M service visit. The data to be reviewed could be referred to as identified clues that are used by the physician performing the E/M service to facilitate discerning the diagnosis of the presenting problem. The various types, or nature, of the data provide information about the complexity of the data to be reviewed. Certainly, the complexity of the data may refer to either individual diagnostic tests that are very complex or to a multitude of ordered diagnostic tests and their review.

- There are six different documentation guidelines regarding the amount and/or complexity of data to be reviewed. These six guidelines address the ordering and scheduling of diagnostic testing, as well as the review of the results of this diagnostic testing. In addition, guidelines address the documentation of any discussion regarding the diagnostic testing results between the physician performing the E/M service visit and the physician who performed the diagnostic testing. Documentation guidelines also address circumstances when the physician performing the E/M service visit independently visualizes the specimen, image, scan, or film. Finally, separate documentation guidelines address circumstances when the physician performing the E/M service visit must request old medical records or collect additional history from a family member, caretaker, or other source. Most significantly, each of the documentation guidelines for the amount and/or complexity of data addresses each of the potential types of data that may be documented in an E/M service visit.

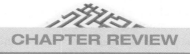

CHAPTER REVIEW

Multiple Choice

Choose the letter that best answers each question or completes each statement.

1. The diagnostic data that could be reviewed during an E/M service visit include
   a. history, physical examination, and medical decision making.
   b. laboratory, pathology, and radiology.
   c. review of systems, history of present illness, and past history.
   d. body areas, organ systems, and general multisystems.

2. Which of the following is NOT an appropriate type of data to be reviewed?
   a. Obtaining and reviewing the patient's old medical records
   b. Reviewing results of diagnostic testing
   c. Collecting additional history from the patient's family or caretaker
   d. Utilizing the physician's senses of sight, hearing, and touch to identify the state of the patient's health

3. What should the medical coder do if any confusion remains about the data to be reviewed?
   a. Make an assumption about what the performing physician did
   b. Ask the physician who performed the E/M service visit to clarify the documentation
   c. Do research online to fill in the blanks left by the documentation

d. Call and ask the patient to tell what happened during the E/M service visit

4. Which of the following best reflects "ordering diagnostic data"?
   a. The physician's review of the results of any diagnostic service intended to assist in diagnosing the patient's presenting problem
   b. The ordering, planning, or scheduling of any diagnostic service intended to assist in diagnosing the patient's presenting problem
   c. Requesting or obtaining the patient's old medical records
   d. Discussion of the results of a diagnostic test with the physician who performed that specific diagnostic test

5. Which of the following best reflects an "independent visualization of specimen, tracing, or image"?
   a. The ordering, planning, or scheduling of any diagnostic service intended to assist in diagnosing the patient's presenting problem
   b. The personal, independent visualization of the radiologic image, tracing, or scan by the physician who is performing the E/M service visit
   c. Requesting or obtaining the patient's old medical records
   d. Discussion of the results of a diagnostic test with the physician who performed that specific diagnostic test

6. During an E/M service visit, Dr. Mike orders a chest X-ray. Which of the following best identifies the amount and/or complexity of data?
   a. Ordering diagnostic testing
   b. Review of diagnostic testing results

c. Independent visualization of image, scan, film

d. Discussion of diagnostic testing results with performing physician

7. During an E/M service visit, Dr. Jude reviews a radiology report that had been recorded 2 days previously and then calls Dr. George, the radiologist who performed the radiology test and dictated the radiology report, to discuss the radiology results. Which of the following best reflects the amount and/or complexity of the data?

a. Ordering diagnostic testing

b. Review of diagnostic testing results

c. Independent visualization of image, scan, film

d. Discussion of diagnostic testing results with physician who performed the test

8. During an E/M service visit, Dr. Smith requests old medical records to review the patient's previous health history, complaints, diagnoses, and treatments. Which of the following best reflects the amount and/or complexity of data?

a. The ordering, planning, or scheduling of any diagnostic service intended to assist in diagnosing the patient's presenting problem

b. Requesting or obtaining the patient's old medical records

c. Discussion of the results of a diagnostic test with the physician who performed that specific diagnostic test

d. Collection of additional history from patient's family, caretaker, or other source

9. During E/M service visit, the patient is not conscious because of previous head trauma. Dr. Jones gathers information from the patient's family, who provide extensive information about the patient. Which of the following best reflects the amount and/or complexity of data?

a. Collection of additional history from patient's family, caretaker, or other source

b. Requesting or obtaining the patient's old medical records

c. Review of physical examination data

d. Discussion of the results of a diagnostic test with the physician who performed that specific diagnostic test

10. During an E/M service visit, Dr. Ferrari orders a urinalysis, complete blood count, and rapid strep test. When the results come back, Dr. Ferrari reviews the diagnostic results. Which of the following best reflects the amount and/or complexity of data?

a. Collection of additional history from patient's family, caretaker, or other source and requesting or obtaining the patient's old medical records

b. The physician's review of the results of any diagnostic service intended to assist in diagnosing the patient's presenting problem and discussion of the results of a diagnostic test with the physician who performed that specific diagnostic test

c. The ordering, planning, or scheduling of any diagnostic service intended to assist in diagnosing the patient's presenting problem and physician's review of the results of any diagnostic service intended to assist in diagnosing the patient's presenting problem

d. Discussion of the results of a diagnostic test with the physician who performed that specific diagnostic test and the personal, independent visualization of the radiologic image, tracing, or scan by the physician who is performing the E/M service visit

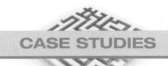

CASE STUDIES

Case Study 10-1

Read the following documentation, and then answer questions 1–5 by identifying the phrase that best supports the amount and/or complexity of data reviewed.

Complaint: I have been asked to consult on James Roberts's abdominal trauma. James Roberts is a 45-year-old new patient who suffered a fall in his home office. Mr. Roberts tripped on the computer cords in his home office and fell onto his office chair, striking his upper abdomen on the armrest of the chair and striking his forehead on the edge of his desk. Patient reports experiencing immediate ULQ pain that he reported as 5/10 at time of fall, but has increased in severity to 7/10. Per patient, there was no LOC. Since that time, he has experienced occasional dizziness and three nosebleeds, each lasting at least 20 minutes. Patient has vomited twice and has noted significant midback pain during each emesis, which he rates at a 7–8/10.

Laboratory: Hemoglobin, 13.5; WBC, 18,000. An abdominal CT scan was reviewed with radiologist; scan showed a small amount of free fluid in ULQ with grade 3 laceration of spleen. Independent visualization of KUB reveals evidence of significant amount of stool within sigmoid and rectum.

Assessment: Hemodynamically stable patient with grade 3 splenic laceration. No immediate correlation between splenic trauma and previous hernia repair is being considered at this time, although Mr. Robert's history of alcoholism could affect treatment of splenic trauma. Contacted patient's primary physician in Charleston, Texas, by phone to discuss pt's previous hernia surgery, complications, alcohol-related conditions, and healthcare management related to long history of alcohol use. Pertinent records to be reviewed upon receipt by fax.

Plan: Patient admitted for overnight observation, IV antibiotics with rehydration. Gastroenterology consultation requested for splenic trauma.

1. Which of the following best reflects the documentation of "hemoglobin, 13.5; WBC, 18,000"?

   a. The ordering, planning, scheduling, or review of any diagnostic service results intended to assist in diagnosing the patient's presenting problem

   b. Requesting or obtaining the patient's old medical records

   c. Discussion of the results of a diagnostic test with the physician who performed that specific diagnostic test

   d. The personal, independent visualization of the radiologic image, tracing, or scan by the physician who is performing the E/M service visit

2. Which of the following best reflects the documentation of "abdominal CT scan was reviewed with radiologist; scan showed a small amount of free fluid"?

   a. Collection of additional history from patient's family, caretaker, or other source

   b. Requesting or obtaining the patient's old medical records

   c. Discussion of the results of a diagnostic test with the physician who performed that specific diagnostic test

   d. The personal, independent visualization of the radiologic image, tracing, or scan by the physician who is performing the E/M service visit

3. Which of the following best reflects the documentation of "contacted patient's primary physician in Charleston, Texas, by phone to discuss pt's previous hernia surgery"?

   a. Collection of additional history from patient's family, caretaker, or other source

   b. The physician's review of the results of any diagnostic service intended to assist in diagnosing the patient's presenting problem

   c. The ordering, planning, or scheduling of any diagnostic service intended to assist in diagnosing the patient's presenting problem

   d. Discussion of the results of a diagnostic test with the physician who performed that specific diagnostic test

4. Which of the following best reflects the documentation of "independent visualization of KUB reveals evidence of significant amount of stool within sigmoid and rectum"?

   a. The ordering, planning, or scheduling of any diagnostic service intended to assist in diagnosing the patient's presenting problem

   b. Requesting or obtaining the patient's old medical records

   c. Discussion of the results of a diagnostic test with the physician who performed that specific diagnostic test

   d. The personal, independent visualization of the radiologic image, tracing, or scan by the physician who is performing the E/M service visit

5. Which of the following best reflects the documentation "pertinent patient medical records to be reviewed upon receipt by fax"?

   a. The physician's review of the results of any diagnostic service intended to assist in diagnosing the patient's presenting problem

   b. The ordering, planning, or scheduling of any diagnostic service intended to assist in diagnosing the patient's presenting problem

   c. Requesting or obtaining the patient's old medical records

   d. Discussion of the results of a diagnostic test with the physician who performed that specific diagnostic test

Case Study 10-2

Read the following documentation, and then answer the questions that follow. You will need to identify the following elements: overall level of history; type of physical examination, referencing one of the three physical examinations; number of diagnoses and/or management options; and amount and/or complexity of data to be reviewed. Remember that Appendix D contains the full content of service worksheet.

Complaint: Frank is well-known to me and presents for sharp left flank pain and dark-orange-colored urine after a fall resulting in blunt abdominal trauma on Saturday afternoon, 2 days ago. He tripped on his dog and fell against the patio railing, striking his upper left abdomen against the decorative wrought iron. Patient reports experiencing immediate stabbing pain across his upper abdomen and down his left flank, which subsided quickly without recurrence. Upon rising on Sunday morning, Frank noticed sharp stabbing pain across ULQ abdomen accompanied by dark, painful bruising in the area of his ULQ where he was struck by the decorative railing. The pain is most severe when he breathes deeply, rating pain at 8/10, and Frank cannot bend his torso without significant pain. Frank reports his urine sample to be very dark and odorous but denies painful urination. He denies any chest pain or racing heartbeat. No reports of tingling of extremities, dizziness, nausea, bloody stool. All other reviews of systems pertinent to this problem are negative. No report of ill contact at work or family, although Frank reports a higher stress level than usual, as budget cuts at work have caused many layoffs, and he is anxious about his employment status at work. There is no history of gastrointestinal disease in family or past medical history.

Physical Exam: T, 97.8; BP, 106/88; P, 68. Eyes clear without jaundice. Head is atraumatic without tenderness, nodules, or swelling. Neck: no thyromegaly. Auscultation of lungs clear without wheezes or rub. No tactile fremitus noted upon palpation of chest. Auscultation of heart reveals regular rate and rhythm with no abnormal sounds noted. No cervical spine tenderness. No thoracic spine tenderness and no lumbar spine tenderness; however, costovertebral tenderness noted upon palpation. No referred pain in left shoulder. Palpation of lower abdomen reveals soft, nontender abdomen, and no hepatomegaly or tenderness upon upper right quadrant palpation or percussion. Upper left abdomen mildly inflamed with dark circular bruise where patient identifies blow to abdomen. Very tender upper left quadrant upon palpation, and patient's pain precludes deep palpation of spleen. No dullness noted upon percussion of left or right flank. Stool sample collected for occult blood test.

Laboratory: CBC reveals white blood count normal; hemoglobin and hematocrit are normal. A FAST scan abdominal CT scan was reviewed with radiologist. Review of KUB revealed significant stool within sigmoid and rectum. Occult blood test negative.

Assessment: It is quite probable that at least one of the lower left ribs has been fractured, although the patient's pain makes it difficult to make a specific rib identification. A splenic injury should be ruled out through CT scan. In my opinion, it would be prudent to begin oral Augmentin treatment at 875 mg twice a day for 7 days and increase fluid intake. Follow-up in 10 days for recheck.

Identify the overall level of history, and explain the supporting rationale for the overall level of history.

1. Overall level of history: _____

2. Explain your rationale. _____
   _____
   _____

Identify the type of physical examination: problem-focused, expanded problem-focused, detailed, or comprehensive.

3. Type of physical examination: _____

4. Which physical examination was referenced: 1995 body area/organ system, 1997 general multisystem, 1997 single organ system? _____

Utilizing the content of service worksheet provided here as a reference, answer the following questions about the medical decision making documented in Case Study 10-2.

5. Number of diagnoses and/or management options:
   _____

   Is this problem new or established?
   _____

   If this is an established problem, is it stable/improving or worsening? _____
   Is a management option documented?
   _____

   If a management option is documented, what is it?
   _____

6. Amount and/or complexity of data to be reviewed:
   _____

   What is the documented data to be reviewed?
   _____

   Identify the complexity of the data to be reviewed:
   _____

Number of Diagnoses and/or Management Options	Established presenting problem, stable or improving	Established presenting problem, worsening	New presenting problem, without workup	New presenting problem, with workup
Amount and/or Complexity of Data to Be Reviewed	Ordering or reviewing diagnostic data	Obtaining old records or additional history from someone other than patient	Discussion of diagnostic results with physician who performed diagnostic testing	Independent visualization of image, tracing, or scan by physician performing the E/M service

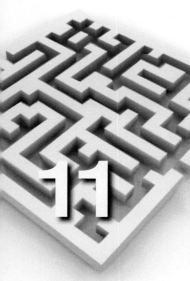

11 Medical Decision Making: Risk of Complication, Comorbidity, or Mortality

Learning Objectives

After completing this chapter, you should be able to do the following:

- Spell and define the key terms and abbreviations presented in this chapter
- Identify the documentation guidelines for the risk of complication, comorbidity, or mortality
- Identify the four levels of risk of complication, comorbidity, and/or mortality
- Identify the three areas of the table of risk: presenting problem, diagnostic procedure ordered, and management option selected

Key Terms

acute myocardial infarction

arterial pH

arterial puncture

arteriogram

assessing the risk

benign prostatic hypertrophy

cardiac catheterization

cardiac electrophysiological tests

cardiac stress test

cataract

colitis

comorbidity

complication

contraindications

contrast medium

culdocentesis

cystitis

diabetic ketoacidosis

drug therapy requiring intensive monitoring for toxicity

echocardiography

effective serum osmolality

electrocardiogram

electroencephalogram

embolus

endoscopies

exacerbation

fetal contraction stress test

incisional biopsy

ketones

lumbar puncture

morbidity

mortality

noninsulin dependent diabetes

percutaneous

peritonitis

pneumonitis

prescription drugs

progressive severe rheumatoid arthritis

pulmonary embolus

pulmonary function tests

pyelonephritis

Reye's syndrome

rhinitis

seizure

serum bicarbonate

severe respiratory distress

table of risk

thoracentesis

tinea corporis

transient ischemic attack

urinary tract infection

venipuncture

well-controlled hypertension

Abbreviations

BPH benign prostatic hyperplasia

MI myocardial infarction

TIA transient ischemic attack

UTI urinary tract infection

INTRODUCTION

The field of medicine is filled with complex language, many different pathologies, and challenging concepts. The physician discerns these multifaceted and connected clinical concerns during the evaluation and management service and documents them as part of the patient's medical record. One of the greatest challenges of medical decision making is distilling the discernment of these complex and nuanced anatomies, pathologies, and diagnostic results. After all, the performing physician has spent years of study to become adept at assessing and diagnosing patients' complaints. Sometimes, the words on paper may not seem to do justice to the effort and skill involved in the physician's clinical judgment; after all, the physician must consider not only the patient's presenting problem, but also any potential ramifications of any diagnostic procedures and any management options on the patient's health. These ramifications represent potential risk to the patient's health as it relates to the diagnosis and management of the patient's presenting problem. This chapter focuses on the documentation of the risk posed by the presenting problem, diagnostic procedures, and management options.

RISK OF COMPLICATION, COMORBIDITY, AND MORTALITY

Risk is the introduction of danger or hazard into any given situation, or the recognition of how a specific situation or action increases a person's vulnerability to danger. For instance, small children are taught to minimize the risk of crossing the street by holding the hand of an adult and looking both ways before stepping off the curb. However, every parent knows that life can be an assessment of risk during the life of the child: Although a parent hopes the child will continue to stop at the corner and look both ways before crossing the street, the parent knows the risk inherent in the child crossing the street alone and assesses the risk of such situations individually. Similarly, when parents discover their child is ill, they assess the risk of their child's illness: Does our child have a fever? If so, has Tylenol reduced the fever? Should we take our child to the doctor's office? Each of these questions addresses the level of risk presented by a specific illness at a specific time.

The determination of risk is very complex and can be difficult to quantify in such a way as to address every conceivable situation. However, the 1995 and 1997 DGs acknowledge that nearly every physician performing an E/M service does assess the risk inherent to a patient. This assessment identifies at least one of three different things: how the presenting problem could get worse, what else is going on in the patient's body aside from the presenting problem, and what could potentially cause the patient's death. These three things are known as complication, comorbidity, and mortality. Each of these areas of risk represents a different aspect of medical decision making and is reflected in the content of service worksheet shown in ■ Figure 11.1. In order to actually determine the risk of complication, comorbidity, and mortality, each area must be clearly understood in the context of an E/M service visit.

Risk of Complication

A **complication** is a pathological development that is not an inherent part of the presenting problem but that occurs in a patient during the management of a patient's presenting problem. This pathological development could be the worsening of a condition because of a secondary disease, such as a secondary

complication a pathological development that is not an inherent part of the presenting problem but that occurs in a patient during the management of a patient's presenting problem

COMPLEXITY OF MEDICAL DECISION-MAKING	Straightforward	Low	Moderate	High
Number of Diagnoses and/or Management Options	Established presenting problem, stable or improving	Established presenting problem, worsening	New presenting problem, without workup	New presenting problem, with workup
Amount and/or Complexity of Data to be Reviewed	Ordering or reviewing diagnostic data	Obtain old records or additional history from someone other than patient	Discussion of diagnostic results with physician who performed diagnostic testing	Independent visualization of image, tracing, or scan by physician performing the evaluation and management service
Risk of Complications, Co-morbidities, and/or Mortality	Minimal	Low	Moderate	High

Figure 11.1 ■ Content of service elements—medical decision making: risk of complications, co-morbidity and/or mortality with complications.

bacterial respiratory infection that develops during a patient's viral influenza. Alternatively, this pathological development could be a negative physiological reaction to a treatment or therapy, for example, the onset of **Reye's syndrome** after a child is given aspirin to treat a fever. Regardless of the cause of the complication, the most essential factor of a complication is the worsening of an existing condition through secondary illness or therapy related to management of the presenting problem. The following example presents a simple illustration of a complication.

Reye's syndrome a disease of unknown cause that prompts a variety of serious pathological effects on several organs, particularly the brain and liver; strongly correlated with aspirin use in children with fevers, although it also has occurred with no associated aspirin use

Example: Documentation of Complication

A patient visits her MD after spraining her left ankle. Her ankle is sore upon weight bearing. The MD places an elastic bandage on her ankle and recommends rest. The next day, after bathing, the patient replaces the bandage on her ankle but puts it on too tightly, which leads to the complication of inflaming the sprained ankle and straining the Achilles tendon.

The complication is the strained Achilles tendon caused by the inflamed ankle, which was caused by an inexpertly placed elastic bandage by the patient.

Risk of Comorbidity

Morbidity denotes a disease, illness, or ill health. Therefore, **comorbidity** is a disease, illness, or ill health that is separate from the presenting problem but that occurs at the same time as the presenting problem. Thus, the risk of comorbidity signifies the risk of an additional disease, illness, or ill health occurring in addition to the presenting problem. Comorbidity differs from complication, which is a pathological reaction that can be traced to the presenting problem; a comorbidity is a separate disease presenting concurrently with the presenting problem.

morbidity a state of disease, illness, or ill health

comorbidity a disease, illness, or ill health that is separate from the presenting problem but that occurs at the same time as the presenting problem

Example: Documentation of Comorbidity

A patient visits her MD reporting head congestion producing thick, green, stringlike mucous, body aches and pains, and a fever of 101.1° F (Fahrenheit). Significant tenderness of maxillary sinuses. Throat culture results negative. Sputum gram stain and culture negative for Streptococcus pneumonia. Urinalysis positive for S. pneumonia antigen. Ordered chest X-ray.

Assessment: Independent visualization of chest X-ray reveals significant inflammation of pleural lining as well as the bronchi.

Diagnosis: Streptococcal pneumonia, pleurisy, and bronchitis.

The comorbidities are the streptococcal pneumonia, pleurisy, and bronchitis, which are three separate, unrelated diseases or pathological reactions. Being diagnosed with one of these diseases does not automatically indicate that the patient will have all three of the conditions.

Risk of Mortality

mortality actual death of the patient or increased potential for death due to the patient's presenting problem, a drastic worsening of the presenting problem, or associated disease process

All humans are mortal, which means all humans are subject to death. **Mortality** is the potential for death, or death itself. Therefore, risk of mortality refers to the actual death of the patient or the increased potential for death due to the patient's presenting problem, complications, or comorbidities.

Example: Documentation of Mortality

A patient visits her MD reporting head congestion producing thick, green, stringlike mucous, body aches and pains, and a fever of 101.1°F. Patient has lost 6 pounds in the past 3 days with severe diarrhea, and she cannot think clearly. Patient has type I diabetes.

ketones chemicals toxic to the function of the body that are built up as a result of low insulin

> **Physical Examination:** Significant tenderness of maxillary sinuses. Throat culture results negative. Sputum gram stain and culture negative for Streptococcus pneumonia. Urinalysis positive for S. pneumonia antigen, positive for **ketones**. Ordered chest X-ray. Blood glucose, 55 mg/dl; **arterial pH**, 7.26; **serum bicarbonate**, 16 mEq/L; **effective serum osmolality** is variable.

arterial pH measurement of the acidity within the blood: levels lower than 7.35 suggesting acidosis and levels higher than 7.45 suggesting alkalosis

> **Assessment:** Mild **diabetic ketoacidosis** per lab report. Independent visualization of chest X-ray reveals significant inflammation of pleural lining as well as the bronchi.

> **Diagnosis:** Streptococcal pneumonia, pleurisy, and bronchitis in a patient with mild diabetic ketoacidosis.

serum bicarbonate also known as HCO3, a component of blood that is tested to measure the metabolic function of the human body; metabolic acidosis indicated by a low level

The risk of mortality has increased for this patient because of the diabetic ketoacidosis. Whereas the patient's three conditions increase the risk inherent in three separate comorbidities, the diabetic ketoacidosis greatly increases her risk of mortality. Although this does not mean the presenting problem will cause imminent death, the comorbidities in combination with the diabetic ketoacidosis have increased her risk of mortality.

---

effective serum osmolality the concentration of chemicals dissolved in the serum of the blood, including sodium, chloride, bicarbonate, proteins, glucose, and others

When creating a plan of care for a patient, the performing physician assesses one or more of these three risks: complication, comorbidity, and mortality. Each of these factors could impact the patient's health or the management of the presenting problem. Since, in general, medical coders are not clinically trained, it can be very difficult for a medical coder to assess the risk to the patient in the documentation. Therefore, both the 1995 and 1997 DGs utilize an organized table classifying the risk of complication, comorbidity, and/or mortality for the physician **assessing the risk** of the presenting problem, the risk of any diagnostic procedures ordered, or the risk of the management option selected.

diabetic ketoacidosis a potentially life-threatening complication due to diabetes mellitus and a lack of insulin in the body

TABLE OF RISK

assessing the risk identifying the level of risk of complication, comorbidity, or mortality posed to the patient by the presenting problem; refers to the ordered or performed diagnostic tests or the management option selected by the performing physician

The 1995 and 1997 DGs provide four distinct levels of risk of complication, comorbidity, and/or mortality to be used in assessing that risk. These four levels—minimal, low, moderate, and high—are presented in the **table of risk**. Organized as an index of the four different levels of risk, the table is based on three different areas of risk that are assessed by the performing physician—presenting problem, diagnostic procedures ordered, and management option selected—any one of which could determine the actual level of risk posed to the patient. For each of these areas, the risk of complication, comorbidity, and/or mortality is considered and documented by the performing physician.

The 1995 and 1997 DGs introduce the table of risk as an objective tool to help determine the level of risk in an easy-to-read form. The table provides specific clinical examples for each area at each level of risk. ■ TABLE 11.1 introduces the format of the table of risk, with the level of risk in the left column and

table of risk an objective tool to determine the level of risk of complication, comorbidity, and/or mortality in an easy-to-read format

■ TABLE 11.1 TABLE OF RISK FORMAT

LEVEL OF RISK	PRESENTING PROBLEM	DIAGNOSTIC ORDERED	MANAGEMENT OPTION
Minimal	• Clinical examples	• Clinical examples	• Clinical examples
Low	• Clinical examples	• Clinical examples	• Clinical examples
Moderate	• Clinical examples	• Clinical examples	• Clinical examples
High	• Clinical examples	• Clinical examples	• Clinical examples

■ TABLE 11.2   TABLE OF RISK: PRESENTING PROBLEM

LEVEL OF RISK	PRESENTING PROBLEM—COMMON EXAMPLES
Minimal	• One self-limited or minor problem—e.g., a cold, insect bite (with no allergic reaction), **tinea corporis**
Low	• Two or more self-limited or minor problems (see above) • One stable chronic illness—e.g., **well-controlled hypertension**, **noninsulin dependent diabetes**, **cataract**, **benign prostatic hypertrophy** • Acute, uncomplicated illness or injury—e.g., cystitis (bladder inflammation), allergic **rhinitis**, simple sprain
Moderate	• One or more chronic illnesses with mild **exacerbation**, progression, or side effects of treatment—e.g., cystitis with UTI, chronic asthma with viral upper respiratory infection • Two or more stable chronic illnesses (see above) • Undiagnosed new problem with uncertain prognosis—e.g., lump in breast • Acute illness with systemic symptoms—e.g., **pyelonephritis**, **pneumonitis**, **colitis** • Acute uncomplicated injury—e.g., head injury with brief loss of consciousness
High	• One or more chronic illnesses with severe exacerbation, progression, or side effects of treatment—e.g., complicated UTI with insulin-dependent diabetes, bacterial pneumonia with COPD • Acute or chronic illnesses or injuries that pose a threat to life or bodily function—e.g., multiple trauma, acute MI, **pulmonary embolus**, **severe respiratory distress**, **progressive severe rheumatoid arthritis**, psychiatric illness with potential threat to self or others, **peritonitis**, acute renal failure. • An abrupt change in neurologic status—e.g., **seizure**, TIA, weakness, or sensory loss

Source: Centers for Medicare and Medicaid, "1995 Documentation Guidelines for Evaluation and Management Services," p. 14, www.cms.gov/Outreach-and-Education/Medicare-Learning-Network-MLN/MLNEdWebGuide/Downloads/95Docguidelines.pdf; "1997 Documentation Guidelines for Evaluation and Management Services," p. 50, www.cms.gov/Outreach-and-Education/Medicare-Learning-Network-MLN/MLNEdWebGuide/Downloads/97Docguidelines.pdf.

a separate column for each of the three areas of risk: presenting problem, diagnostic procedures ordered, and management option selected.

Because the assessment of risk can sometimes be difficult to quantify, the table of risk contains everyday examples that are familiar to most people with minimal clinical knowledge. In this way, the table provides suggestions and guidelines rather than an absolute measurement of risk, which is best assessed by the performing physician.

Presenting Problem

In the table of risk, the presenting problem reflects the risk of complication, comorbidity, and/or mortality posed to the patient not only at the current visit, but also in the interval of time between the current visit and the subsequent visit. Within the context of risk, the presenting problem asks "How risky is this presenting problem, and how risky could it become?" The 1995 and 1997 DGs state that any comorbidity or pathology that increases the complexity of the medical decision making should be documented by the physician to clearly reflect his or her energies and expertise.

There is a wide range of conditions and circumstances that could increase the risk of the presenting problem, and determining that level of risk requires critical thinking and an ability to synthesize clinical information. However, to provide guidance and clarity, the 1995 and 1997 DGs provide 12 different examples that span the four levels of risk. ■ TABLE 11.2 gives the common, everyday examples listed in the presenting problem area of the table of risk.

Notice that the pathological severity increases along with the increasing level of risk. For instance, in the low, moderate, and high levels, **urinary tract infection (UTI)** or **cystitis** has been identified in different stages of severity. Simple cystitis, or inflammation of the bladder, is considered a low level

tinea corporis fungal infection of the skin, also known as ringworm

well-controlled hypertension high blood pressure that is responding well to treatment

noninsulin dependent diabetes commonly referred to as "type II" diabetes; requires no insulin therapy and can be managed through lifestyle and diet

cataract a disease of the eye that causes clouding of the ocular lens

benign prostatic hypertrophy enlargement of the cells within the prostate; also known as benign prostatic hyperplasia

rhinitis inflammation of the mucosal lining of the nasal cavity

exacerbation worsening in severity of a disease, syndrome, or any symptoms thereof

pyelonephritis inflammation of the kidney and/or renal pelvis, otherwise known as the junction of the kidney and the ureter, or tube that carries urine from the kidney into the bladder; most commonly caused by an infection

pneumonitis inflammation of the lung tissue

colitis inflammation of the colon, or large intestine

pulmonary embolus obstruction of the pulmonary artery or part of the branches of the pulmonary artery; caused by the presence of an embolus

severe respiratory distress extremely difficult breathing that could cause very serious pathological damage unless treated immediately

progressive severe rheumatoid arthritis the most severe, debilitating form of rheumatoid arthritis; a chronic, painful, inflammatory disorder that affects the synovial joints of the human body and encompasses a variety of symptoms throughout the body, including the skin, heart, liver, lungs, and kidneys; requires long-term treatment and managed care

peritonitis inflammation of the lining of the peritoneum, the membrane lining the inside of the abdominal cavity and all the internal organs within the peritoneal cavity

seizure sudden convulsion, contraction, or uncontrolled movements caused by interruptions of the electric impulses of the brain; may also manifest in sensory disturbances or periods of altered consciousness

urinary tract infection (UTI) infectious process involving the urethra, bladder, ureters, or any other part of the urinary tract

cystitis inflammation of the bladder

lumbar puncture an invasive diagnostic procedure that requires the placement of a needle between two spinal vertebrae for the purpose of extracting cerebrospinal fluid; may also be used for therapeutic purposes

contrast medium a substance that is relatively impenetrable by X-rays or other forms of radiation; used in diagnostic radiology such as arteriograms, X-rays, and magnetic resonance imaging

of risk as an acute, uncomplicated illness or injury, whereas pyelonephritis, a complicated UTI that has caused an infection of at least one of the kidneys, is considered a moderate level of risk as an acute illness with systemic symptoms. However, emphysematous pyelonephritis in a patient with type I diabetes is an extremely dangerous condition that causes gas to build up in the kidneys during an infectious process and would be considered a chronic illness with a severe exacerbation due to the type I diabetes.

Diagnostic Procedures Ordered

In certain circumstances, diagnostic procedures are an integral part of discerning the diagnosis; they are considered in the number of diagnoses or management options as well as the amount of data to be reviewed. However, the table of risk considers a different aspect of diagnostic procedures: the risk they pose to the patient.

Although diagnostic procedures are intended to provide specific data about the internal anatomy and physiopathology of the patient's body, every diagnostic procedure poses a certain amount of risk to the patient. Any child who has experienced a strep throat swab would attest to the risk of the throat swab. However, a throat swab poses less risk to a patient than a **lumbar puncture**, which involves the collection of cerebrospinal fluid through a needle inserted into the space between the vertebrae. Since certain diagnostic procedures carry a higher level of risk than others do, the physician who performs the E/M service and has ordered a particular diagnostic procedure should document the level of risk it poses.

There is a wide spectrum of diagnostic procedures, ranging from a urinalysis, which identifies the chemical or microbial content of urine, to an intravenous pyelogram, which uses a **contrast medium** delivered intravenously and radiology imaging to provide a radiologic image of the structures of the urinary tract, including the bladder, ureters, and kidneys. Each diagnostic procedure allows the physician performing the E/M service to identify findings that cannot be seen with the naked eye. For instance, a physician cannot identify the blood chemistry of a patient by palpating the patient's arms; however, the laboratory results of a complete blood count allow that physician to identify the patient's white blood count, the lipid panel, and more. Likewise, a physician would not be able to visualize the bladder, ureters, or kidneys by looking at the patient's lower back; however, with the findings from the intravenous pyelogram, that physician can identify anatomic, physiologic, or pathologic findings that could be helpful in diagnosing the presenting problem.

As with the presenting problem area of the table of risk, the diagnostic procedures ordered area identifies the four different levels of risk and gives common examples of diagnostic procedures that present a specific level of risk to the patient during and immediately after the diagnostic procedure (see ■ TABLE 11.3).

Notice that there are fewer specific examples provided for the levels of risk of diagnostic procedures ordered than for the presenting problem; the reason is that the condition of the patient will often determine the risk posed by the diagnostic procedure. For instance, the risk posed by an upper gastric endoscopy will be different depending on the underlying health and condition of the patient, so the presenting problem should be clearly documented by the physician performing the E/M service. On the other hand, a lumbar puncture procedure poses a higher level of risk regardless of the underlying condition; however, that level of risk may be even more severe depending on the presenting problem.

Certain diagnostic procedures may be performed during the E/M service visit and should be clearly documented along with any findings determined by the procedures. Other diagnostic procedures must be scheduled for another time and performed at a separate location or in a surgical environment, whereas certain clinical circumstances require the diagnostic procedures to be performed immediately because of an emergent health crisis. The physician performing the E/M service who has ordered the diagnostic procedures should document them precisely, which allows their risk to be determined. The type of every diagnostic procedure ordered should be documented and should specify whether the procedure is of a surgical or invasive nature.

Management Option Selected

Consider a toddler who runs to her parent after falling on the playground. The parent assesses the crying child to determine the extent of any injuries and perhaps learns the circumstance of the fall through visual or verbal cues from the child. Then, once the situation has been identified, the parent selects the best way to manage the situation. This management will depend on the health of the child, the circumstances surrounding the parent and child, and the parent's knowledge about the child.

In the same way, the physician performing the E/M service has intimate knowledge about the presenting problem from the collected findings about the patient's history, the physical examination of the patient, and any diagnostic procedures the physician has deemed necessary to discern the diagnosis. With this information, the performing physician identifies and selects at least one specific approach to manage the treatment of the patient's presenting problem. This selection of a management option requires an assessment of the risk posed to the patient, which remains dependent upon the risk of complication,

■ TABLE 11.3   TABLE OF RISK: DIAGNOSTIC PROCEDURES ORDERED

LEVEL OF RISK	DIAGNOSTIC PROCEDURES ORDERED—COMMON EXAMPLES
Minimal	• Laboratory tests requiring **venipuncture**—e.g., blood tests • Chest X-rays • EKG/EEG (**electrocardiogram** or **electroencephalogram**) • Urinalysis • Ultrasound—e.g., **echocardiography** • KOH prep (used to facilitate observations of fungal skin infections)
Low	• Physiologic tests not under stress—e.g., **pulmonary function tests** • Noncardiovascular imaging studies with contrast—e.g., barium enema • Superficial needle biopsies • Clinical laboratory tests requiring **arterial puncture** • Skin biopsies
Moderate	• Physiologic tests under stress—e.g., **cardiac stress test**, **fetal contraction stress test** • Diagnostic **endoscopies** with no identified risk factors • Deep needle or **incisional biopsy** • Cardiovascular imaging studies with contrast and no identified risk factors—e.g., **arteriogram**, **cardiac catheterization** • Obtaining fluid from body cavity—e.g., lumbar puncture, **thoracentesis**, **culdocentesis**
High	• Cardiovascular imaging studies with contrast with identified risk factors • **Cardiac electrophysiological tests** • Diagnostic endoscopies with identified risk factors

Source: Centers for Medicare and Medicaid, "1995 Documentation Guidelines for Evaluation and Management Services," p. 14, www.cms.gov/Outreach-and-Education/Medicare-Learning-Network-MLN/MLNEdWebGuide/Downloads/95Docguidelines.pdf; "1997 Documentation Guidelines for Evaluation and Management Services," p. 50, www.cms.gov/Outreach-and-Education/Medicare-Learning-Network-MLN/MLNEdWebGuide/Downloads/97Docguidelines.pdf.

comorbidity, and/or mortality during and immediately following the management option. Nearly every E/M service results in some management of the presenting problem, regardless of whether the management is as simple as recommending rest or as serious as recommending emergency surgery.

The table of risk identifies the same four levels of risk for the management option selected—minimal, low, moderate, and high—and lists 20 different examples across those levels. These examples range from simply gargling to the difficult decision not to resuscitate a patient. Rather than being strict rules, these examples form guidelines that can help identify the level of risk posed by the management option selected by the physician performing the E/M service (see ■ TABLE 11.4).

Some of the examples listed in this section are self-explanatory, such as "rest" for the minimal level of risk and "emergency major surgery" for the high level of risk. However, other examples may be less obvious. For instance, OTC drugs—such as Tylenol, Advil, and Tums—are an inherent part of the modern world and are available at nearly every pharmacy or grocery store without a prescription. These drugs are taken to cause a positive effect in a person's condition, such as to reduce the severity of a headache or to alleviate nasal congestion. However, the introduction of any substance into the human body causes changes in the body and can affect the health of the body, and OTC drugs are no exception. Unpleasant or unwanted effects caused by OTC drugs are known as "side effects" and are commonly listed on the packaging of the drugs, along with a list of indicators, signs, or symptoms that require immediate medical attention. The possibility that unpleasant side effects could result from taking OTC drugs places the level of risk for this selected management option at low.

Prescription drugs, which can be obtained only with a physician's order and dispensed by a pharmacist, are substances that require the clinical management and oversight of a physician, nurse practitioner,

---

venipuncture puncturing the walls of a vein with a hypodermic needle for the purpose of drawing blood; can also be used in the delivery of therapeutic treatment

electrocardiogram a graphic recording of the electric activity of the heart through the placement of electrodes along the surface of the skin

electroencephalogram a graphic record of the electric waves of the brain through the placement of electrodes along the surface of the scalp

echocardiography the graphic recording of the electric activity of the heart, utilizing ultrasound to create images of the heart

pulmonary function tests a thorough evaluation and assessment of the respiratory function through the collection of patient history, physical examination data, chest X-ray, laboratory blood analysis, and intensive respiratory testing, including spirometry and oxygen desaturation during a 6-mile walk on a treadmill

arterial puncture puncturing the walls of an artery with a hypodermic needle for the purpose of drawing blood; like venipuncture, may also be used in the delivery of therapeutic treatment

cardiac stress test measurement of the heart function and the ability to respond to stress caused by physical activity or pharmacologic stimulation in a controlled clinical environment

fetal contraction stress test ultrasound measurement of the fetal heartbeat during uterine contractions prior to birth

endoscopies internal observation of the structure of the human body, organs, vessels, tubes, or cavities, using an instrument known as an endoscope

incisional biopsy the incision and removal of part of a lesion for the purpose of diagnosis

arteriogram a radiologic view of the arterial structure achieved by injecting contrast medium into the artery and using X-rays

cardiac catheterization the insertion of a catheter into a chamber of the heart for the purpose of diagnosis, measurement, and investigation; may be accomplished through an incision in the femoral artery in the groin

thoracentesis an invasive diagnostic procedure that requires the placement of a needle or tube into the space between the two layers of the pleural lining of the chest for the purpose of extracting collected pleural fluid for diagnostic or therapeutic purposes

culdocentesis an invasive diagnostic procedure that requires the placement of a needle in the rectouterine pouch, or the space between the uterus and the rectum, for the purpose of extracting fluid

cardiac electrophysiological tests invasive and noninvasive diagnostic testing to determine and understand any abnormal heart rhythms; cardiac electrophysiological treatments may also be used for therapeutic purposes

prescription drugs any medication prescribed by a physician and dispensed by a pharmacist

percutaneous referring to the introduction of surgical, therapeutic, or diagnostic devices through the skin

■ TABLE 11.4 TABLE OF RISK: MANAGEMENT OPTION SELECTED

LEVEL OF RISK	MANAGEMENT OPTION SELECTED—COMMON EXAMPLES
Minimal	• Rest • Gargling • Elastic bandages • Superficial bandages
Low	• OTC drugs • Minor surgery with no identified risk factors • Physical therapy • Occupational therapy • Intravenous (IV) fluids without additives
Moderate	• Minor surgery with identified risk factors • Elective major surgery (open, **percutaneous**, or endoscopic) • Prescription drug management • Therapeutic nuclear medicine • Intravenous (IV) fluids with additives • Closed treatment of fracture or dislocation without manipulation
High	• Elective major surgery (open, percutaneous, or endoscopic) with identified risk factors • Emergency major surgery (open, percutaneous, or endoscopic) • Parental-controlled substances • Drug therapy requiring intensive monitoring for toxicity • Decision not to resuscitate or to de-escalate care because of poor prognosis

Source: Centers for Medicare and Medicaid, "1995 Documentation Guidelines for Evaluation and Management Services," p. 14, www.cms.gov/Outreach-and-Education/Medicare-Learning-Network-MLN/MLNEdWebGuide/Downloads/95Docguidelines.pdf; "1997 Documentation Guidelines for Evaluation and Management Services," p. 50, www.cms.gov/Outreach-and-Education/Medicare-Learning-Network-MLN/MLNEdWebGuide/Downloads/97Docguidelines.pdf.

or other qualified clinician. Antibiotics are a good example of a prescription medication. Remember that the introduction of any substance into the body changes the body and has the potential to cause unwanted or unpleasant side effects. The physician performing the E/M service is familiar with the patient's medical history and has performed a physical examination before the prescription medication will be introduced into the patient's body. Therefore, that physician can utilize his or her extensive knowledge and expertise to identify any potential side effects or **contraindications**, that is, medical reasons the patient should not take a specific prescription medication. For example, from previously obtained information, the performing physician may know that the patient is currently taking a different prescription that interacts negatively with a specific antibiotic, thus informing the physician's selection of a management option. Similarly, the performing physician may understand that the patient has an underlying condition or comorbidity that precludes the use of a specific antibiotic. Sometimes a patient may have an unidentified allergy to a specific antibiotic, which increases the risk of complication, comorbidity, or mortality for the patient. Regardless of the specific prescription drug, the overall risk of complication, comorbidity, or mortality for this management option has been identified as moderate.

However, certain prescription medications are more complicated because of their potential side effects—for instance, the anticoagulant warfarin, which is used to reduce the risk of blood clots and is available by prescription under many different brand names, such as Coumadin, Jantoven, and Warrant. One of the most common side effects of warfarin is hemorrhage, which can pose a varying risk of complication, comorbidity, and/or mortality depending on the nature of the hemorrhage. Therefore, all warfarin medications are considered to have a high risk of toxicity and thus to be a **drug therapy requiring intensive monitoring** of a trained healthcare clinician. Accordingly, the level of risk for a warfarin anticoagulant is considered to be high. Likewise, insulin is an important, complicated medication that requires physician discernment, expertise, and knowledge for proper dosing. Because of the need for monitoring insulin dosages, the level of risk of complication, comorbidity, and/or mortality is higher than that of a prescription drug that does not require the same intensive monitoring. Therefore, the management option of insulin therapy is considered to pose a high level of risk.

These three examples illustrate the differences among the four levels of risk for the management option selected; the distinctions can be applied to the other examples listed. Since the performing physician has the extensive training, expertise, and experience to identify the most appropriate management option, there may be times when more than one management option is selected. In that case, the management option with the highest level of risk determines the level of risk for the selected management options. Regardless of the number of management options selected, the physician performing the E/M service should document the selected management option(s) and thus the level of risk.

The Complete Table of Risk

The table of risk allows full consideration of the risk of the presenting problem, the diagnostic procedures ordered, and the management option selected. In a simple-to-read chart, the table provides for an easy review of all four levels of risk, as shown in ■ TABLE 11.5.

In order to identify the overall level of risk, the levels of the presenting problem, diagnostic procedures ordered, and management option selected should all be identified. The highest of the three areas of risk determines the overall level of risk of complication, comorbidity, and mortality posed to the patient.

contraindications physiologic, diagnostic, or medical reasons that indicate that a specific medication, therapy, treatment, or plan of care would be undesirable, unwise, or impossible to prescribe for a patient's health

drug therapy requiring intensive monitoring for toxicity any prescription drug with a significantly higher risk of potentially harmful side effects that may require regular monitoring for appropriate dosing and identification of the onset of potentially harmful side effects or contraindications

---

Example: Documentation of Overall Level of Risk for Sprained Ankle

A patient visits her doctor after spraining her left ankle. Her ankle is sore upon weight bearing. The physician places an elastic bandage on her ankle and recommends rest. The next day, after bathing, the patient replaces the bandage on her ankle but puts it on too tightly, which leads to the complication of inflaming the sprained ankle and straining the Achilles tendon. Physical therapy is prescribed for 3 weeks to reduce the swelling and prevent future injury.

> Presenting problem—one self-limited or minor problem, minimal level of risk
>
> Diagnostic procedures ordered—No diagnostic procedure ordered, minimal level of risk
>
> Management option selected—physical therapy, low level of risk
>
> Overall level of risk—low (determined by the management option selected)

Notice that no diagnostic procedure has been ordered in the previous example, which limits the level of risk posed by the diagnostic procedures ordered to minimal.

Example: Documentation of Overall Level of Risk for Pneumonia, Pleurisy, Bronchitis

A patient visits her MD reporting head congestion producing thick, green, stringlike mucous, body aches and pains, and a fever of 101.1°F. Throat culture results negative. Sputum gram stain and culture negative for Streptococcus pneumonia. Urinalysis positive for S. pneumonia antigen. Ordered chest X-ray.

Diagnosis: Streptococcal pneumonia, pleurisy, and bronchitis.

Plan: Azithromycin prescribed.

> Presenting problem—acute, uncomplicated illness or injury, low level of risk
>
> Diagnostic procedures ordered—urinalysis, sputum culture, and X-ray, minimal level of risk
>
> Management option selected—prescription drug management, moderate level of risk
>
> Overall level of risk—moderate (determined by the management option selected)

Although the sputum culture ordered in the previous example is not listed among the examples of the table of risk, the nonbronchoscopy sputum culture falls within the examples listed under the minimal level of risk for the diagnostic procedures ordered. It is worth noticing that although three different diseases are identified—pneumonia, pleurisy, and bronchitis—each is represented as an acute, uncomplicated illness.

■ TABLE 11.5 COMPLETE TABLE OF RISK

LEVEL OF RISK	PRESENTING PROBLEM	DIAGNOSTIC PROCEDURES ORDERED	MANAGEMENT OPTION SELECTED
Minimal	• One self-limited or minor problem—e.g., cold, insect bite (with no allergic reaction), tinea corporis	• Laboratory tests requiring venipuncture—e.g., blood tests • Chest X-rays • EKG/EEG (electrocardiogram or electroencephalogram) • Urinalysis • Ultrasound—e.g., echocardiography • KOH prep (used to facilitate observations of fungal skin infections)	• Rest • Gargling • Elastic bandages • Superficial bandages
Low	• Two or more self-limited or minor problems (see above) • One stable chronic illness—e.g., well-controlled hypertension, noninsulin dependent diabetes, cataract, benign prostatic hypertrophy • Acute, uncomplicated illness or injury—e.g., cystitis (bladder inflammation), allergic rhinitis, simple sprain	• Physiologic tests not under stress—e.g., pulmonary function tests • Noncardiovascular imaging studies with contrast—e.g., barium enema • Superficial needle biopsies • Clinical laboratory tests requiring arterial puncture • Skin biopsies	• OTC drugs • Minor surgery with no identified risk factors • Physical therapy • Occupational therapy • Intravenous (IV) fluids without additives
Moderate	• One or more chronic illnesses with mild exacerbation, progression, or side effects of treatment—e.g., cystitis with UTI, chronic asthma with viral upper respiratory infection • Two or more stable chronic illnesses (see above) • Undiagnosed new problem with uncertain prognosis—e.g., lump in breast • Acute illness with systemic symptoms—e.g., pyelonephritis, pneumonitis, colitis • Acute uncomplicated injury—e.g., head injury with brief loss of consciousness	• Physiologic tests under stress—e.g., cardiac stress test, fetal contraction stress test • Diagnostic endoscopies with no identified risk factors • Deep needle or incisional biopsy • Cardiovascular imaging studies with contrast and no identified risk factors—e.g., arteriogram, cardiac catheterization • Obtaining fluid from body cavity—e.g., lumbar puncture, thoracentesis, culdocentesis	• Minor surgery with identified risk factors • Elective major surgery (open, percutaneous, or endoscopic) • Prescription drug management • Therapeutic nuclear medicine • Intravenous (IV) fluids with additives • Closed treatment of fracture or dislocation without manipulation
High	• One or more chronic illnesses with severe exacerbation, progression, or side effects of treatment—e.g., complicated UTI with insulin-dependent diabetes, bacterial pneumonia with COPD • Acute or chronic illnesses or injuries that pose a threat to life or bodily function—e.g., multiple trauma, acute MI, pulmonary embolus, severe respiratory distress, progressive severe rheumatoid arthritis, psychiatric illness with potential threat to self or others, peritonitis, acute renal failure • An abrupt change in neurologic status—e.g., seizure, TIA, weakness, or sensory loss	• Cardiovascular imaging studies with contrast with identified risk factors • Cardiac electrophysiological tests • Diagnostic endoscopies with identified risk factors	• Elective major surgery (open, percutaneous, or endoscopic) with identified risk factors • Emergency major surgery (open, percutaneous, or endoscopic) • Parental-controlled substances • Drug therapy requiring intensive monitoring for toxicity • Decision not to resuscitate or to de-escalate care because of poor prognosis

Source: Centers for Medicare and Medicaid, "1995 Documentation Guidelines for Evaluation and Management Services," p. 14, www.cms.gov/Outreach-and-Education/Medicare-Learning-Network-MLN/MLNEdWebGuide/Downloads/95Docguidelines.pdf; "1997 Documentation Guidelines for Evaluation and Management Services," p. 50, www.cms.gov/Outreach-and-Education/Medicare-Learning-Network-MLN/MLNEdWebGuide/Downloads/97Docguidelines.pdf.

> **Example: Documentation of Overall Level of Risk for Pneumonia, Pleurisy, Bronchitis with Mild Diabetic Ketoacidosis**
>
> A patient visits her MD reporting head congestion producing thick, green, stringlike mucous, body aches and pains, and a fever of 101.1°F. Throat culture results negative. Sputum gram stain and culture negative for Streptococcus pneumonia. Urinalysis positive for S. pneumonia antigen, positive for ketones. Ordered chest X-ray. Blood glucose, 55 mg/dl; arterial pH, 7.26; serum bicarbonate, 16 mEq/L; effective serum osmolality is variable.
>
> > **Assessment:** Sputum gram stain and culture positive for Streptococcus pneumonia. Urinalysis positive for S. pneumonia antigen. Mild diabetic ketoacidosis per lab report. Independent visualization of chest X-ray reveals significant inflammation of pleural lining as well as the bronchi.
> >
> > **Diagnosis:** Streptococcal pneumonia, pleurisy, and bronchitis in a patient with mild diabetic ketoacidosis.
> >
> > **Plan:** Admission for IV rehydration; IV doxycycline 100 mg every 12 hours; IV insulin therapy.
> >
> > > Presenting problem—one or more chronic illnesses with severe exacerbation, progression, or side effects of treatment, high level of risk
> > >
> > > Diagnostic procedures ordered—chest X-ray, minimal level of risk
> > >
> > > Management option selected—drug therapy requiring intensive monitoring for toxicity, high level of risk
> > >
> > > Overall level of risk high (determined by both the presenting problem and the management option selected)

Identifying the overall risk of complication, comorbidity, and/or mortality requires identifying the risks of the presenting problem, any ordered diagnostic procedures, and the selected management option and then integrating the levels of risk for these three areas into one overall level of risk.

Exercise 11.1 Overall Level of Risk for Sinus Infection

Using the table of risk, identify the level of risk for the presenting problem, diagnostic procedures ordered, and management option selected in the following medical documentation. Once the respective levels of risk have been identified, identify the overall level of risk and the area of risk that determined the overall level of risk.

History: Patient returns for worsening sinus pressure. The right side of the patient's head hurts so much that she feels she cannot hold her head up due to the throbbing pain. Patient states every part of her hurts now. Patient recognizes flu is likely but is concerned about strep throat.

Exam: Patient is very pale and appears very tired. Conjunctivae red, swollen, and inflamed. Exquisite pain upon palpation of face, particularly the forehead and maxillary sinuses. Copious production of thick, white/brown mucus per nares. Patient unable to open mouth due to pain.

Laboratory: Rapid antigen test negative; throat swab sent for culture. Influenza swab deferred per patient.

Assessment: Sinus infection, probable influenza.

Plan: Azithromycin. Increased fluids, rest. Per patient's request, note written for employer indicating need for 3-day release from work for bed rest.

1. Presenting problem: _____
   Level: _____
2. Diagnostic procedures ordered: _____
   Level: _____
3. Management option selected: _____
   Level: _____
4. Overall level of risk is _____
   Determined by _____

Exercise 11.2 Overall Level of Risk for Rule Out Appendiceal Abscess

Using the table of risk, identify the level of risk for the presenting problem, diagnostic procedures ordered, and management option selected in the following medical documentation. Once the respective levels of risk have been identified, identify the overall level of risk and the area of risk that determined the overall level of risk.

Timmy is a 12-year-old established patient and presents for recurrent abdominal pain. Timmy's pain is localized in the right lower quadrant. Since Timmy's previous visit, his abdominal pain has increased in severity and frequency, preventing him from attending school and requiring him to take pain relievers.

continued

Exercise 11.2 *continued*

Review of systems: Diarrhea has subsided, and negative for bloody stools. Negative for dysuria, hematuria. Negative for fevers, sick contact, or trauma other than the goal-side tackle reported during Timmy's previous visit dated 09/23. All other ROS pertaining to this problem are negative.

Assessment: The severity of the pain makes it prudent to rule out appendiceal abscess.

Plan: Recommend abdominal CT scan, KUB, complete blood panel, and urinalysis. Timmy will return tomorrow morning to provide urine and blood samples for workup. Radiology scheduled for tomorrow afternoon. Return for recheck in 2 days after receipt of radiology scans.

1. Presenting problem: _____
   Level: _____
2. Diagnostic procedures ordered: _____
   Level: _____
3. Management option selected: _____
   Level: _____
4. Overall level of risk is _____
   Determined by _____

Exercise 11.3 Overall Level of Risk for Lower Back Pain

Using the table of risk, identify the level of risk for the presenting problem, diagnostic procedures ordered, and management option selected in the following medical documentation. Once the respective levels of risk have been identified, identify the overall level of risk and the area of risk that determined the overall level of risk.

Joan is an established patient who presents for lower back pain. Her lower back hurts, down by beltline, and pain is sometimes very severe. The pain is sporadic, mostly when standing up after sitting in one place for an extended period. Ibuprofen used to help, but now it does not help back pain anymore. At its worst, low back pain is sharp and throbbing. Joan has had occasional back pain for about 20 years, since first in the service, but she first noticed this particular low back pain shortly after playing touch football with adult children this past Thanksgiving. Patient denies any other joint pain than this low back pain. Patient denies double vision or dizziness, and no chest pain or shortness of breath. Patient denies tobacco or alcohol use. Pain has not affected her work as a fifth-grade teacher.

Plan: Recommend physical therapy, NSAID as needed for inflammation. Follow-up in 6 weeks.

1. Presenting problem: _____
   Level: _____
2. Diagnostic procedures ordered: _____
   Level: _____
3. Management option selected: _____
   Level: _____
4. Overall level of risk is _____
   Determined by _____

Ultimately, the risk of complication, comorbidity, and/or mortality is the medical decision-making element that is most difficult to categorize and clearly represent because the level of risk is completely dependent upon the documentation of the physician who performs the E/M service. The documentation reflects the effort, expertise, and clinical work of that physician.

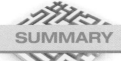

SUMMARY

- The third element of medical decision making is known as the risk of complication, comorbidity, and/or mortality. Each of these represents a different aspect of risk posed to the patient by the three areas of risk: presenting problem, diagnostic procedures ordered, and the management option selected.
- There are four recognized levels of risk of complication, comorbidity, and/or mortality: minimal, low, moderate, and high. Each level reflects a different constellation of hazards to which

the patient is exposed because of the presenting problem, diagnostic procedures ordered, or management option selected.
- The 1995 and 1997 DGs list an organized chart known as the table of risk, which identifies the risk of complication, comorbidity, and/or mortality in the three areas. In order to determine the overall level of risk, the level of risk should be determined for each of the three areas; the highest level of risk among the three areas determines the overall level of risk.

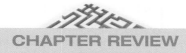

CHAPTER REVIEW

Multiple Choice

Choose the letter that best answers each question or completes each statement.

1. Which of the following best defines a complication?

   a. A disease, illness, or ill health that is separate from the presenting problem but that occurs at the same time as the presenting problem

   b. A pathological development that is not an inherent part of the presenting problem but that occurs in a patient during the management of the patient's presenting problem

   c. The actual death of the patient, or increased potential for death, due to the patient's presenting problem, a drastic worsening of the presenting problem, or associated disease process

   d. A state of disease, illness, or ill health

2. Which of the following best defines a comorbidity?

   a. The actual death of the patient, or increased potential for death, due to the patient's presenting problem, a drastic worsening of the presenting problem, or associated disease process

   b. A state of disease, illness, or ill health

   c. A disease, illness, or ill health that is separate from the presenting problem but that occurs at the same time as the presenting problem

   d. A pathological development that is not an inherent part of the presenting problem but that occurs in a patient during the management of the patient's presenting problem

3. Which of the following best defines mortality?

   a. A pathological development that is not an inherent part of the presenting problem but that occurs in a patient during the management of the patient's presenting problem

   b. A disease, illness, or ill health that is separate from the presenting problem but that occurs at the same time as the presenting problem

   c. A state of disease, illness, or ill health

   d. The actual death of the patient, or increased potential for death, due to the patient's presenting problem, a drastic worsening of the presenting problem, or associated disease process

4. Which of the following best reflects an example of the risk of a selected management option?

   a. The risk posed to the patient by the chief complaint, illness, or disease that brought him or her into the clinic, especially in relation to the interval of time between the current visit and the subsequent visit

   b. The risk posed to the patient by any testing that has been ordered by the physician who performs the E/M service and is intended to help that physician diagnose the complaint

   c. An objective tool to determine the level of risk of complication, comorbidity, and/or mortality in an easy-to-read format

   d. The risk posed to the patient by the therapeutic, resuscitative, or maintenance plan of care selected by the physician performing the E/M service

5. Which of the following best reflects an example of the risk of an ordered diagnostic procedure?

   a. An objective tool to determine the level of risk of complication, comorbidity, and/or mortality in an easy-to-read format

   b. The risk posed to the patient by the chief complaint, illness, or disease that brought him or her into the clinic, especially in relation to the interval of time between the current visit and the subsequent visit

   c. The risk posed to the patient by the therapeutic, resuscitative, or maintenance plan of care selected by the physician performing the E/M service

   d. The risk posed to the patient by any testing that has been ordered by the physician who performs the E/M service and that is intended to help that physician diagnose the complaint

6. Which of the following levels of risk indicates the overall level for the following three areas of risk:

   Presenting problem—undiagnosed new problem with uncertain prognosis

   Diagnostic procedures ordered—deep needle or incisional biopsy

   Management option selected—elective major surgery with no identified risk factors

   a. Minimal

   b. Low

   c. Moderate

   d. High

7. Which of the following best describes how to determine the overall level of risk of complication, comorbidity, and/or mortality?

   a. The area with the lowest level of risk determines the overall level of risk of complication, comorbidity, and/or mortality.

   b. The average risk of all three areas of risk determines the overall level of risk of complication, comorbidity, and/or mortality.

   c. The area with the highest level of risk determines the overall level of risk of complication, comorbidity, and/or mortality.

   d. The performing physician must identify the level of risk in the documentation of the E/M service.

8. In the table of risk, which level of risk is supported by the example "parental-controlled substances"?

   a. Minimal

   b. Low

   c. Moderate

   d. High

9. Which of the following indicates the overall level for the following:

Presenting problem—undiagnosed new problem with uncertain prognosis

Diagnostic procedures ordered—chest X-ray, noncardiovascular imaging studies with contrast (CT scan), diagnostic endoscopies with no identified risk factors

Management option selected—prescription drug management
   a. Minimal
   b. Low
   c. Moderate
   d. High

10. Which of the following indicates the overall level for the following:

Presenting problem—acute, uncomplicated illness or injury

Diagnostic procedures ordered—urinalysis

Management option selected—prescription drug management
   a. Minimal
   b. Low
   c. Moderate
   d. High

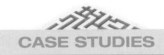

CASE STUDIES

Case Study 11-1

Review the following excerpts from one documented E/M service visit. Using the table of risk, answer questions 1–7 to determine the risk of complication, comorbidity, and/or mortality.

Complaint: I have been asked to consult on James Roberts's abdominal trauma. James Roberts is a 45-year-old new patient who suffered a fall in his home office. Mr. Roberts tripped on the computer cords in his home office and fell onto his office chair, striking his upper abdomen on the armrest of the chair and striking his forehead on the edge of his desk. Patient reports experiencing immediate ULQ pain that he reported as 5/10 at time of fall, but has increased in severity to 7/10. Per patient, there was no LOC. Since that time, he has experienced occasional dizziness and three nosebleeds, each lasting at least 20 minutes. Patient has vomited twice and has noted significant midback pain during each emesis, which he rates at a 7–8/10.

Laboratory: Hemoglobin, 13.5; WBC, 18,000. An abdominal CT scan was reviewed with radiologist; scan showed a small amount of free fluid in ULQ with grade 3 laceration of spleen. Evidence of significant amount of stool within sigmoid and rectum.

Assessment: Patient is hemodynamically stable with splenic laceration no higher than grade 3. No immediate correlation between splenic trauma and previous hernia repair is being considered at this time, although Mr. Roberts's history of alcoholism could affect treatment of splenic trauma. Contacted patient's primary physician in Charleston, Texas, by phone to discuss patient's previous hernia surgery, complications, alcohol-related conditions, and healthcare management related to long history of alcohol use. Pertinent records to be reviewed upon receipt by fax.

Plan: Patient admitted for overnight observation, IV antibiotics with rehydration. Gastroenterology consultation requested for splenic trauma.

1. Which area of risk best reflects the words "patient is hemodynamically stable with splenic laceration no higher than grade 3"?
   a. Presenting problem
   b. Diagnostic procedures ordered
   c. Management option selected
   d. Part of the physical examination

2. What level of risk best reflects the words "patient is hemodynamically stable with splenic laceration no higher than grade 3"?
   a. Minimal
   b. Low
   c. Moderate
   d. High

3. What area of risk best reflects these words: "Hemoglobin, 13.5; WBC, 18,000. An abdominal CT scan was reviewed with radiologist; scan showed a small amount of free fluid in ULQ with grade 3 laceration of spleen. There is evidence of significant amount of stool within sigmoid and rectum"?
   a. Documentation of the physical examination
   b. Presenting problem
   c. Diagnostic procedures ordered
   d. Management option selected

4. What level of risk best reflects these words: "Hemoglobin, 13.5; WBC, 18,000. An abdominal CT scan was reviewed with radiologist; scan showed a small amount of free fluid in ULQ with grade 3 laceration of spleen. There is evidence of significant amount of stool within sigmoid and rectum"?
   a. Minimal
   b. Low
   c. Moderate
   d. High

5. What area of risk best reflects the phrase "patient admitted for overnight observation, IV antibiotics with rehydration"?
   a. Not part of the medical decision making
   b. Presenting problem
   c. Diagnostic procedures ordered
   d. Management option selected

6. What level of risk best reflects the phrase "patient admitted for overnight observation, IV antibiotics with rehydration"?
   a. Minimal
   b. Low
   c. Moderate
   d. High

7. Which of the following levels best reflects the documented overall level of risk of complication, comorbidity, and/or mortality?
   a. Minimal
   b. Low
   c. Moderate
   d. High

Case Study 11-2

Read the following documentation, and then answer questions 1–4 to identify the following elements: overall level of history; type of physical examination, referencing one of the three physical examinations; number of diagnoses and/or management options; amount and/or complexity of data to be reviewed; and level of risk. Remember that Appendix D contains the full content of service worksheet.

Complaint: Frank is well-known to me and presents for sharp left flank pain and dark-orange-colored urine after a fall resulting in blunt abdominal trauma on Saturday afternoon, 2 days ago. He tripped on his dog and fell against the patio railing, striking his upper left abdomen against the decorative wrought iron. Patient reports experiencing immediate stabbing pain across his upper abdomen and down his left flank, which subsided quickly without recurrence. Upon rising on Sunday morning, Frank noticed sharp stabbing pain across ULQ abdomen accompanied by dark, painful bruising in the area of his ULQ where he was struck by the decorative railing. The pain is most severe when he breathes deeply, rating pain at 8/10, and Frank cannot bend his torso without significant pain. Frank reports his urine sample to be very dark and odorous but denies painful urination. He denies any chest pain or racing heartbeat. No reports of tingling of extremities, dizziness, nausea, bloody stool. All other reviews of systems pertinent to this problem are negative. No report of ill contact at work or family, although Frank reports a higher stress level than usual, as budget cuts at work have caused many layoffs, and he is anxious about his employment status at work. There is no history of gastrointestinal disease in family or past medical history.

Physical Exam: T, 97.8F; BP, 106/88; P, 68. Eyes clear without jaundice. Head is atraumatic without tenderness, nodules, or swelling. Neck: no thyromegaly. Auscultation of lungs clear without wheezes or rub. No tactile fremitus noted upon palpation of chest. Auscultation of heart reveals regular rate and rhythm with no abnormal sounds noted. No cervical spine tenderness. No thoracic spine tenderness and no lumbar spine tenderness; however, costovertebral tenderness noted upon palpation. No referred pain in left shoulder. Palpation of lower abdomen reveals soft, nontender abdomen, and no hepatomegaly or tenderness upon upper right quadrant palpation or percussion. Upper left abdomen mildly inflamed with dark circular bruise where patient identifies blow to abdomen. Very tender upper left quadrant upon palpation, and patient's pain precludes deep palpation of spleen. No dullness noted upon percussion of left or right flank. Stool sample collected for occult blood test.

Laboratory: CBC reveals white blood count normal; hemoglobin and hematocrit are normal. A FAST scan abdominal CT scan was reviewed with radiologist. Review of KUB revealed significant stool within sigmoid and rectum. Occult blood test negative.

Assessment: It is quite probable that at least one of the lower left ribs has been fractured, although the patient's pain makes it difficult to make a specific rib identification. A splenic injury should be ruled out through CT scan. In my opinion, it would be prudent to begin oral Augmentin treatment at 875 mg twice a day for 7 days and increase fluid intake. Follow-up in 10 days for recheck.

Utilizing prior knowledge, identify the overall level of history, and explain the supporting rationale for the overall level of history:

1. Overall level of history: _____

2. Explain your rationale._____

_____

Utilizing prior knowledge, identify the physical examination, using either the 1995 body area/organ system guidelines, the general multisystem guidelines, or the single organ–system guidelines.

3. Type of physical examination:_____

4. Which physical examination was referenced: 1995 body area/organ system, 1997 general multisystem, or 1997 single organ system? _____

Utilizing the content of service worksheet that follows, answer questions 5–7 about the medical decision making documented in Case Study 11-2.

	Established presenting problem, stable or improving	Established presenting problem, worsening	New presenting problem, without workup	New presenting problem, with workup
Number of Diagnoses and/or Management Options				
Amount and/or Complexity of Data to Be Reviewed	Ordering or reviewing diagnostic data	Obtaining old records or additional history from someone other than patient	Discussion of diagnostic results with physician who performed diagnostic testing	Independent visualization of image, tracing, or scan by physician performing the E/M service
Risk of Complication, Comorbidity, and/or Mortality	Minimal	Low	Moderate	High

5. Number of diagnoses and/or management options:

   _____

   Is this problem new or established?

   _____

   If this is an established problem, is it stable/improving or worsening? _____

   Is a management option documented?

   _____

   If a management option is documented, what is it?

   _____

6. Amount and/or complexity of data to be reviewed:

   _____

   What documented data have been reviewed?

   _____

Identify the complexity of the data to be reviewed:

   _____

7. Risk of complication, comorbidity, and/or mortality:

   _____

   Presenting problem:_____

   Level of risk:_____

   Diagnostic procedures ordered:_____

   Level of risk:_____

   Management option selected:_____

   Level of risk:_____

   Overall level of risk of complication, comorbidity, and/or mortality:_____

   Determined by_____

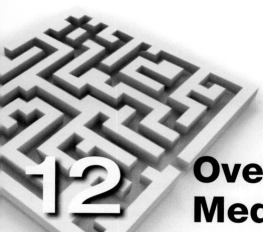

12 Overall Complexity of Medical Decision Making

Learning Objectives

After completing this chapter, you should be able to do the following:

- Spell and define the key terms and abbreviations presented in this chapter
- Identify the four levels of overall medical decision-making complexity
- Recognize the guidelines for selecting the overall medical decision-making complexity
- Utilize the three elements of medical decision making to determine the overall medical decision-making complexity.

Key Terms

anteroposterior

apical

arterial blood gases

bowel obstruction

diaphragmatic

gastroschisis

high medical decision making

hyperextended

intra-abdominal adhesions

intussusception

kyphoplasty

low medical decision making

moderate medical decision making

pleuritic

pneumothorax

positive bone scan

prone

straightforward medical decision making

supine

thoracoabdominal

INTRODUCTION

Every patient is different, which means medical decision making can be a complex process, requiring consideration of each decision-making element. Identifying the levels of all three elements of medical decision making provides clinical insight into the patient's presenting problem, possible diagnosis, and potential plan of care. However, the findings for these three elements reflect only the individual building blocks that produce the complexity of the overall medical decision making. The process of selecting the overall medical decision-making level requires compliance with specific guidelines intended to stream-line this important, multifaceted component of the documented E/M service visit. This chapter examines those guidelines.

THE FOUR LEVELS OF MEDICAL DECISION-MAKING COMPLEXITY

Assigning a quantifiable label to medical decision making can be a difficult task. After all, the decision-making process is inherently complex because of the intricacies of human anatomy, pathologies, and the diagnostic and treatment options through which the physician must sift. However, the 1995 and 1997 DGs classify medical decision making according to four different levels of complexity—straightforward, low, moderate, and high—which indicate an increasing degree of decision-making complexity.

- The straightforward level of medical decision-making complexity is clear, simple, and distinct, involving little or no ambiguity. Even though **straightforward medical decision making** may still be a little complicated, this level of complexity reflects a direct course of evidence that facilitates the physician's final diagnosis of the presenting problem and decision for treatment.
- A low level of medical decision-making complexity involves a more complicated combination of elements, but **low medical decision making** still does not warrant a significant or substantial level of medical decision making on the part of the performing physician.
- **Moderate medical decision making** reflects a complexity that requires a much greater amount of complicated coordination on the part of the performing physician but does not pose an excessive risk to the patient.
- **High medical decision making** indicates a complexity that involves a very intricate process of difficult or extreme decisions, difficult coordination of diagnostic tests or results, complex diagnosis or diagnoses, or convoluted management options, any of which may involve a high risk to the patient.

GUIDELINES FOR SELECTING THE LEVEL OF MEDICAL DECISION MAKING

Each of the four levels of medical decision-making complexity reflects a different constellation of the three elements involved in medical decision making: the number of diagnoses and/or management options, the amount and/or complexity of data to be reviewed, and the risk of complication, comorbidity, and/or mortality. The 1995 and 1997 DGs present these four levels of medical decision-making complexity as shown in ■ FIGURE 12.1, illustrating the complicated process involved in selecting an overall level of medical decision-making complexity.

The top row of Figure 12.1 identifies the levels of medical decision making; the individual elements of medical decision making are identified in the rows below. The format of the figure may seem similar to that of the overall history selection chart, but that similarity is in appearance only, and the similarities end

---

straightforward medical decision making the lowest of the four levels of medical decision making, which reflects a relatively uncomplicated process of medical decision making

low medical decision making one of the four levels of medical decision making that reflects a more complicated combination of medical decision-making elements but does not warrant a significant or substantial level of medical decision making

moderate medical decision making one of the four levels of medical decision making that reflects more complicated coordination on the part of the physician performing the E/M service but does not pose an excessive risk to the patient

high medical decision making one of the four levels of medical decision making that reflects a very intricate process of difficult or extreme decisions, difficult coordination of diagnostic tests or results, complex diagnosis or diagnoses, or convoluted management options, all of which may involve a high risk to the patient

---

Level of Medical Decision-Making Complexity	Straightforward	Low	Moderate	High
Number of Diagnoses and/or Management Options	Established presenting problem, stable or improving	Established presenting problem, worsening	New presenting problem, without workup	New presenting problem, with workup
Amount and/or Complexity of Data to Be Reviewed	Ordering or reviewing diagnostic data	Obtaining old records or additional history from someone other than patient	Discussion of diagnostic results with physician who performed diagnostic testing	Independent visualization of image, tracing, or scan by physician performing the E/M service
Risk of Complication, Comorbidity, and/or Mortality	Minimal	Low	Moderate	High

Figure 12.1 ■ Content of service element: overall medical decision-making complexity.

there. Whereas the selection of the overall history level is determined by the lowest individual history element, the selection of the medical decision-making complexity is determined in a different manner. The 1995 and 1997 DGs state that to determine the level of overall medical decision-making complexity, "two of the three elements in the table must be either met or exceeded."[1]

UTILIZING THE THREE ELEMENTS IN SELECTING THE LEVEL OF MEDICAL DECISION MAKING

The significant complexity of medical decision making stems from the myriad of possible circumstances faced by the physician performing the E/M service. These circumstances are documented in the number of diagnoses and/or management options, the amount and/or complexity of the data to be reviewed, and the risk of complication, comorbidity, and/or mortality. The requirement that only two of the three elements must be met or exceeded to justify the selection of that overall level of complexity results in quite a variety of possible combinations of the individual medical decision-making elements. ■ FIGURE 12.2 shows some of those possible combinations to justify a low level of overall medical decision-making complexity.

Notice that in each of the five examples listed in Figure 12.2, a low level of overall medical decision-making complexity has been met or exceeded by the individual elements of medical decision making. In this way, the intricate and involved medical decision-making process of the physician performing the E/M service can be portrayed in an equitable manner that respects the varying possibilities of the many clinical circumstances that could face the physician.

Exercise 12.1 Overall Level of Medical Decision-Making Complexity for Sinus Pressure

Using the medical decision-making selection chart provided, identify the level of medical decision-making complexity documented in the following case.

History: Patient returns for worsening sinus pressure. The right side of the patient's head hurts so much that she feels she cannot hold her head up due to the throbbing pain. Patient states every part of her hurts now. Patient recognizes flu is likely but is concerned about strep throat.

Exam: Patient is very pale and appears very tired. Conjunctivae are red, swollen, and inflamed bilaterally, with greenish mucus along ducts. Exquisite pain upon palpation of face, particularly the forehead and maxillary sinuses.

Copious production of thick, white/brown mucus per nares. Patient is unable to open mouth due to pain. Pleural rub noted upon auscultation of lungs. Tactile fremitus identified upon palpation.

Laboratory: CBC panel reveals elevated WBC at 11,000. Rapid antigen test negative; throat swab sent for culture.

Assessment: Sinus infection, probable influenza with secondary pneumonia infection.

Plan: Azithromycin prescribed for pneumonia; hydrocodone polystirex prescribed for cough suppression. Increased fluids, rest. Per patient's request, note written for employer indicating need for 3-day release from work for bed rest.

Level of Medical Decision-Making Complexity	Straightforward Complexity	Low Complexity	Moderate Complexity	High Complexity
Number of Diagnoses and/or Management Options	Minimal	Limited	Moderate	Extensive
Amount and/or Complexity of Data to Be Reviewed	Minimal or none	Limited	Moderate	Extensive
Risk of Complication, Comorbidity, and/or Mortality	Minimal	Low	Moderate	High

Identify the overall complexity of medical decision making: _____

_____   _____

---

[1]Centers for Medicare and Medicaid Services, "1995 Documentation Guidelines for Evaluation and Management Services," p. 11, www.cms.gov/Outreach-and-Education/Medicare-Learning-Network-MLN/MLNEdWebGuide/Downloads/95Docguidelines.pdf; "1997 Documentation Guidelines for Evaluation and Management Services," p. 46, www.cms.gov/Outreach-and-Education/Medicare-Learning-Network-MLN/MLNEdWebGuide/Downloads/95Docguidelines.pdf.

Example 1: Low Medical Decision-Making Complexity

Level of Medical Decision-Making Complexity	Straightforward Complexity	Low Complexity	Moderate Complexity	High Complexity
Number of Diagnoses and/or Management Options	Minimal	Limited	Moderate	Extensive
Amount and/or Complexity of Data to Be Reviewed	Minimal or none	Limited	Moderate	Extensive
Risk of Complication, Comorbidity, and/or Mortality	Minimal	Low	Moderate	High

Example 2: Low Medical Decision-Making Complexity

Level of Medical Decision-Making Complexity	Straightforward Complexity	Low Complexity	Moderate Complexity	High Complexity
Number of Diagnoses and/or Management Options	Minimal	Limited	Moderate	Extensive
Amount and/or Complexity of Data to Be Reviewed	Minimal or none	Limited	Moderate	Extensive
Risk of Complication, Comorbidity, and/or Mortality	Minimal	Low	Moderate	High

Example 3: Low Medical Decision-Making Complexity

Level of Medical Decision-Making Complexity	Straightforward Complexity	Low Complexity	Moderate Complexity	High Complexity
Number of Diagnoses and/or Management Options	Minimal	Limited	Moderate	Extensive
Amount and/or Complexity of Data to Be Reviewed	Minimal or none	Limited	Moderate	Extensive
Risk of Complication, Comorbidity, and/or Mortality	Minimal	Low	Moderate	High

Example 4: Low Medical Decision-Making Complexity

Level of Medical Decision-Making Complexity	Straightforward Complexity	Low Complexity	Moderate Complexity	High Complexity
Number of Diagnoses and/or Management Options	Minimal	Limited	Moderate	Extensive
Amount and/or Complexity of Data to Be Reviewed	Minimal or none	Limited	Moderate	Extensive
Risk of Complication, Comorbidity, and/or Mortality	Minimal	Low	Moderate	High

Example 5: Low Medical Decision-Making Complexity

Level of Medical Decision-Making Complexity	Straightforward Complexity	Low Complexity	Moderate Complexity	High Complexity
Number of Diagnoses and/or Management Options	Minimal	Limited	Moderate	Extensive
Amount and/or Complexity of Data to Be Reviewed	Minimal or none	Limited	Moderate	Extensive
Risk of Complication, Comorbidity, and/or Mortality	Minimal	Low	Moderate	High

Figure 12.2 ■ Five examples of low medical decision-making complexity.

Exercise 12.2 **Overall Level of Medical Decision-Making Complexity for Rule Out Appendiceal Abscess**

Using the medical decision-making selection chart provided, identify the level of medical decision-making complexity documented in the following case.

Timmy is a 12-year-old who presents to the emergency room for severe abdominal pain. Patient's most severe pain is localized in the right lower quadrant, but entire belly hurts. Patient tackled during soccer game 1 week ago, and pain has steadily increased in severity since that day. Patient reports diarrhea for 2 days after tackle, followed by fatigue and loss of appetite. Low-grade fever developed 2 days ago. Patient awakened by severe abdominal pain, and father noted high temperature, patient's distress, and brought his son to the ER.

ROS: Negative for bloody stools, dysuria, hematuria. All other ROS pertaining to this problem are negative.

Past medical history: **Gastroschisis** at birth, repaired at 2 days. No history of small **bowel obstruction, intra-abdominal adhesions**, or **intussuseption**. No family history of abdominal problems.

Physical exam: T, 38.4°C. Timmy is very uncomfortable and clearly in distress. Significant guarding of tense abdomen and exquisite pain precluded any prolonged abdominal exam. Extreme pain when asked to cough.

Diagnostic: WBC, 22,000; CRP, 150 mg/L. KUB reveals free air.

Exercise 12.2 *continued*

Assessment: Possible intra-abdominal adhesions with likely ruptured appendix.

Plan: Emergency appendectomy for rupture with suspected intra-abdominal adhesions.

Level of Medical Decision-Making Complexity	Straightforward Complexity	Low Complexity	Moderate Complexity	High Complexity
Number of Diagnoses and/or Management Options	Minimal	Limited	Moderate	Extensive
Amount and/or Complexity of Data to Be Reviewed	Minimal or none	Limited	Moderate	Extensive
Risk of Complication, Comorbidity, and/or Mortality	Minimal	Low	Moderate	High

Identify the overall complexity of medical decision making: _____

Exercise 12.3 Overall Level of Medical Decision-Making Complexity for Lower Back Pain

Using the medical decision-making selection chart provided, identify the level of medical decision-making complexity documented in the following case.

Joan is an established patient who presents for lower back pain. Her lower back hurts, down by beltline, and pain is sometimes very severe. The pain is sporadic, mostly when standing up after sitting in one place for an extended period. Ibuprofen used to help, but now it does not help back pain anymore. At its worst, low back pain is sharp and throbbing. Joan has had occasional back pain for about 20 years, since first in the service, but she first noticed this particular low back pain shortly after playing touch football with adult children this past Thanksgiving. Patient denies any other joint pain than this low back pain. Patient denies double vision or dizziness, and no chest pain or shortness of breath. Patient denies tobacco or alcohol use. Pain has not affected her work as a fifth-grade teacher.

Plan: Suspected vertebral fracture between T12 and L2 vertebrae. MRI scheduled to rule out vertebral fracture. Request for consult made to Dr. Backouch of Southwestern Pain Management. NSAID as needed for inflammation with recommendation of light activity prior to MRI.

Level of Medical Decision-Making Complexity	Straightforward Complexity	Low Complexity	Moderate Complexity	High Complexity
Number of Diagnoses and/or Management Options	Minimal	Limited	Moderate	Extensive
Amount and/or Complexity of Data to Be Reviewed	Minimal or none	Limited	Moderate	Extensive
Risk of Complication, Comorbidity, and/or Mortality	Minimal	Low	Moderate	High

Identify the overall complexity of medical decision making: _____

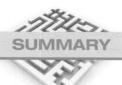

SUMMARY

- The four levels of complexity identified in the 1995 and 1997 DGs are straightforward, low, moderate, and high. Each level reflects an assorted constellation of the individual elements of medical decision making: number of diagnoses and/or management options, amount and/or complexity of data to be reviewed, and risk of complication, comorbidity, and/or mortality.

- Determination of the overall medical decision-making complexity requires two of the three elements in the table to be either met or exceeded. This guideline recognizes an inherent amount of variation among and within the individual decision-making elements.

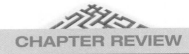

CHAPTER REVIEW

Multiple Choice

Choose the letter that best answers each question or completes each statement.

1. Which of the following reflects the guideline defined by the 1995 and 1997 DGs to determine the overall level of medical decision-making complexity?
   a. To qualify for a given level, all three of the elements in the table must be met.
   b. To qualify for a given level, at least two of the three elements in the table must be met or exceeded.
   c. To qualify for a given level, the highest element determines the overall level.
   d. To qualify for a given level, specific elements identified by a bullet must be documented.

2. Which of the following reflects the four levels of overall medical decision-making complexity defined in the 1995 and 1997 DGs?
   a. Problem-focused, expanded problem-focused, detailed, comprehensive
   b. Straightforward, low, moderate, high
   c. Minimal, low, moderate, extensive
   d. None, pertinent, extended, complete

3. Which of the following levels of overall medical decision-making complexity reflects a direct course of evidence that facilitates the final decision with little or no ambiguity?
   a. Straightforward complexity
   b. Low complexity
   c. Moderate complexity
   d. High complexity

4. Which of the following levels of overall medical decision-making complexity reflects a higher, but not excessive, amount of complexity facing the physician performing the E/M service?
   a. High complexity
   b. Low complexity
   c. Straightforward complexity
   d. Moderate complexity

5. Which of the following levels of overall medical decision-making complexity reflects a more complicated constellation of decision-making elements facing the performing physician but does not pose excessive risk to the patient?
   a. Moderate complexity
   b. Low complexity
   c. Straightforward complexity
   d. High complexity

6. Which of the following levels of overall medical decision-making complexity reflects an intricate process of difficult or extreme decisions that involve a high risk to the patient?
   a. High complexity
   b. Low complexity
   c. Straightforward complexity
   d. Moderate complexity

7. Identify the overall level of medical decision-making complexity for the following clinical excerpt:

   A new patient presents for an E/M service in a physician's office with complaints of recent, extreme headaches and recent dizziness. Physical exam reveals numbness in the fingers of the patient's right hand and little response during the Babinski test. Complete blood and urinalysis workup ordered, CT scan of the patient's head, and referral made to neurologist for peripheral numbness and suspected previous transient ischemic attack.

   a. Straightforward complexity
   b. Low complexity
   c. Moderate complexity
   d. High complexity

8. Identify the overall level of medical decision-making complexity for the following clinical excerpt:

   An 85-year-old woman presents to orthopedic surgeon due to confirmed fracture of L1 vertebra. Orthopedic surgeon recommends **balloon kyphoplasty**. No diagnostic testing required; however, orthopedic surgeon independently reviewed images of **positive bone scan**. Extensive discussion with patient regarding risks of surgery, potential complications, and postsurgical expectations. Patient agrees to kyphoplasty. Surgery scheduled for next week.

   a. Straightforward complexity
   b. Low complexity
   c. Moderate complexity
   d. High complexity

9. The medical documentation of an E/M service visit supports the following levels of medical decision-making elements:

   Number of diagnoses and/or management options: extensive (new problem with workup)

   Amount and/or complexity of data reviewed: minimal (ordered X-ray, reviewed lab tests)

   Risk of complication, comorbidity, and/or mortality: moderate (undiagnosed new problem with uncertain prognosis)

   Which of the following levels best reflects the overall medical decision-making complexity?

   a. Straightforward complexity
   b. Low complexity
   c. Moderate complexity
   d. High complexity

10. The medical documentation of an E/M service visit supports the following levels of medical decision-making elements:

    Number of diagnoses and/or management options: established problem, stable

Amount and/or complexity of data reviewed: positive rapid strep test

Risk of complication, comorbidity, and/or mortality: flulike symptoms, no additional data other than rapid strep test; antibiotics prescribed

Which of the following levels best reflects the overall medical decision-making complexity?

a. Straightforward complexity

b. Low complexity

c. Moderate complexity

d. High complexity

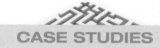

Case Study 12-1

Review the following excerpts from one documented E/M service visit. Using the table of risk, answer questions 1–7 to determine the risk of complication, comorbidity, and/or mortality.

Complaint: James Roberts is a well-known patient who presents for recent abdominal trauma that occurred 2 days ago. James fell in his bathroom after stepping out of the shower and slipping on the wet tile floor. He fell heavily against the edge of the sink, **hyperextended** his right wrist, and sprained his left ankle during the process. Patient reports hearing cracks and experiencing immediate, extreme upper abdominal pain that he reported as 9/10 at time of fall. His pain lessened significantly directly after his fall but has increased in severity to 7/10 as the weekend progressed. Per patient, there was no LOC as a direct result of the fall, although he reports dizzy spells over the last 24 hours, especially after rising from a **supine** or **prone** position. His wife wrapped an elastic bandage around his chest because James assumed he had cracked some ribs due to his pain while breathing. His pain increased over the weekend, and this morning, when he removed the bandage, he noted significant upper abdominal bruising and tenderness, as well as swollen left ankle and weak, swollen right wrist. His primary concern is his abdomen and painful respiration. James reports no nausea or vomiting, no bloody stool, blood in urine, or painful urination. No episodes of syncope, only the dizziness noted above. James reports breathing causes severe pain, especially when lying prone. James's wife was present during visit and reported that James's dyspnea interfered with sleep, causing him to vocalize during the night, which James does not remember. His wife reports notation of significant swelling of bruised area of upper abdomen this morning.

Physical examination: Abdomen tender; however, significant guarding noted. Patient describes excruciating **pleuritic** chest pain upon palpation and when asked to cough.

Laboratory: Complete blood count reveals normal results, specifically hemoglobin, hematocrit, and WBC. **Arterial blood gases** reveal decreased oxygen.

Imaging: Anteroposterior chest X-ray demonstrates three left lateral lower rib fractures of 8–11 with small **apical pneumothorax** on the left.

Assessment: Patient has fracture of at least three ribs between ribs 8 and 11. Patient's dyspnea recommends rule out of **diaphragmatic** injury. CT scan scheduled to rule out diaphragmatic injury, as well as identify any splenic trauma. Patient sent to hospital for immediate CT scan with Dr. Bellyoch.

Plan: CT scan scheduled to rule out diaphragmatic injury, as well as identify any splenic trauma. After telephone conference with general surgeon Dr. Smothbell, patient sent to hospital for immediate **thoracoabdominal** CT scan. Spoke directly with radiologist Dr. Radyo regarding CT scan and the potential urgency of patient's pathology. Request for consultation submitted to Dr. Smothbell of general surgery upon completion of abdominal CT scan. Tylenol recommended for pain caused by rib fracture; a prescription for Tylenol 3 will be available in the event traumatic diaphragmatic injury is ruled out.

1. Which of the following best reflects the number of diagnoses and/or management options?
   a. Minimal (established problem, stable)
   b. Limited (established problem, worsening)
   c. Moderate (new problem requiring no diagnostic workup)
   d. Extensive (new problem requiring diagnostic workup)

2. Which of the following best reflects the amount and/or complexity of data to be reviewed?
   a. Minimal or none (either no data reviewed, or only diagnostic laboratory tests reviewed or ordered)
   b. Limited (order/review of diagnostic laboratory tests, order/review of diagnostic radiology tests, collection of history from someone other than patient)
   c. Moderate (order/review of diagnostic laboratory tests, order/review of diagnostic radiology tests, collection of history from someone other than patient, independent review of radiology scan)
   d. Extensive (order/review of diagnostic laboratory tests, order/review of diagnostic radiology tests, collection of history from someone other than patient, independent review of radiology scan, discussion of presenting problem with another clinician, specifically general surgeon and radiologist)

3. Using the table of risk, which of the following best reflects the risk of complication, comorbidity, and/or mortality posed by the presenting problem(s)?
   a. Minimal
   b. Low
   c. Moderate
   d. High

4. Using the table of risk, which of the following best reflects the risk of complication, comorbidity, and/or mortality posed by the diagnostic procedures ordered?

   a. Minimal

   b. Low

   c. Moderate

   d. High

5. Using the table of risk, which of the following best reflects the risk of complication, comorbidity, and/or mortality posed by the management options selected?

   a. Minimal

   b. Low

   c. Moderate

   d. High

6. Which of the following best reflects the risk of complication, comorbidity, and/or mortality? (Hint: Remember the highest level of risk determines the overall risk of complication, comorbidity, and/or mortality.)

   a. Minimal

   b. Low

   c. Moderate

   d. High

7. Using the following medical decision-making selection chart, which of the following best reflects the overall level of medical decision-making complexity?

   a. Straightforward complexity

   b. Low complexity

   c. Moderate complexity

   d. High complexity

Level of Medical Decision-Making Complexity	Straightforward Complexity	Low Complexity	Moderate Complexity	High Complexity
Number of Diagnoses and/or Management Options	Minimal	Limited	Moderate	Extensive
Amount and/or Complexity of Data to Be Reviewed	Minimal or none	Limited	Moderate	Extensive
Risk of Complication, Comorbidity, and/or Mortality	Minimal	Low	Moderate	High

Case Study 12-2

Read the following documentation, and then answer the questions that follow, identifying the specified content of service elements. Remember that Appendix D contains the full content of service worksheet.

Complaint: Frank is well-known to me and presents for sharp left flank pain and dark-orange-colored urine after a fall resulting in blunt abdominal trauma on Saturday afternoon, 2 days ago. He tripped on his dog and fell against the patio railing, striking his upper left abdomen against the decorative wrought iron. Patient reports experiencing immediate stabbing pain across his upper abdomen and down his left flank, which subsided quickly without recurrence. Upon rising on Sunday morning, Frank noticed sharp stabbing pain across ULQ abdomen accompanied by dark, painful bruising in the area of his ULQ where he was struck by the decorative railing. The pain is most severe when he breathes deeply, rating pain at 8/10, and Frank cannot bend his torso without significant pain. Frank reports his urine sample to be very dark and odorous but denies painful urination. He denies any chest pain or racing heartbeat. No reports of tingling of extremities, dizziness, nausea, bloody stool. All other reviews of systems pertinent to this problem are negative. No report of ill contact at work or family, although Frank reports a higher stress level than usual, as budget cuts at work have caused many layoffs, and he is anxious about his employment status at work. There is no history of gastrointestinal disease in family or past medical history.

Physical Exam: T, 97.8F; BP, 106/88; P, 72. Eyes clear without jaundice. Head is atraumatic without tenderness, nodules, or swelling. Neck: no thyromegaly. Auscultation of lungs clear without wheezes or rub. No tactile fremitus noted upon palpation of chest. Auscultation of heart reveals regular rate and rhythm with no abnormal sounds noted. No cervical spine tenderness. No thoracic spine tenderness and no lumbar spine tenderness; however, costovertebral tenderness noted upon palpation. No referred pain in left shoulder. Palpation of lower abdomen reveals soft, nontender abdomen, and no hepatomegaly or tenderness upon upper right quadrant palpation or percussion. Upper left abdomen mildly inflamed with dark circular bruise where patient identifies blow to abdomen. Very tender upper left quadrant upon palpation, and patient's pain precludes deep palpation of spleen. No dullness noted upon percussion of left or right flank. Stool sample collected for occult blood test.

Laboratory: CBC reveals white blood count normal; hemoglobin and hematocrit are normal. A FAST scan abdominal CT scan was reviewed with radiologist. Review of KUB revealed significant stool within sigmoid and rectum. Occult blood test negative.

Assessment: It is quite probable that at least one of the lower left ribs has been fractured, although the patient's pain makes it difficult to make a specific rib identification. A splenic injury should be ruled out through CT scan. In my opinion, it would be prudent to begin oral Augmentin treatment at 875 mg twice a day for 7 days and increase fluid intake. Follow-up in 10 days for recheck.

Utilizing prior knowledge, identify the overall level of history, and explain the supporting rationale for it.

1. Overall level of history: _____

2. Explain your rationale. _____

   Utilizing prior knowledge, identify the type of physical examination, using the 1995 body area/organ system guidelines, the general multisystem guidelines, or the single organ–system guidelines.

3. Type of physical examination: _____

4. Which physical examination was referenced: 1995 body area/organ system, 1997 general multisystem, or 1997 single organ system? _____

Level of Medical Decision-Making Complexity	Straightforward Complexity	Low Complexity	Moderate Complexity	High Complexity
Number of Diagnoses and/or Management Options	Minimal	Limited	Moderate	Extensive
Amount and/or Complexity of Data to Be Reviewed	Minimal or none	Limited	Moderate	Extensive
Risk of Complication, Comorbidity, and/or Mortality	Minimal	Low	Moderate	High

Utilizing prior knowledge, identify the complexity of medical decision making.

5. Number of diagnoses and/or management options:

_____

Is this problem new or established?_____

If this is an established problem, is it stable/improving or worsening?_____

Is a management option documented? _____

If a management option is documented, what is the management option?_____

6. Amount and/or complexity of data to be reviewed:

_____

What documented data have been reviewed?_____

Identify the complexity of the data to be reviewed:

_____

7. Risk of complication, comorbidity, or mortality:

Presenting problem: _____

Level of risk: _____

Diagnostic procedures ordered: _____

Level of risk: _____

Management options selected: _____

Level of risk: _____

Overall level of risk of complication, comorbidity, or mortality:

_____

Determined by_____

8. Overall complexity of medical decision making:

_____

gastroschisis a congenital defect that is identified at birth, characterized by a defect in the abdominal wall that allows intestinal contents to protrude outside the abdominal cavity; requires surgical intervention to return intestinal contents to the abdominal cavity and repair the abdominal wall

bowel obstruction anything that prevents the normal flow and function of the small or large intestines; may be caused by a foreign body, a pathological process, anatomical defect, or abnormal collection of waste

intra-abdominal adhesions fibrous bands that form between organs and/or tissues within the abdominal cavity, most commonly after an injury or during postoperative recovery; often referred to as internal scar tissue

intussusception an intestinal condition in which part of the small intestine folds in on itself, thereby creating a telescope-like compression as the walls of the small intestine rub together; requires emergency intervention

kyphoplasty a percutaneous surgical procedure that utilizes fluoroscopic radiologic guidance and is used to repair collapsed or fractured vertebrae; involves the placement of a small balloon into which a specific kind of cement is injected, thereby reducing the deformity caused by the fracture or the collapse (sometimes referred to as "balloon kyphoplasty")

positive bone scan a specific kind of diagnostic test that utilizes X-rays to measure the calcium content in the bone, often in the lumbar region of the back

hyperextended bentto an extreme angle farther than the normal range of motion

supine lying on the back; often refers to blood pressure that is taken when the patient is lying down

prone lying face down

pleuritic related to pleurisy

arterial blood gases the oxygen and carbon dioxide content of the blood as measured in diagnostic laboratory tests

anteroposterior view from the front to the back of the body, as in the direction of an X-ray image

apical referring to the tip, as in an apical pneumothorax, which is the accumulation of air or gas in the pleural cavity at the tip of the lung

pneumothorax an abnormal presence of air or gas within the pleural cavity, which can cause pain, difficult breathing, or lung collapse; may be the result of an injury or illness or could be surgically induced as a form of treatment

diaphragmatic related to the diaphragm, the sheet of muscle that separates the organs within the chest cavity from the organs within the abdominal cavity

thoracoabdominal related to the thorax and the abdomen

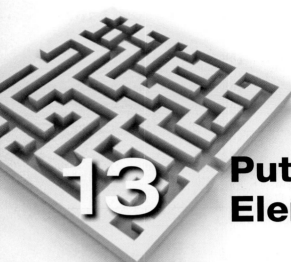

13 Putting Components and Elements Together

Learning Objectives

After completing this chapter, you should be able to do the following:

- Spell and define the key terms and abbreviations presented in this chapter
- Utilize all of the components and elements of the content of service together
- Recognize the site of service and patient type from the language used in the clinical documentation
- Identify the contributing components: counseling and coordination of care
- Recognize the elements of time and the nature of the presenting problem
- Identify the two types of intraservice time
- Identify the typical time requirements for specific E/M service visit codes

Key Terms

coordination of care

counseling

diagnostic laparoscopy

face-to-face time

intraservice time

site of service

typical time

unit/floor time

INTRODUCTION

The 1995 and 1997 DGs present specific guidelines for the documentation of the various elements of the E/M content of service—the history, physical examination, and medical decision making. Each one of these elements is made up of different components, all of which function together to clearly reflect the performed E/M service, as shown in Appendix C: The Anatomy of the Evaluation and Management Medical Documentation. However, the documentation of the service varies, depending on the needs of the patient, the nature of the presenting problem, and the place of service. Therefore, it is important to recognize how to utilize the elements of the content of service together, as well as identify any additional components that augment, support, or supersede these components. On the strong foundation of content of service comprehension, further knowledge about E/M service visits can build a clear awareness about the wide-ranging E/M service visit codes. This chapter builds on previous knowledge and introduces the components of counseling, coordination of care, and the element of time that contribute to identifying the level of the E/M service visit.

UTILIZING ALL OF THE CONTENT OF SERVICE ELEMENTS: HISTORY, PHYSICAL EXAMINATION, AND MEDICAL DECISION MAKING

The individual elements have all been introduced and studied: the history elements, the three different physical examinations, and the medical decision-making elements. The 1995 and 1997 DGs give specific guidelines for the documentation of the content of service through the guidelines for each of these key components and their composite elements. Those guidelines extend to identifiable numeric indicators for the levels of each component; these individual elements function in concert to identify the overall complexity of the performed E/M service visit. ■ FIGURE 13.1 shows the five numeric levels of overall content of service complexity and the individual component levels for each of those five levels.

Remember that each of the three components utilizes definite levels to reflect a particular level of documentation. The individual levels of these components then support the level of the E/M service. ■ FIGURE 13.2 illustrates how the individual component levels determine the overall level of service for a detailed overall history, detailed physical examination, and a low level of medical decision making. The manner in which the levels of the individual components determine the overall level of service is remarkably similar to the selection of the overall history, or the overall level of medical decision-making complexity. This figure illustrates a simple example because all of the individual component levels are the same.

However, what happens if the individual component levels are disparate, as in ■ FIGURE 13.3, which shows a comprehensive history, detailed physical examination, and straightforward medical decision

Content of Service	Level 1	Level 2	Level 3	Level 4	Level 5
History	Problem-focused	Expanded problem-focused	Detailed	Comprehensive	Comprehensive
Physical Examination	Problem-focused	Expanded problem-focused	Detailed	Comprehensive	Comprehensive
Medical Decision Making	Straightforward	Straightforward	Low	Moderate	Comprehensive

Figure 13.1 ■ Levels of the key components within the overall levels of service.

Content of Service	Level 1	Level 2	Level 3	Level 4	Level 5
History	Problem-focused	Expanded problem-focused	Detailed	Comprehensive	Comprehensive
Physical Examination	Problem-focused	Expanded problem-focused	Detailed	Comprehensive	Comprehensive
Medical Decision Making	Straightforward	Straightforward	Low	Moderate	Comprehensive

Figure 13.2 ■ How individual levels determine the overall level of service.

Content of Service	Level 1	Level 2	Level 3	Level 4	Level 5
History	Problem-focused	Expanded problem-focused	Detailed	Comprehensive	Comprehensive
Physical Examination	Problem-focused	Expanded problem-focused	Detailed	Comprehensive	Comprehensive
Medical Decision Making	Straightforward	Straightforward	Low	Moderate	Comprehensive

Figure 13.3 ■ Varying levels for the individual content of service components.

making? In the case of varying levels for the components, certain specific questions must be asked about the site of service and patient type in order to determine the parameters for the specific E/M service visit. These questions address the location in which the E/M service visit took place and the status of the patient as a new or established patient. Both site of service and patient type significantly impact the professional relationship between the physician and the patient and consequently also impact the overall level of E/M service.

SITE OF SERVICE AND PATIENT TYPE

In reviewing the documentation of an E/M service visit, several factors must be considered: where this service visit occurred and whether this physician has treated this patient before. These two factors address the site of service and the patient type.

Site of Service

site of service the location in which an E/M service visit occurs

E/M services occur in many different locations, such as the physician's office, an emergency room, hospital inpatient, and home service, to name a few. Each of these different locations is known as a **site of service**, or the location in which an E/M service visit occurs. Each different kind of site presents a different set of parameters, requirements, and circumstances that influence the E/M service visit as a whole. Therefore, the specific site of service should be documented; it illustrates the environment and conditions in which that specific E/M service visit occurred. After all, an emergency room site of service would present a very different environment from a home, with a completely different set of conditions for the physician, nurse practitioner, or other qualified healthcare professional.

The CPT manual provides an exhaustive list of numerical codes that represent the many different E/M service visits. These numerical codes are separated into different categories, each of which represents a different site of service. One specific list of codes represents the E/M service visits performed in an office or other outpatient setting, whereas a completely different series of codes represents the visits performed in an emergency department. For each category, a different set of guidelines offers specific rules, parameters, and expectations for the E/M services performed in that specific site of service. Included in these guidelines are the requirements for the content of service, specifically the documented levels for the history, physical examination, and medical decision making. The guidelines and requirements provide clear parameters for the required levels of each key component of the content of service. It is important to note that this text specifically addresses the guidelines and requirements identified in the CPT manual.

Patient Type: New Patient versus Established Patient

Not only are there many different sites of service in which E/M service visits occur, but there are two different circumstances in which a physician can see a patient for an E/M service visit. These two different circumstances address the patient type. The patient type identifies whether the patient is a new patient or an established patient, using the same distinctions made in determining the past, family, and social history. In order for the patient type to meet a new patient definition, the patient must not have received any professional, medical, or other healthcare services from the performing physician, or another physician of the exact same specialty and subspecialty who also belongs to the same group practice, during the 3 years prior to the E/M service visit in question. On the other hand, to qualify as an established patient, the patient must have received professional, medical, or other healthcare services from the performing physician, or another physician of the exact same specialty and subspecialty who also belongs to the same group practice, during the 3 years prior to the E/M service visit in question. The rationale for this distinction is quite logical and bears great significance.

New Patient Type

Two people approach one another for their very first meeting. By definition, the phrase "very first meeting" suggests that neither person knows anything about the other, which means that initial introductory questions are required to become familiar with one another. Interrogative questions inform each person about the other, thereby providing a foundation of understanding and familiarity with one another.

Consider a similar situation between a physician and a patient during an E/M service visit. The patient's history, individual anatomy, medical history, pathological presentations, and any underlying comorbidities are unidentified and unfamiliar to the physician. In recognition of this unfamiliarity, the content of service requirements tend to be more rigorous for a new patient E/M service visit because it is expected that the physician must collect much more information and findings. Fortunately, the AMA has provided in the CPT manual easily identifiable requirements for the series of numeric codes that represent the new patient type of any given category of E/M service visit. The following example provides some illustrations of new patients and the site of service in which they may be seen.

Examples of Documentation for New Patients

99381-99387—New preventive medicine service: Jodie is a 26-year-old woman who has just moved to the area and presents to the clinic for her first annual exam. Jodie has not been seen in this clinic before, nor has she received medical, clinical, or professional services from this specific physician or any physicians of a similar specialty in the clinic.

99201-99205—New office or other outpatient service: Mark is a 67-year-old man who presents for a persistent cough. His previous healthcare clinic closed, and he needs a new primary care provider.

99221-99223—New hospital services: Francis presents to the hospital for dizziness and difficulty breathing. The hospital physician identifies Francis's condition and admits the patient to the hospital for treatment and care.

One of the most common requirements for the new patient type of service is the consideration of all three key components when determining the overall level of service, similar to the manner of determining the overall level of history. Therefore, in selecting the level of E/M service for a new patient, the key component with the lowest level determines the overall level of service. ■ FIGURE 13.4 provides a visual aid for determining the overall level of service.

Established Patient Type

Consider two people who are very familiar with one another, meeting at a restaurant. The nature of the interrogative questions between these two people is limited to the events since their last meeting, since each of the two people is familiar with the past history and personal habits of the other person. In the same way, an established patient type visit acknowledges the previous experience and familiarity with the patient gained by the physician over repeated E/M service visits, which may have occurred as recently as the last week or month or within the last year or two. In addition, past medical history, underlying or associated conditions, and the patient's individual anatomical structure are all familiar to the physician. In recognition of this familiarity, the CPT manual identifies a distinct series of numeric codes and individualized requirements for the established patient within each category of service. The following example provides some illustrations of established patients and the site of service in which they may be seen.

Examples of Documentation for Established Patients

99391-99397—Established preventive medicine service: Jodie is a 26-year-old woman who presents to the clinic for her annual exam. Jodie has been a patient at this clinic for 2 years.

99211-99215—Established office or other outpatient service: Mark is a 67-year-old man who presents for a persistent cough. He has been a patient at this clinic for 10 years and presents to be seen by his primary care provider.

99231-99233—Established hospital services: Francis admitted to the hospital 2 nights ago for dizziness and difficulty breathing, and on the third day of admission, she is seen by the attending physician, Dr. Nerdowell.

Content of Service	Level 1: New Patient	Level 2: New Patient	Level 3: New Patient	Level 4: New Patient	Level 5: New Patient
History	Problem-focused	Expanded problem-focused	Detailed	Comprehensive	Comprehensive
Physical Examination	Problem-focused	Expanded problem-focused	Detailed	Comprehensive	Comprehensive
Medical Decision Making	Straightforward	Straightforward	Low	Moderate	Comprehensive

Figure 13.4 ■ Content of service level requirements for a new patient.

Content of Service	Level 1: Established Patient	Level 2: Established Patient	Level 3: Established Patient	Level 4: Established Patient	Level 5: Established Patient
History	Problem-focused	Expanded problem-focused	Detailed	Comprehensive	Comprehensive
Physical Examination	Problem-focused	Expanded problem-focused	Detailed	Comprehensive	Comprehensive
Medical Decision Making	Straightforward	Straightforward	Low	Moderate	Comprehensive

Figure 13.5 ■ Content of service level requirements for an established patient.

The most common requirement for selecting the overall level of service for an established patient is that two of the three key components must be met or exceeded. Consequently, the process of selecting the overall level of service is most similar to the selection of medical decision-making complexity; only two of the three key components—history, physical examination, and medical decision making—are required, and their grouping is not predetermined. Therefore, one established patient E/M service visit may utilize the physical examination and medical decision making to qualify for a given overall level of service, whereas a different established patient service may employ history and medical decision making. ■ FIGURE 13.5 provides a visual aid for selecting the overall level of service for an established patient.

Exercise 13.1 Overall Level of E/M Service for Sinus Pressure

Read the following medical documentation, and then answer the questions that follow.

History: Joanie Smith is a new patient who presents for increased sinus pressure, sore throat, and a cough. The right side of the patient's head hurts so much that she feels she cannot hold her head up due to the throbbing pain. The patient states that her teeth began to ache last night, and this morning every part of her hurts. Although the patient recognizes flu is likely, she is concerned about a sinus infection. Appetite greatly reduced, no reports of nausea, vomiting, or diarrhea. No reports of heart palpitations or shortness of breath. Other than feeling chilled all the time, she reports no other health problems. The patient is a preschool teacher, and she provides multiple reports of ill contact at work.

Exam: Patient is very pale and appears very tired. Conjunctivae are red, swollen, but not inflamed. The patient reports exquisite pain and associated dizziness upon palpation of face, particularly the forehead and maxillary sinuses. The patient loses her balance easily when asked to tip her head forward. Minimal phlegm production per nares is noted. Oropharynx is red and minimally inflamed, and patient reports feeling that she has something tickling her throat. No rub or fremitus noted upon auscultation of lungs.

Assessment: Sinus infection, without impaction.

Plan: Azithromycin prescribed for sinus infection. Increased fluids, recommended rest.

1. Which patient type is represented, new or established? Please support your answer._____

_____

2. Identify the level of service documented by circling the appropriate elements and the overall content of service on the selection chart provided here.

Content of Service	Level 1	Level 2	Level 3	Level 4	Level 5
History	Problem-focused	Expanded problem-focused	Detailed	Comprehensive	Comprehensive
Physical Examination	Problem-focused	Expanded problem-focused	Detailed	Comprehensive	Comprehensive
Medical Decision Making	Straightfoward	Straightfoward	Low	Moderate	High

Exercise 13.2 Overall Level of E/M Service to Rule Out Appendiceal Abscess

Please read the following medical documentation, and then answer the questions that follow.

Timmy is a 12-year-old who presents to the emergency room for severe abdominal pain. Patient's most severe pain is localized in the right lower quadrant, but entire belly hurts. Patient tackled during soccer game 1 week ago, and pain has steadily increased in severity since that day. Patient reports diarrhea for 2 days after tackle, followed by fatigue and loss of appetite. Low-grade fever

Exercise 6.1 *continued*

developed 2 days ago. Patient awakened by severe abdominal pain, and father noted high temperature, patient's distress, and brought his son to the ER.

ROS: Negative for bloody stools, dysuria, hematuria. All other ROS pertaining to this problem are negative.

Past medical history: Gastroschisis at birth, repaired at 2 days. No history of small bowel obstruction, intra-abdominal adhesions, or intussusception. No family history of abdominal problems.

Physical exam: T, 102.5. Timmy is very uncomfortable and clearly in distress. Significant guarding of tense abdomen and exquisite pain precluded any prolonged abdominal exam. Extreme pain when asked to cough.

Diagnostic: WBC, 22,000; CRP, 150 mg/L. KUB reveals free air.

Assessment: Possible intra-abdominal adhesions with likely ruptured appendix.

Plan: Emergency appendectomy for rupture with suspected intra-abdominal adhesions.

1. Which patient type is represented, new or established? Please support your answer._____

   _____

2. Identify the level of service documented by circling the appropriate elements and the overall content of service on the selection chart provided here.

Content of Service	Level 1	Level 2	Level 3	Level 4	Level 5
History	Problem-focused	Expanded problem-focused	Expanded problem-focused	Detailed	Comprehensive
Physical Examination	Problem-focused	Expanded problem-focused	Expanded problem-focused	Detailed	Comprehensive
Medical Decision Making	Straightforward	Low	Moderate	Moderate	High

Exercise 13.3 Overall Level of E/M Service for Lower Back Pain

Read the following medical documentation, and then answer the questions that follow.

Joan is an established patient who presents for lower back pain. Her lower back hurts, down by beltline, and pain is sometimes very severe. The pain is sporadic, mostly when standing up after sitting in one place for an extended period. Ibuprofen used to help, but now it does not help back pain anymore. At its worst, low back pain is sharp and throbbing. Joan has had occasional back pain for about 20 years, since first in the service, but she first noticed this particular low back pain shortly after playing touch football with adult children this past Thanksgiving. Patient denies any other joint pain than her low back pain. Patient denies double vision or dizziness, and no chest pain or shortness of breath. Patient denies tobacco or alcohol use. Pain has not affected her work as a fifth-grade teacher.

Plan: Suspected vertebral fracture between T12 and L2 vertebrae. MRI scheduled to rule out vertebral fracture. Request for consult made to Dr. Backouch of Southwestern Pain Management. NSAID as needed for inflammation with recommendation of light activity prior to MRI.

1. Which patient type is represented, new or established? Please support your answer._____

   _____

2. Identify the level of service documented by circling the appropriate elements and the overall content of service on the selection chart provided here.

Content of Service	Level 1	Level 2	Level 3	Level 4	Level 5
History	Problem-focused	Problem-focused	Expanded problem-focused	Detailed	Comprehensive
Physical Examination	Problem-focused	Problem-focused	Expanded problem-focused	Detailed	Comprehensive
Medical Decision Making	Straightforward	Straightforward	Low	Moderate	High

CONTRIBUTING COMPONENTS: COUNSELING AND COORDINATION OF CARE

The documentation of an E/M service visit represents the various elements of the clinical visit between a physician and a patient: the collection of history elements, the performance of the physical examination, and the level of medical decision-making complexity. However, every patient is a unique individual with different symptoms, experiences, and needs; and some circumstances warrant a different element of evaluation and management during the visit. Although some of these additional elements of interaction may be difficult to quantify in a specific numerical context, they can contribute a tremendous amount of clinical support, promote healing, and provide good quality care for the patient. Their documentation reflects the physician's attention to detail during the E/M service.

Certain circumstances may warrant an extensive discussion between the physician and the patient regarding the disease process or one or more selected treatment options, such as a child who is experiencing abnormal abdominal pains with no specific defined, diagnosed cause. Other circumstances may require the physician to coordinate a specific plan of care for the patient by contacting another specialist or other healthcare professional; for example, a physician might coordinate specialists for a patient experiencing unexplained, recurrent bloody noses and unexplained shortness of breath, nausea, and dizziness. When these contributing components are considered in concert with the other elements of the documented E/M service, the complete content of service becomes a full portrait of the service visit. Documentation of any of these extra components contributes additional insight into the care provided by the physician performing the E/M service.

Counseling

counseling the dialogue between the physician and the patient during which the physician provides additional information regarding the disease process, expected prognosis, diagnostic procedures or results, treatment or management options, the necessity for compliance, or any other unanswered questions from the patient and/or family

Providing counsel indicates an offer of advice, guidance, encouragement, or direction. When a patient presents for an E/M service because of an illness, the patient is seeking the professional knowledge and medical expertise necessary to diagnose the presenting problem and identify any needed treatment plan or management option. While the physician collects the history, performs the physical examination, and determines the most appropriate medical decision for managing the patient's presenting problem, specific issues or needs may require additional explanation by or discussion with the physician. When the physician addresses these specific needs or issues for the patient, or the patient's family, the physician is providing **counseling**. Counseling during an E/M service generally involves the physician's sharing of wisdom, advice, or guidance during a regular healthcare appointment. This wisdom or advice may be in the form of additional information about a disease process, diagnostic results, or treatment plan. Counseling may involve answering questions from the patient and/or family members about the expected prognosis or the risks posed by a selected management option. On the other hand, counseling may involve the physician's instructions regarding a treatment plan or emphasis on the importance of complying with a specific treatment or management plan. Even though each of these aspects of counseling seems to be inherent in the care provided by a physician during the regular performance of an E/M service, counseling involves a more concerted or precise direction of clinical support for the patient or the patient's family. Every E/M service requires the performing physician to provide a certain amount of counseling to the patient, but when certain circumstances require counseling that is above the expected amount, the physician should document the performance of this additional counseling to thoroughly reflect the quality of care provided to the patient.

Coordination of Care

coordination of care managed sharing of medical findings, management options, and treatment plans between two or more participants in the patient's healthcare

diagnostic laparoscopy an invasive surgical procedure that involves an incision in the abdominal wall and inflation of the abdominal cavity to allow the insertion of a small scope for examining the abdominal cavity and internal organs

During an E/M service visit, diagnostic procedures or management options may require coordination with other healthcare professionals. **Coordination of care** can be simply defined as organized sharing between two or more parties who happen to be involved in providing a patient's healthcare, medical findings, or management options. This coordination goes beyond ordering diagnostic laboratory tests or a radiology scan. Coordinating the care for a patient may involve a recommendation for an invasive diagnostic procedure such as a **diagnostic laparoscopy** or lumbar puncture. Coordinating management options requires that the physician performing the E/M service know about any other medical management currently being employed by the patient. For instance, a certain prescription medication may interact negatively with other medications or even an OTC drug. Therefore, gathering the list of medications and/or drugs being taken by the patient can inform the physician's decision regarding coordination of the patient's future care. Treatment plans also require coordination of care, as the introduction of any treatment or therapy could not only bring about a positive change in the patient's current condition, but might also affect the patient's anatomy or pathology in unexpected ways.

Coordination of care includes anyone involved in the patient's care. For instance, the coordination of care for a relatively healthy person dealing with an acute, uncomplicated illness may involve the physician, the clinical laboratory, and the pharmacist. However, coordination of care for a patient dealing with a chronic illness, multiple underlying conditions, or a combination thereof, becomes more complex because of the number of participants involved in the management and treatment of the patient's conditions. These different participants can include different physicians, nurses, and pharmacists, as well as clinical support staff, nurse practitioners, physical or occupational therapists, mental healthcare professionals, dietitians, even the patient's family members who may assist in maintaining or managing the patient's healthcare. Documentation of this coordination of care becomes an important part of the patient's medical record.

TIME AND THE NATURE OF THE PRESENTING PROBLEM

The CPT manual identifies two important characteristics of an E/M service: the identifiable problem for which the patient seeks healthcare and the time spent during a service visit. Each one of these factors plays an important role in the delivery of healthcare.

The Nature of the Presenting Problem

When a patient makes an appointment to see a physician, often a healthcare problem has prompted the appointment. This problem is considered the presenting problem, which is sometimes known as the chief complaint, the current complaint, or the reason for the patient's visit. This presenting problem is the disease, traumatic injury, medical condition, illness, undefined symptom, undiagnosed complaint, or any other reason for the E/M service visit. Not only is this range of possibilities broad, but every patient is a unique individual, and categorizing the presenting problem into quantifiable types can be difficult; after all, is the presenting problem the result of an injury, a disease, or an illness? To alleviate confusion in the medical documentation, the presenting problem is discussed in terms of the nature of the presenting problem. By identifying the *nature* of the presenting problem, the CPT manual is able to sort the wide-ranging possibilities into five different types of presenting problems: minimal, self-limited or minor, low severity, moderate severity, and high severity. ■ TABLE 13.1 presents the definitions for each of the five presenting problem types.

Notice that the severity of the presenting problem increases with each type. Given previous information about the content of service, a presenting problem of high severity would inherently require a more detailed or comprehensive documentation than a self-limited or minor type of presenting problem would. It would stand to reason that the higher the severity of the presenting problem, the more intensive the amount of time spent by the physician performing the E/M service visit.

In order to provide greater clarity and continuity, the CPT manual correlates specific types of presenting problems with specific levels of E/M services. ■ FIGURE 13.6 illustrates the correlation of specific types of presenting problems with specific levels of E/M services performed for a new patient in an office or other outpatient setting.

■ TABLE 13.1   FIVE TYPES OF PRESENTING PROBLEM

Minimal severity	A problem that may not require the presence of the physician, but service is provided under the physician's supervision
Self-limited or minor severity	A problem that runs a definite and prescribed course, is transient in nature, and either is not likely to permanently alter health status or has a good prognosis with management and compliance
Low severity	A problem for which the risk of morbidity without treatment is low, there is little to no risk of mortality without treatment, and full recovery without functional impairment is expected
Moderate severity	A problem for which the risk of morbidity without treatment is moderate, there is a moderate risk of mortality without treatment, and there is an uncertain prognosis OR increased probability of prolonged functional impairment
High severity	A problem for which the risk of morbidity without treatment is high to extreme, there is a moderate to high risk of mortality without treatment, OR there is a high probability of severe, prolonged functional impairment

Office or Other Outpatient Site: New Patient	Level 1	Level 2	Level 3	Level 4	Level 5
History	Problem-focused	Expanded problem-focused	Detailed	Comprehensive	Comprehensive
Physical Examination	Problem-focused	Expanded problem-focused	Detailed	Comprehensive	Comprehensive
Medical Decision Making	Straightforward	Straightforward	Low	Moderate	High
Presenting Problem	Self-limited or minor severity	Low to moderate severity	Moderate severity	Moderate to high severity	Moderate to high severity

Office or Other Outpatient Site: Established Patient	Level 1	Level 2	Level 3	Level 4	Level 5
History	Problem-focused	Problem-focused	Expanded problem-focused	Detailed	Comprehensive
Physical Examination	Problem-focused	Problem-focused	Expanded problem-focused	Detailed	Comprehensive
Medical Decision Making	Straightforward	Straightforward	Low	Moderate	High
Presenting Problem	Minimal severity	Self-limited or minor severity	Moderate severity	Moderate to high severity	Moderate to high severity

Figure 13.6 ■ Correlating types of presenting problems for new patient, office or other outpatient site, and for established patient, office or other outpatient site, for E/M services.

The Element of Time

Clearly, the nature of the presenting problem may introduce a level of complication and complexity that can be difficult to express in the documentation. For instance, a presenting problem of high severity may require a significant coordination of care, which then may necessitate an equally significant amount of counseling to ensure that the patient understands the nature of the presenting problem as well as any ordered diagnostic procedures and/or management options. In cases when a higher amount of counseling and/or coordination of care is required to provide good quality healthcare during an E/M service, documentation of the necessary coordination of care and/or required counseling provides a strong reflection of the care provided by the performing physician.

But how do the content of service components—history, physical examination, and medical decision making—fit into cases when the coordination of care or counseling dominates the E/M service visit? The 1995 and 1997 DGs list one simple guideline specifically for these circumstances when counseling and/or coordination of care might occupy a majority of the E/M service visit. This guideline states that circumstances that require more than 50 percent of the E/M service visit to be spent in providing counseling and/or coordination of care, time "should be considered the key or controlling factor to qualify for a particular level of E/M service."[1] In simple terms, if the provision of counseling and/or coordination of care occupies more than half of the entire time spent in the service visit, then the time spent in the visit becomes the overwhelmingly important element that determines the level of the E/M service. In such a case, the controlling factor of time becomes more important even than the individual content of service components themselves.

INTRASERVICE TIME

intraservice time the amount of time the physician spends performing an E/M service

The 1995 and 1997 DGs suggest that there are specific standards of time for certain E/M service visit codes, which is very true. The CPT manual defines the amount of time spent during an E/M service as **intraservice** time, which refers to the services performed during the entire E/M service. Further, the CPT manual provides lengthy explanations regarding the nature of the intraservice time, identifying two distinct types of intraservice time. These two types are defined by the context in which the E/M service occurs, and their titles offer a hint as to the respective settings: *face-to-face* and *unit/floor*.

[1]Centers for Medicare and Medicaid Services, "1995 Documentation Guidelines for Evaluation and Management Services," p. 15, www.cms.gov/Outreach-and-Education/Medicare-Learning-Network-MLN/MLNEdWebGuide/Downloads/95Docguidelines.pdf; "1997 Documentation Guidelines for Evaluation and Management Services," p. 51, www.cms.gov/Outreach-and-Education/Medicare-Learning-Network-MLN/MLNEdWebGuide/Downloads/95Docguidelines.pdf.

Face-to-Face Intraservice Time

The CPT manual states that **face-to-face** time occurs during office or other outpatient E/M service visits and during consultations that occur in an office or other outpatient setting. An office or other outpatient setting is considered a physician's office, outpatient hospital setting, or an ambulatory facility, which means the patient is not only physically able to walk away, but is healthy enough to do so. As a result, face-to-face intraservice time involves the physician's personal interaction with the patient—collecting history, performing the physical examination, making the medical decisions, providing counseling to the patient, and/or coordinating care while in the presence of the patient. If the physician reviews diagnostic results or independently visualizes a scan, image, or specimen while face-to-face with the patient, then this review or independent visualization would constitute face-to-face intraservice time. However, CPT manual makes clear that if the physician reviews diagnostic results or independently visualizes a scan, image, or specimen before the E/M service begins or after the service ends, this would not constitute face-to-face intraservice time. The work performed before or after the E/M service has been calculated into the total work of these specific visits.

face-to-face time the time the physician spends in the presence of the patient collecting history, performing the physical examination, determining the medical decision making, providing counseling to the patient, and/or coordinating care during the E/M service

Unit/Floor Intraservice Time

The CPT manual defines **unit/floor** time as occurring in inpatient settings, including services such as hospital observation, inpatient hospital care, initial inpatient hospital consultations, and care in a nursing facility. Generally, a patient's departure from these settings may be medically contraindicated because of illness, symptom, injury, or disease, and the patient's presence in these settings is of a more urgent or emergent nature. As a result, the parameters for unit/floor intraservice time are very different, including the time that the physician is present on the patient's hospital unit or floor as well as the time the physician spends at the patient's bedside. However, like the face-to-face intraservice time, any time spent off the patient's unit or floor—even reviewing diagnostic results or independently visualizing an image, scan, or specimen—is not considered to be part of the total unit/floor intraservice time. This effort is not considered intraservice time because it has been calculated into the total work of these E/M service visits.

unit/floor time the time the physician spends on the patient's hospital unit or floor, as well as the time the physician spends at the patient's bedside, collecting history, performing the physical examination, making medical decisions, providing counseling to the patient and/or family, and/or coordinating care during the E/M service

TYPICAL TIME FOR SPECIFIC E/M SERVICES

Typical time is considered the amount of time during which physicians usually perform the E/M service. Typical time represents the specific intraservice time, unit/floor or face-to-face, the physician spends during a particular E/M service visit. The CPT manual provides standards that represent the typical time during which one of these specific E/M services is performed. These recorded standards of typical intraservice time are averages taken over years of study and provide an appropriate representation of the time required to perform an E/M service in one of these six categories: hospital observation, inpatient hospital care, inpatient consultations, office or other outpatient services, or office or other outpatient consultations. These levels of typical time provide clear parameters for dealing with the cases when counseling and/or coordination of care makes up more than 50 percent of the intraservice. ■ FIGURE 13.7 illustrates the typical time spent face-to-face with new patients during an office or other outpatient E/M service. The 1995 and 1997 DGs, as well as the CPT manual, each provide the standards, guidelines, and requirements for the many E/M services that are performed in many different settings.

typical time the standardized amount of intraservice time usually spent by a physician performing this specific E/M service

Office or Other Outpatient: New Patient	Level 1	Level 2	Level 3	Level 4	Level 5
History	Problem-focused	Expanded problem-focused	Detailed	Comprehensive	Comprehensive
Physical Examination	Problem-focused	Expanded problem-focused	Detailed	Comprehensive	Comprehensive
Medical Decision Making	Straightforward	Straightforward	Low	Moderate	High
Presenting Problem	Self-limited or minor severity	Low to moderate severity	Moderate severity	Moderate to high severity	Moderate to high severity
Face-to-Face Intraservice Time	10 minutes face-to-face with the patient and/or family	20 minutes face-to-face with the patient and/or family	30 minutes face-to-face with the patient and/or family	45 minutes face-to-face with the patient and/or family	60 minutes face-to-face with the patient and/or family

Figure 13.7 ■ Typical time spent face-to-face with a new patient during an office or other outpatient E/M service.

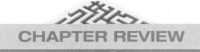

SUMMARY

- The E/M service is performed and then documented in the patient's medical record. The documented content of service components—history, physical examination, and medical decision making—reflect the services and care provided during the E/M service and then documented by the clinician. The levels of these key components support the documented content of service for the E/M service. The manner in which the levels of the individual components determine the overall level of service is remarkably similar to the selection of the overall history or the overall medical decision-making complexity. Different E/M services list different requirements for the content of service, which are found in the CPT manual.

- The site of service is the location in which an E/M service visit occurs, and each site presents a different set of parameters, requirements, and circumstances that influence the E/M service visit. The CPT manual provides an exhaustive list of numerical codes that represent the many different categories of E/M service visits; each category of codes represents a different site of service. The patient type defines whether the patient has received clinical, medical, or professional services from the performing physician, or another physician of the exact same specialty and subspecialty who also belongs to the same group practice, during 3 years prior to the E/M service in question. New patients have *not* received such services and require that all three of the key components be considered to determine the level of E/M service. Established patients *have* received such services and require only that two of the three key components be met or exceeded for the E/M service to qualify for a particular level.

- Counseling and coordination of care are two components that contribute significantly to the performance of the E/M service. Counseling is a dialogue the physician facilitates for the patient and/or family concerning the disease process, expected prognosis, diagnostic results, treatment plan, risk factors, or some other aspect of care. Coordination of care is an organized sharing, between two or more parties who happen to be involved in the provision of the patient's healthcare, of medical findings about and management options for a specific patient. Coordination of care may include different physicians, nurses, and pharmacists, as well as clinical support staff, nurse practitioners, physical or occupational therapists, mental healthcare professionals, dietitians, even the patient's family members who may assist in maintaining or managing the patient's healthcare.

- The presenting problem is the disease, traumatic injury, medical condition, illness, undefined symptom, undiagnosed complaint, or any other reason for the E/M service visit. The nature of the presenting problem represents an identification of the level of severity involved in the disease, traumatic injury, medical condition, illness, undefined symptom, or undiagnosed complaint. There are five different levels of presenting problem severity: minimal, self-limited or minor, low, moderate, and high. The CPT manual correlates specific types of presenting problem with specific levels of E/M services. When the nature of the presenting problem, counseling, and coordination of care require that more than 50 percent of the E/M service visit be spent in providing counseling and/or coordination of care, time becomes the controlling factor in determining the level of the E/M service. Intraservice time is the amount of time the physician spends providing clinical, medical, or professional service during an E/M service.

- There are two types of intraservice time: face-to-face and unit/floor. Face-to-face time occurs during office or other outpatient E/M service visits and during consultations that occur in an office or other outpatient setting. Face-to-face time deals with the services provided while the physician is face-to-face with the patient, collecting history, performing the physical examination, making the medical decisions, providing counseling to the patient, and/or coordinating care while in the presence of the patient. Unit/floor time addresses services provided in inpatient settings, such as hospital observation services, inpatient hospital care, initial inpatient hospital consultations, and care in nursing facilities. Unit/floor intraservice time differs from face-to-face time because unit/floor intraservice time includes the time that the physician is present on the patient's hospital unit or floor as well as the time the physician spends at the patient's bedside.

- The CPT manual, published by the AMA, identifies the typical time an E/M service requires in one of these six categories: hospital observation, inpatient hospital care, inpatient consultations, office or other outpatient services, or office or other outpatient consultations. Each level of E/M services performed in these six categories lists a typical amount of intraservice time spent by the physician. These levels provide clear parameters for dealing with the cases when counseling and/or coordination of care makes up more than 50 percent of the intraservice time.

CHAPTER REVIEW

Multiple Choice

Choose the letter that best answers each question or completes each statement.

1. Which of the following best reflects a presenting problem?

   a. A problem that may not require the presence of the physician, but medical service is provided under the physician's supervision

   b. The disease, traumatic injury, medical condition, illness, undefined symptom, undiagnosed complaint, or any other reason for the visit

   c. Managed sharing of medical findings, management options, and treatment plans between two or more participants in the patient's healthcare

   d. The location in which an E/M service visit occurs

2. Which of the following best reflects counseling?

   a. Whether the patient has received, or has not received, any professional, medical, or other healthcare services from the physician during the 3 years prior to the E/M service visit in question

   b. Managed sharing of medical findings, management options, and treatment plans between two or more participants in the patient's healthcare

   c. The dialogue between the physician and the patient and/or family during which the physician provides additional information regarding the disease process, expected prognosis, diagnostic procedures or results, treatment or management options, the necessity for compliance, or any other unanswered questions from the patient and/or family

   d. A problem that runs a definite and prescribed course, is transient in nature, and is not likely to permanently alter health status or has a good prognosis with management and compliance

3. Which of the following best reflects coordination of care?

   a. The dialogue between the physician and the patient and/or family during which the physician provides additional information regarding the disease process, expected prognosis, diagnostic procedures or results, treatment or management options, the necessity for compliance, or any other unanswered questions from the patient and/or family

   b. A problem for which the risk of comorbidity without treatment is low, there is little to no risk of mortality without treatment, and full recovery without functional impairment is expected

   c. The time the physician spends on the patient's hospital unit or floor as well as the time the physician spends at the patient's bedside collecting history, performing the physical examination, making the medical decisions, providing counseling to the patient and/or family, and/or coordinating care during the E/M service

   d. Managed sharing of medical findings, management options, and treatment plans between two or more participants in the patient's healthcare

4. Which of the following best reflects the site of service?

   a. Whether the patient has received, or has not received, any professional, medical, or other healthcare services from the performing physician, or another physician of the exact same specialty and subspecialty who also belongs to the same group practice, during the 3 years prior to the E/M service visit in question

   b. The location in which an E/M service visit occurs

   c. The disease, traumatic injury, medical condition, illness, undefined symptom, undiagnosed complaint, or any other reason for the E/M service visit

   d. The standardized amount of intraservice time usually spent by a physician performing this specific E/M service

5. Which of the following best reflects the patient type?

   a. The patient has never received any professional, medical, or other healthcare services from the physician or physician group

   b. The patient has received professional, medical, or other healthcare services from the physician or physician group during 3 years prior to the E/M service visit in question

   c. Whether the patient has received, or has not received, any professional, medical, or other healthcare services from the performing physician, or another physician of the exact same specialty and subspecialty who also belongs to the same group practice, during 3 years prior to the E/M service visit in question

   d. The patient has not received professional, medical, or other healthcare services from the physician or physician group during 3 years prior to the E/M service visit in question

6. Which of the following best completes the following sentence?

   Unit/floor time is the intraservice time the physician spends _____ collecting history, performing the physical examination, making the medical decisions, providing counseling to the patient and/or family, and/or coordinating care during the E/M service

   a. on the patient's hospital unit or floor as well as at the patient's bedside

   b. in the presence of the patient

   c. performing an E/M service

   d. independently reviewing the scan or image with the radiologist

7. Which of the following best completes the following sentence?

   Face-to-face time is the intraservice time the physician spends _____ collecting history, performing the physical examination, making the medical decisions, providing counseling to the patient and/or family, and/or coordinating care during the E/M service

   a. treating a problem for which the risk of comorbidity without treatment is low

   b. on the patient's hospital unit or floor as well as at the patient's bedside

   c. performing an E/M service

   d. in the presence of the patient

8. Which of the following best completes the following sentence?

   When counseling and/or coordination of care makes up more than _____ of the intraservice time, time should be considered the controlling factor for determining the level of E/M service.

   1. 25%

   2. 10%

   3. 33.3%

   4. 50%

9. The physician documents a comprehensive history, expanded problem-focused physical examination, and a moderate level of medical decision-making complexity for a new patient. Using the following overall level selection chart, on the following page, identify the correct level for this service.

   a. Level 2

   b. Level 3

   c. Level 4

   d. Level 5

Content of Service	Level 1	Level 2	Level 3	Level 4	Level 5
History	Problem-focused	Expanded problem-focused	Detailed	Comprehensive	Comprehensive
Physical Examination	Problem-focused	Expanded problem-focused	Detailed	Comprehensive	Comprehensive
Medical Decision Making	Straight-forward	Straightforward	Low	Moderate	High

10. The physician documents a problem-focused history, detailed physical examination, and moderate level of medical decision-making complexity for an established patient. Using the following overall level selection chart, identify the correct level for this service.

    a. Level 1
    b. Level 2
    c. Level 3
    d. Level 4

Content of Service	Level 1	Level 2	Level 3	Level 4	Level 5
History	Problem-focused	Expanded problem-focused	Detailed	Comprehensive	Comprehensive
Physical Examination	Problem-focused	Expanded problem-focused	Detailed	Comprehensive	Comprehensive
Medical Decision Making	Straight-forward	Straightforward	Low	Moderate	High

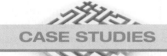

CASE STUDIES

Case Study 13-1

Utilizing the overall level selection chart provided with each case, identify the overall level of service for the following documentations.

1. A new patient presents for an E/M service in a physician's office with complaints of extreme headaches and recent dizziness, which began suddenly 3 days ago. Patient is obese but reports no cardiac problems, respiratory issues, or nausea. Remainder of review negative in detail. Father died of massive stroke at 58. Patient retired school janitor. Physical exam reveals numbness in the fingers of the patient's right hand and little response during the Babinski test. Complete blood and urinalysis workup ordered, CT scan of the patient's head, and referral made to neurologist for peripheral numbness and suspected previous TIA. More than half of this 30-minute visit spent in counseling and coordinating care with the patient's family, especially identifying the s/s of stroke, the need to prevent future falls, and compliance with recommended treatment, especially medication regimen.

    a. Level 1
    b. Level 2
    c. Level 3
    d. Level 4

Content of Service	Level 1	Level 2	Level 3	Level 4	Level 5
History	Problem-focused	Expanded problem-focused	Detailed	Comprehensive	Comprehensive
Physical Examination	Problem-focused	Expanded problem-focused	Detailed	Comprehensive	Comprehensive
Medical Decision Making	Straight-forward	Straightforward	Low	Moderate	High
Face-to-Face Time	10 minutes	20 minutes	30 minutes	45 minutes	60 minutes

2. An 85-year-old woman presents to orthopedic surgeon due to confirmed fracture of L1 vertebra. Detailed history collected, and physical examination performed. Orthopedic surgeon recommends balloon kyphoplasty. No diagnostic testing required;

however, orthopedic surgeon independently reviewed images of positive bone scan. Orthopedic surgeon recommends kyphoplasty. More than half of this visit spent in extensive discussion with patient regarding risks of surgery, potential complications, and postsurgical expectations. Patient agrees to kyphoplasty. Surgery scheduled for next week.

a. Level 2
b. Level 3
c. Level 4
d. Level 5

Content of Service	Level 1	Level 2	Level 3	Level 4	Level 5
History	Problem-focused	Expanded problem-focused	Detailed	Comprehensive	Comprehensive
Physical Examination	Problem-focused	Expanded problem-focused	Detailed	Comprehensive	Comprehensive
Medical Decision Making	Straight-forward	Straight-forward	Low	Moderate	High
Face-to-Face Time	10 minutes	20 minutes	30 minutes	45 minutes	60 minutes

Case Study 13-2

Review this case and identify the content of service elements that follow. Remember that Appendix D contains the full content of service worksheet.

Complaint: James Roberts is a new patient who presents for recent abdominal trauma that occurred 2 days ago. James recently moved to the area and, while staying at a local hotel, fell in his bathroom after stepping out of the shower and slipping on the wet tile floor. He fell heavily against the edge of the sink, hyperextended his right wrist, and sprained his left ankle during the process. Patient reports hearing cracks and experiencing immediate, extreme upper abdominal pain that he reported as 9/10 at time of fall. His pain lessened significantly directly after his fall but increased in severity to 7/10 as the weekend progressed. Per patient, there was no LOC as a direct result of the fall, although he reports dizzy spells over the last 24 hours, especially after rising from a supine or prone position. His wife wrapped an elastic bandage around his chest because James assumed he had cracked some ribs due to his pain while breathing. His pain increased over the weekend, and this morning when he removed the bandage, he noted significant upper abdominal bruising and tenderness, as well as swollen left ankle and weak, swollen right wrist. His primary concern is his abdomen and painful respiration. James reports no nausea or vomiting, no bloody stool, blood in urine, or painful urination. No episodes of syncope, only the dizziness noted here. James reports breathing causes severe pain, especially when lying prone. James's wife was present during visit and reported that James's dyspnea interfered with sleep, causing him to vocalize during the night, which James does not remember. His wife reports notation of significant swelling of bruised area of upper abdomen this morning.

Physical examination: Abdomen tender; however, significant guarding noted. Patient describes excruciating pleuritic chest pain upon palpation and when asked to cough.

Laboratory: Complete blood count reveals normal results, specifically hemoglobin, hematocrit, and WBC. Arterial blood gases reveal decreased oxygen.

Imaging: Anteroposterior chest X-ray demonstrates three left lateral lower rib fractures of 8–11 with small apical pneumothorax on the left.

Assessment: Patient has fracture of at least three ribs between ribs 8 and 11. Patient's dyspnea recommends rule-out of diaphragmatic injury. CT scan scheduled to rule out diaphragmatic injury, as well as identify any splenic trauma.

Plan: Chest wrapped to minimize pain of rib fractures. CT scan scheduled to rule out diaphragmatic injury, as well as identify any splenic trauma. Patient is reluctant to have a general surgery consultation regarding potential diaphragmatic injury. Tylenol recommended for pain caused by rib fracture, with a prescription for Tylenol 3 available in the event the traumatic diaphragmatic injury is ruled out. More than half of this 75-minute office visit was spent in providing face-to-face counseling to the patient regarding his probable splenic laceration, the importance of avoiding OTC NSAIDs such as Aleve, Advil, Motrin, or ibuprofen. The danger of a potential diaphragmatic injury was stressed with the patient and the patient's wife, and the patient was urged to visit the general surgeon, Dr. Smothbelly, at the scheduled appointment.

1. According to the documentation, is this a new patient or an established patient?

   _____

   Utilizing prior knowledge, identify the overall level of history, and explain the supporting rationale for it.
2. Overall level of history: _____
   Explain your rationale. _____

Utilizing prior knowledge, identify the type of physical examination, using either the 1995 body area/organ system guidelines, the general multisystem guidelines, or the single organ–system guidelines.

3. Which type of physical examination was referenced: 1995 body area/organ system, 1997 general multisystem, 1997 single organ system? _____
4. Type of physical examination—problem-focused, expanded problem-focused, detailed, or comprehensive: _____

Utilizing prior knowledge, identify the complexity of medical decision making.

5. Number of diagnoses and/or management options: _____
   Is this problem new or established? _____
   If this is an established problem, is it stable/improving or worsening? _____

Is a management option documented? _____

If a management option is documented, what is the management option? _____

6. Amount and/or complexity of data to be reviewed: _____

   What documented data have been reviewed? _____

   Identify the complexity of the data to be reviewed: _____

7. Risk of complication, comorbidity, and/or mortality: _____

   What is the presenting problem? _____

   Level of risk: _____

   What is (are) the diagnostic procedure(s) ordered? _____

   Level of risk: _____

   What is (are) the management option(s) selected? _____

   Level of risk: _____

Overall level of risk of complication, comorbidity, and/or morality: _____

Determined by _____

8. Overall complexity of medical decision making: _____

9. Has intraservice (face-to-face) time been documented in this case study? _____

   If yes, how much time has been documented? _____

10. Has any counseling and/or coordination of care been documented in this case study? _____

    If yes, summarize: _____

11. Using the content of service requirement worksheet provided here, determine what level of service best reflects this case study documentation. _____

Content of Service	Level 1	Level 2	Level 3	Level 4	Level 5
History	Problem-focused	Expanded problem-focused	Detailed	Comprehensive	Comprehensive
Physical Examination	Problem-focused	Expanded problem-focused	Detailed	Comprehensive	Comprehensive
Medical Decision Making	Straight-forward	Straight-forward	Low	Moderate	High
Face-to-Face Time	10 minutes	20 minutes	30 minutes	45 minutes	60 minutes

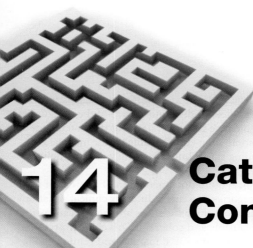

14 Categories Requiring Content of Service

Learning Objectives

After completing this chapter, you should be able to do the following:

- Spell and define the key terms and abbreviations presented in this chapter
- Identify the E/M categories that require content of service and contributing components
- Understand office or other outpatient services
- Identify hospital observation services
- Recognize hospital inpatient services
- Understand inpatient and outpatient consultations
- Identify emergency department services
- Recognize nursing facility services
- Understand domiciliary, rest home, or custodial care services
- Identify home services

Key Terms

activities of daily living (ADLs)

admission

admitting physician

ambulatory healthcare facility

annual nursing facility assessment

beneficiary

convalescent care

day management

fee-for-service program

intermediate care facility

long-term care facility

Medicaid

Medicare

observation status

partial hospital setting

per diem

rehabilitative care

skilled nursing facility

subsequent

supervising physician

transfer of care

Abbreviation

EOMI extra-ocular movements intact

INTRODUCTION

Guidelines provide the overarching structure for the E/M services. Even as definitive guidelines inform the documentation of the content of an E/M service, specific guidelines distinguish each of the categories of E/M services. The 1995 and 1997 DGs impart valuable guidance for understanding the documented E/M services, and each of the individual guidelines conveys something equally valuable for medical coders. Fully understanding the guidelines requires not only reading them, but also being willing to deliberate on the nuances of patient care.

Of the many categories of E/M services, nearly half of them require documentation of content of service and the contributing components. Each of these E/M categories presents a different clinical situation with unique characteristics. When these distinctions are understood, the differences among the categories become stark, and the logic of the guidelines becomes more plausible and coherent. This chapter presents an introduction to the guidelines for each of the categories listed in the CPT manual and reinforces the strong foundation of the content of service and contributing components.

CATEGORIES, SUBCATEGORIES, AND CODES

The nature of the E/M service can provide insight into the logic of the guidelines for each specific category of service. Each of the categories discussed in this chapter requires documentation of the content of service, and many of the category guidelines identify contributing components as significant factors in the selection of the E/M service code.

Guidelines dictate the constituents essential to reporting the content of an E/M service. Each of the individual category guidelines also provides cross-references to other categories to direct, channel, and lead coders to the category of service that most appropriately reflects the care provided to the patient. Remember that accurate reflection of the care provided to the patient is the primary concern of each aspect of medical documentation. The same is true for the selection of specific categories, subcategories, and individual codes.

OFFICE OR OTHER OUTPATIENT SERVICES

An outpatient service is considered any service that is not an inpatient service. Even though this may seem to be counterintuitive, common sense underlies the reasoning. The term *outpatient* refers to any patient who does not reside at the healthcare facility and is not required to spend the night at the healthcare facility for medical care. Examples of an outpatient setting include, but are not limited to, a physician's clinic office, an emergency department, and an **ambulatory healthcare facility**. The most important aspect of an outpatient service is that the patient can walk away from the E/M service on his or her own accord by the end of the calendar day. This distinction becomes very important when considering the context of the E/M service because the final decision for an outpatient status falls to the medical decision making of the physician performing the E/M service.

Since the definition of *outpatient* suggests the patient's ability to walk away, the term *ambulatory* has been closely associated with the office or other outpatient category. The evolution of healthcare has created various settings of outpatient service. With the advent of greater medical technology have come more opportunities for patient treatment in ambulatory settings, where the patient can receive medical care and return home the same day. Therefore, the most important factor of the office or other outpatient category of E/M service is the concept that the patient is able to return home that day after receiving the service. In the event that the medical decision making of the physician determines that admission to a hospital or nursing facility is necessary, the guidelines for office or other outpatient services give direction to the appropriate inpatient category. Therefore, when reviewing the documented office or other outpatient service, the guidelines for this same service category should be carefully reviewed and considered.

ambulatory healthcare facility any healthcare facility that provides same-day care for the patient

Office or Other Outpatient Service Subcategories: New and Established Patient

The office or other outpatient service category contains two subcategories: new patient and established patient. Each of these subcategories lists the required components and elements specific to each category. ■ TABLES 14.1 and 14.2 illustrate the specific requirements for each subcategory of the office or other outpatient E/M service.

■ TABLE 14.1   OFFICE OR OTHER OUTPATIENT SERVICES: NEW PATIENT REQUIREMENTS

OFFICE OR OTHER OUTPATIENT SERVICES: NEW PATIENT REQUIREMENTS	99201	99202	99203	99204	99205
History	Problem-focused	Expanded problem-focused	Detailed	Comprehensive	Comprehensive
Physical Examination	Problem-focused	Expanded problem-focused	Detailed	Comprehensive	Comprehensive
Medical Decision Making	Straightforward	Straightforward	Low	Moderate	High
Intraservice Time	10 minutes of face-to-face time with patient and/or family	20 minutes of face-to-face time with patient and/or family	30 minutes of face-to-face time with patient and/or family	45 minutes of face-to-face time with patient and/or family	60 minutes of face-to-face time with patient and/or family
Nature of Presenting Problem	Self-limited or minor severity	Low to moderate severity	Moderate severity	Moderate to high severity	Moderate to high severity

■ TABLE 14.2   OFFICE OR OTHER OUTPATIENT SERVICES: ESTABLISHED PATIENT REQUIREMENTS

OFFICE OR OTHER OUTPATIENT SERVICES: ESTABLISHED PATIENT	99211	99212	99213	99214	99215
History	No defined level of history required and may not require the presence of a physician	Problem-focused	Expanded problem-focused	Detailed	Comprehensive
Physical Examination	No defined level of physical examination required and may not require the presence of a physician	Problem-focused	Expanded problem-focused	Detailed	Comprehensive
Medical Decision Making	No defined level of medical decision making required and may not require the presence of a physician	Straightforward	Low	Moderate	High
Intraservice Time	5 minutes of face-to-face time with patient and/or family	10 minutes of face-to-face time with patient and/or family	15 minutes of face-to-face time with patient and/or family	25 minutes of face-to-face time with patient and/or family	40 minutes of face-to-face time with patient and/or family
Nature of Presenting Problem	Minimal severity	Self-limited or minor severity	Low to moderate severity	Moderate to high severity	Moderate to high severity

Understanding the content of service, the nature of the presenting problem, and the intraservice time required allows the reviewer to focus on the specific medical decision made by the performing physician: If the patient can walk away from the E/M service, this is an office or other outpatient service.

HOSPITAL OBSERVATION SERVICES

Generally, an observation is made when information must be gathered to make a decision or identify something. In healthcare, observation means that findings are recorded, inferences made, and measurements or tests performed not only for diagnosing the presenting problem, but also for determining the best course of action for the patient. As a result, hospital observation is a service that is provided for a patient, rather than a specific site of service, so the physician performing the E/M service must make the designation of observation care. Once the physician makes the clinical decision to observe the patient, this performing physician becomes the **supervising physician** of the patient's observation care.

supervising physician specific physician who may not be the only clinician involved in the observation of this patient, but who is responsible for the observation service provided for the patient

observation status the designation given when the patient's clinical presentation requires the physician performing the E/M service to closely monitor the patient's health before a final determination can be made

Hospital observation services may occur within a designated area of the facility or as a specific type of admission, which designates this patient as having **observation status**. Often, observation status is associated with an emergency room setting, when the severity of the presenting problem remains unclear. In such a case, the presenting problem does not immediately meet the clinical criteria for immediate admission into the hospital for treatment, but the acute or emergent nature of the presenting problem prevents the patient from walking away from the E/M service. Therefore, the CPT manual states that a hospital observation service occurs when the patient's clinical presentation requires the physician performing the E/M service to closely monitor the patient's health before a final determination of care can be made. Hospital observation is divided into three subcategories: initial observation care, subsequent observation care, and observation care discharge services.

Initial Observation Care: New or Established Patient

The period of observation begins at the moment the supervising physician identifies and documents the need for observation. It is important to recognize the word "supervising" since this specific physician may not be the only clinician involved in the observation status of this patient, but the supervising physician is responsible for the observation service provided for the patient. The period of observation may commence when the patient is put in a specific area of the hospital or placed in a hospital bed "for observation" or when the physician documents the observation of the patient. The CPT manual gives specific directions for the appropriate category and code selection for the E/M service, depending on the presentation of the patient, the decisions documented by the supervising physician, and the time of any potential hospital admission. Remember that according to the CPT manual, hospital observation is a service provided to determine the most appropriate plan of treatment for the presenting problem. Therefore, like an intersection of several different paths, hospital observation provides a crossroads of various options available for the treatment of the patient, providing the physician the opportunity to weigh each possible option before making the final clinical selection.

In the CPT manual, the subcategory of initial observation care focuses on the first clinical interaction between the supervising physician and the patient, when the physician makes the determination that an observation service should be performed to identify the most appropriate course of treatment. Initial observation care identifies no difference between an established patient and a new patient: This initial observation care is the same service regardless of the patient type. Therefore, regardless of whether the supervising physician has provided clinical, medical, or professional services for the patient during the previous 3 years, the preliminary observation care service provided by the supervising physician will always be considered an initial observation care service.

An initial observation service may be initiated in an emergency department, a physician's clinic office, a nursing care facility, or even a hospital. In these cases, any E/M services provided in conjunction with the commencement of observation care are included in the initial observation service. Regardless of the amount of time the physician spends with the patient, initial observation care services are considered "per day," or **per diem**. For example, if the patient receives E/M care in the emergency department just prior to the supervising physician initiating observation status, the care provided in the emergency department is included with the initial observation service care. However, the CPT manual has included intraservice time in the guidelines for initial observation care services, which affects the documented content of service when selecting the initial observation care code. ■ TABLE 14.3 illustrates the required components for the selection of the appropriate initial observation care code.

per diem measurement by day, per day, or according to the passage of 1 day

■ TABLE 14.3 **INITIAL OBSERVATION CARE: NEW OR ESTABLISHED PATIENT REQUIREMENTS**

HOSPITAL OBSERVATION SERVICE: INITIAL OBSERVATION CARE	99218	99219	99220
History	Detailed or comprehensive	Comprehensive	Comprehensive
Physical Examination	Detailed or comprehensive	Comprehensive	Comprehensive
Medical Decision Making	Straightforward or low	Moderate	High
Intraservice Time	Although this is a per diem code, physicians typically spend 30 minutes at the bedside *and* on the patient's floor or unit.	Although this is a per diem code, physicians typically spend 50 minutes at the bedside *and* on the patient's floor or unit.	Although this is a per diem code, physicians typically spend 70 minutes at the bedside *and* on the patient's floor or unit.
Nature of Presenting Problem	Low severity	Moderate severity	High severity

■ TABLE 14.4   SUBSEQUENT OBSERVATION CARE REQUIREMENTS

HOSPITAL OBSERVATION SERVICE: SUBSEQUENT OBSERVATION CARE	99224	99225	99226
History	Problem-focused	Expanded problem-focused	Detailed
Physical Examination	Problem-focused	Expanded problem-focused	Detailed
Medical Decision Making	Straightforward or low	Moderate	High
Intraservice Time	Although this is a per diem code, 15 minutes of unit/floor intraservice time is typical.	Although this is a per diem code, 25 minutes of unit/floor intraservice time is typical.	Although this is a per diem code, 35 minutes of unit/floor intraservice time is typical.
Nature of Presenting Problem	Severity is not defined, but generally the patient is stable, recovering, or improving.	Severity is not defined, but generally the patient is responding inadequately to therapy, or a minor complication has developed.	Severity is not defined, but generally the patient is unstable or has developed a significant complication or a significant new problem.

The CPT manual states that there are certain circumstances when initial observation care services should not be reported. As stated, any E/M services that are directly related to the commencement of an initial observation care service should not be reported separately. In addition, observation care services may not be reported for any postoperative recovery periods, since a certain amount of observation is inherently required because of the nature of the procedure.

The CPT guidelines provide direct assistance and guidance regarding the various clinical encounters that may arise during and surrounding an initial observation care service. It is important to remember that the guidelines acknowledge that clinical circumstances vary depending on the nature of the encounter, and the guidelines provide specific direction for category selection. Therefore, if there is any doubt about whether to select an initial observation care service code, the CPT guidelines should be carefully reviewed.

Subsequent Observation Care

The term **subsequent** suggests that an event, task, or procedure is preceded by a different essential event, task, or procedure. This is true for subsequent observation care. This service includes the review of the patient's medical record and any diagnostic testing results, changes in the patient's status, physical examination findings, and medical decision-making findings. The CPT manual identifies requirements for a subsequent observation care service visit, which are different from an initial observation care service because the patient has received clinical, medical, or professional services from the performing physician while the patient has been in observation status (see ■ TABLE 14.4).

subsequent provided after the initial E/M service

As with the initial observation care service codes, the subsequent observation care codes are per diem, and any E/M services related to observation care services are considered part of the subsequent observation care service.

Hospital Observation Care Discharge Services   Unlike initial observation care and subsequent observation care services, observation care discharge services do not require content of service or any of the contributing components. The CPT manual states that observation care discharge services occur when the supervising physician makes the determination that observation care services can be concluded. The observation care discharge service can be reported only on a day *other than* the day that initial observation service commenced. Since observation care discharge service includes any management services related to the cessation of observation care provided by the physician, the observation care discharge service is considered a day management. **Day management** refers to the inclusion of any services provided to the patient during the entire process of discharging the patient from observation care status. It is worth noting that in the event that a hospital observation care discharge service is performed on the same date as an admission to a nursing facility, both services can be reported separately.

day management refers to the inclusion of any services provided to the patient during the entire process of discharging the patient from observation care status

HOSPITAL INPATIENT SERVICES

The word *inpatient* suggests that either a patient has been formally admitted to a medical facility and has remained in the hospital overnight for treatment or the patient resides in the medical facility. Hospital inpatient services include E/M services provided to patients who have been formally admitted to the

admission the formal acceptance of the patient's care by the hospital, nursing home, domiciliary care provider, boarding or rest home, or other healthcare facility where the patient will remain overnight

admitting physician physician responsible for completion of documentation specific to the hospital inpatient setting, including documentation intended to facilitate coordination of care with other physicians, nurses, and any other clinical staff who will provide care and treatment for the patient

hospital. When a patient is formally admitted to the hospital, the period of time the patient remains in the hospital can be referred to as one specific **admission**. As with hospital observation care services, hospital inpatient services do not identify the typical patient type, new or established, but instead recognize two different subcategories—initial hospital care service and subsequent hospital care service—plus two sub-subcategories of subsequent care.

Initial Hospital Care: New or Established

The word *initial* designates the beginning of a series of events or procedures. Initial hospital care services reflect the first E/M services provided for a patient in an inpatient hospital setting. The physician who performs an initial hospital care service becomes the **admitting physician**. That physician is responsible for completion of documentation specific to the hospital inpatient setting, including documentation of services to facilitate coordination of care with other physicians, nurses, and any other clinical staff who will provide care and treatment for the patient. Since the intent of an initial hospital care service is the admission of the patient into the hospital, the inpatient hospital care service does not distinguish between a new patient and an established patient. Instead, the encounter is recognized as a new inpatient hospital admission.

A hospital admission is a completely different circumstance from a physician office visit. However, there may be circumstances when a patient is admitted to the hospital during the course of an E/M service or encounter in a different site of service, such as a physician's clinic office, an emergency department, nursing facility, or even home care. In the event the patient is admitted to the hospital from a different site of service, the E/M services provided by that physician in conjunction with the hospital admission are considered part of the initial hospital care service. Therefore, to reflect the time and effort involved in completing a new admission to the hospital, initial inpatient care services are considered to be per diem services and report the E/M services provided during the day of admission. The documentation requirements reflect the inclusive nature of these guidelines. TABLE ■ 14.5 illustrates the content of service and contributing component requirements for initial hospital care services.

Certain clinical circumstances pose inherent complications, either because of the nature of the presenting problem or the situation surrounding the encounter. For instance, admissions of a neonate, or an infant younger than 28 days of age, require different documentation requirements and therefore must be reported with a different category of E/M service. As with every category and subcategory of E/M service, the guidelines should be reviewed.

Subsequent Hospital Care

Every subsequent E/M service performed during a patient's stay in the hospital is reported on a per diem basis. This per diem reporting includes the review of diagnostic testing results, the patient's medical record for the continued coordination of care for the patient, and any changes in status since the most recent physician assessment during the hospital day. As such, the documentation requirements for a subsequent hospital care service are slightly less stringent than those for the initial hospital care. ■ TABLE 14.6 illustrates the documentation requirements for subsequent hospital care services.

Observation or Inpatient Care Services (Including Admission and Discharge Services)   These E/M services are a very specific type: observation or inpatient care provided to patients who have been admitted and discharged on the same date of service—that is, they have been admitted for at least 9 hours but less than 24 hours. For example, the supervising physician at the hospital admits

■ TABLE 14.5   **INITIAL HOSPITAL CARE REQUIREMENTS**

HOSPITAL INPATIENT SERVICE: INITIAL HOSPITAL CARE	99221	99222	99223
History	Detailed or comprehensive	Comprehensive	Comprehensive
Physical Examination	Detailed or comprehensive	Comprehensive	Comprehensive
Medical Decision Making	Straightforward or low	Moderate	High
Intraservice Time	30 minutes of unit/floor time	50 minutes of unit/floor time	70 minutes of unit/floor time
Nature of Presenting Problem	Low severity	Moderate severity	High severity

■ TABLE 14.6   SUBSEQUENT HOSPITAL CARE SERVICE REQUIREMENTS

HOSPITAL INPATIENT SERVICE: SUBSEQUENT HOSPITAL CARE	99231	99232	99233
History	Problem-focused	Expanded problem-focused	Detailed
Physical Examination	Problem-focused	Expanded problem-focused	Detailed
Medical Decision Making	Straightforward or low	Moderate	High
Intraservice Time	15 minutes of unit/floor time	Although a per diem code, typically 25 minutes of unit/floor time	Although a per diem code, typically 35 minutes of unit/floor time
Nature of Presenting Problem	Severity is not defined, but generally the patient is recovering, or the patient's condition is stable or improving.	Severity is not defined, but generally the patient is responding inadequately to therapy or has developed a minor complication.	Severity is not defined, but generally the patient is unstable or has developed a significant complication or a significant new problem.

Jack into hospital observation at 7:30 a.m. to determine whether he should be admitted for inpatient treatment. Over the course of the day, Jack's condition is observed and assessed, and management options are reviewed. After 13 hours of observation or inpatient care services, the supervising physician discharges him home. Because all of the aspects of this subsubcategory of services—admission, observation care, and discharge—have occurred in less than 24 hours, these services are treated differently from other hospital observation care services, which require discharge to occur on a different date from that of service initiation.

It is important to note, however, that the admission aspect of this subsubcategory of services is consistent with the guidelines for initial hospital observation care services because this subsubcategory reflects a specific type of care rather than a specific location in which the care is provided. As a result, if an observation service has been initiated in another site of service, the E/M services performed in conjunction with that initiated observation service are considered to be part of that observation service as long as the E/M services are performed on the same date as the documented observation service. For example, Julie presents for treatment to the emergency department, which is a specific site of service, at 7:00 a.m., and the supervising physician there admits her to observation, which is a specific type of care, where her condition is observed and assessed and management options are reviewed. After 10 hours of observation, the supervising physician discharges Julie home. Because the emergency department is a separate site of service, the E/M services provided throughout the day would be considered part of the initial hospital observation care service rather than an example of this subsubcategory.

Consistent with all other E/M services requiring documentation of content of service, this subsubcategory—observation or inpatient care services (including admission and discharge services)—has specific requirements for the documented content of service. ■ TABLE 14.7 illustrates the requirements stipulated by the guidelines.

■ TABLE 14.7   OBSERVATION OR INPATIENT CARE SERVICES (INCLUDING ADMISSION AND DISCHARGE SERVICES) REQUIREMENTS

HOSPITAL INPATIENT SERVICE: OBSERVATION OR INPATIENT CARE SERVICES (INCLUDING ADMISSION AND DISCHARGE SERVICES)	99234	99235	99236
History	Detailed or comprehensive	Comprehensive	Comprehensive
Physical Examination	Detailed or comprehensive	Comprehensive	Comprehensive
Medical Decision Making	Straightforward or low	Moderate	High
Intraservice Time	As a per diem code, intraservice time is not applicable, but counseling and coordination of care are appropriate to the patient's presenting problem and the needs of the family.	As a per diem code, intraservice time is not applicable, but counseling and coordination of care are appropriate to the patient's presenting problem and the needs of the family.	As a per diem code, intraservice time is not applicable, but counseling and coordination of care are appropriate to the patient's presenting problem and the needs of the family.
Nature of Presenting Problem	Low severity	Moderate severity	High severity

Hospital Discharge Services At the conclusion of a patient's stay in the hospital, the patient must be discharged from the inpatient facility. The process of discharging a patient from an inpatient hospital stay requires time to allow for the documentation of any final examination of the patient and preparation of prescriptions, referral forms, or coordination of care. If any discussion regarding the hospital stay occurs between the discharging physician and the patient, the content of this discussion may be documented as well, which may include instructions for the patient regarding future care. In addition, since the patient has been admitted to an inpatient facility, the discharging physician must prepare the discharge records. Because of this required documentation, the hospital discharge services report the total amount of time spent by the physician in discharging the patient from the inpatient facility. The guidelines determine the following allotments of time for hospital discharge services: less than 30 minutes of time spent by the physician or more than 30 minutes of time spent by the physician. In the event that a hospital discharge service is performed on the same date as an admission to a nursing facility, both services may be reported separately.

CONSULTATIONS

The category of consultations reflects a specific kind of E/M service: one physician performs an E/M service at the request of another physician for the sole purpose of providing a professional opinion on the patient's presenting problem. One physician or appropriate source must request the professional opinion of a different physician; a physician, physician assistant, nurse practitioner, insurance company, or other specific source listed in the consultation guidelines of the CPT manual can initiate this request.

The documentation of this request for opinion sets in motion the performance of the consultation service. Once the written or verbal request has been made and the consultation service performed, the consulting physician's opinion, findings, and any pertinent results or performed services should be documented in the patient's medical record and conveyed to the source of the consultation request. Given the strict documentation requirements for consultations, no distinction is made between a new patient and an established patient. As a result, there are only two subcategories of consultations, which reflect the site of service in which the consultation is performed: office or other outpatient consultations and hospital inpatient consultations. Although the content of service requirements for both subcategories are the same, the requirements for the contributing components are very different.

Office or Other Outpatient Consultations

Consultations performed in an office or other outpatient setting include consultations performed in a physician's office as well as those performed in an outpatient setting or an ambulatory facility. These office or other outpatient consultations may be performed during a hospital observation service or in a rest home, an emergency department, or any other facility where the patient does not currently reside or has not been admitted as an inpatient. ■ TABLE 14.8 illustrates the documentation requirements for consultations performed in an office or other outpatient setting.

■ **TABLE 14.8** **OFFICE OR OTHER OUTPATIENT CONSULTATION REQUIREMENTS**

CONSULTATIONS: OFFICE OR OTHER OUTPATIENT	99241	99242	99243	99244	99245
History	Problem-focused	Expanded problem-focused	Detailed	Comprehensive	Comprehensive
Physical Examination	Problem-focused	Expanded problem-focused	Detailed	Comprehensive	Comprehensive
Medical Decision Making	Straightforward	Straightforward	Low	Moderate	High
Intraservice Time	15 minutes of face-to-face time with patient and/or family	30 minutes of face-to-face time with patient and/or family	40 minutes of face-to-face time with patient and/or family	60 minutes of face-to-face time with patient and/or family	80 minutes of face-to-face time with patient and/or family
Nature of Presenting Problem	Self-limited or minor severity	Low severity	Moderate severity	Moderate to high severity	Moderate to high severity

An important distinction must be made between a consultation and a **transfer of care**. Whereas a consultation service documents the request for professional opinion from the physician performing the consultation service, a transfer of care is a process that begins when a physician who has previously provided E/M services for one or more issues related to a patient's care relinquishes the responsibility for some or all of the patient's care to a different physician, who has not previously provided either any healthcare services for the patient or a consultation on the patient's condition. In order for the transfer of care to be completed, it is important that the new physician explicitly accept responsibility for the patient's care, at which point the original physician is no longer responsible for the care of these specific transferred problems. This does not mean that the original physician will not provide any care for the patient, but it does indicate that the original physician has relinquished care of the specific problems that have been transferred to the other physician. This distinction creates a stark difference between a consultation, in which the original physician requests a professional opinion regarding a patient's specific presenting problem, and a transfer of care, in which the original physician relinquishes all care regarding a patient's specific presenting problem to a different physician, who agrees to accept responsibility for treating the patient's specific presenting problem.

Inpatient Consultations

Inpatient consultations include consultation services provided to patients who reside in a facility or have been admitted to an inpatient hospital. These inpatient settings include nursing facilities, hospitals, and **partial hospital settings**. As with office or other outpatient consultations, inpatient consultations are intended to obtain an opinion on the patient's presenting problem from a different physician. This request for a consultation, which may be verbal or written, then leads to the requested physician's rendering of his or her professional opinion. That opinion must then be documented in the patient's medical record by the physician who performed the consultation and must be communicated to the physician who made the consultation request.

In contrast to office or other outpatient consultations, when an inpatient consultation is performed on the same date as the patient's admission into a hospital or nursing facility, all of the E/M services provided by the consulting physician that relate to the inpatient admission are included in the consultation service. Given the extensive requirements for the performance of an inpatient consultation, the documentation requirements are equally stringent, as shown in ▪ TABLE 14.9.

Although the guideline regarding transfer of care applies equally to inpatient consultations and to office or other outpatient consultations, the specific guidelines pertinent to inpatient settings should be reviewed in the CPT manual.

Special Circumstances   As of January 2010, the Centers for **Medicare** and **Medicaid** Services no longer recognized consultations as a valid E/M service and eliminated payment of consultation services performed for a **beneficiary** of any Medicare **fee-for-service program** or any government Medicare or Medicaid program. Although this has affected the reporting of consultation services, the CPT manual continues to include these services in the numeric list of E/M services.

transfer of care the process that occurs when a patient's primary care physician relinquishes the responsibility of some or all of the patient's care to a different physician who has not previously provided any consultation services for the patient

partial hospital setting a healthcare facility that offers intensive therapeutic treatment or support for a patient whose condition does not warrant admission into an inpatient facility; most commonly provides psychiatric and mental healthcare

Medicare a federal program that provides healthcare insurance for people of the United States over the age of 65 and for those with disabilities or anyone with end-stage renal disease; founded in 1965 and administered by the Center for Medicare and Medicaid Services

Medicaid a healthcare program that works in cooperation with each of the states to provide assistance for low-income children and adults, as well as individuals with disabilities; founded in 1965 and monitored by the Center for Medicare and Medicaid Services

▪ TABLE 14.9   INPATIENT CONSULTATION REQUIREMENTS

CONSULTATIONS: INPATIENT	99251	99252	99253	99254	99255
History	Problem-focused	Expanded problem-focused	Detailed	Comprehensive	Comprehensive
Physical Examination	Problem-focused	Expanded problem-focused	Detailed	Comprehensive	Comprehensive
Medical Decision Making	Straightforward	Straightforward	Low	Moderate	High
Intraservice Time	20 minutes of unit/floor time at the patient's bedside or on the floor/unit	40 minutes of unit/floor time at the patient's bedside or on the floor/unit	55 minutes of unit/floor time at the patient's bedside or on the floor/unit	80 minutes of unit/floor time at the patient's bedside or on the floor/unit	110 minutes of unit/floor time at the patient's bedside or on the floor/unit
Nature of Presenting Problem	Self-limited or minor severity	Low severity	Moderate severity	Moderate to high severity	Moderate to high severity

■ **TABLE 14.10 EMERGENCY DEPARTMENT SERVICE REQUIREMENTS**

EMERGENCY DEPARTMENT SERVICES	99281	99282	99283	99284	99285
History	Problem-focused	Expanded problem-focused	Expanded problem-focused	Detailed	Comprehensive
Physical Examination	Problem-focused	Expanded problem-focused	Expanded problem-focused	Detailed	Comprehensive
Medical Decision Making	Straightforward	Low	Moderate	Moderate	High
Intraservice Time	Time is not a contributing component because it is difficult to quantify the amount of time spent face-to-face with one specific patient.	Time is not a contributing component because it is difficult to quantify the amount of time spent face-to-face with one specific patient.	Time is not a contributing component because it is difficult to quantify the amount of time spent face-to-face with one specific patient.	Time is not a contributing component because it is difficult to quantify the amount of time spent face-to-face with one specific patient.	Time is not a contributing component because it is difficult to quantify the amount of time spent face-to-face with one specific patient.
Nature of Presenting Problem	Self-limited or minor severity	Low to moderate severity	Moderate severity	High severity and requiring urgent medical attention but not posing a threat to life or physiologic function	High severity and posing imminent threat to life and/or bodily function, therefore requiring immediate medical attention

beneficiary an individual who receives the benefit of a service or program; most commonly used in reference to private, state, and federal health and/or medical insurance policies

fee-for-service program in healthcare, a specific service that establishes a standard of payment, acknowledging the amount of work involved in the provision of that service, care, or treatment

EMERGENCY DEPARTMENT SERVICES

Not every unforeseen, serious situation that occurs suddenly can be considered an emergency. However, an unforeseen, serious situation that occurs suddenly and results in a presenting problem that requires immediate medical attention would be considered an emergency. An emergency department is any section of a hospital facility that is specifically staffed with medical professionals trained in emergency medical care, equipped to respond to and treat medical emergencies, and remains open 24 hours a day. Since medical emergencies occur without warning, no distinction is made between a new patient and an established patient in the guidelines for emergency department services, regardless of the number of times a patient has received professional or medical services at that specific emergency department during the 3 years prior to the emergency department service in question. Because of the inherently unpredictable nature of medical emergencies, the documentation requirements are stringent, even though there is no intraservice guideline for emergency department services. ■ Table 14.10 illustrates the documentation requirements for emergency department services.

It is important to distinguish between the E/M services provided for a patient in an emergency department setting and E/M services provided for a patient for whom initial observation care has been initiated. This distinction is best identified in the physician's documentation of the performed service.

Exercise 14.1 E/M Category, Subcategory, and Level for Sinus Pressure

Read the following medical documentation, and then answer the following questions.

History: Joanie Smith presents to the clinic for increased sinus pressure, sore throat, and a cough. Patient has recently moved to the area. The right side of the patient's head hurts so much that she feels she cannot hold her head up due to the throbbing pain. The patient states that her teeth began to ache last night, and this morning every part of her hurts. Although the patient recognizes flu is likely, she is concerned about a sinus infection.

Appetite greatly reduced, no reports of nausea, vomiting, or diarrhea. No reports of heart palpitations or shortness of breath. Other than feeling chilled all the time, she reports no other health problems. The patient is a preschool teacher, and she provides multiple reports of ill contact at work.

Exam: Patient is very pale and appears very tired. Conjunctivae are red, swollen, but are not inflamed. The patient reports exquisite pain and associated dizziness upon palpation of face, particularly the forehead and maxillary sinuses. The patient loses her balance easily when asked to tip her head forward.

Exercise 14.1 *continued*

Minimal phlegm production per nares is noted. Oropharynx is red and minimally inflamed, and patient reports feeling that she has something tickling her throat. No rub or fremitus noted upon auscultation of lungs.

Assessment: Sinus infection, without impaction.

Plan: Azithromycin prescribed for sinus infection. Increased fluids, recommended rest.

1. Which category best reflects the E/M service provided? Explain your rationale.

   _____

   _____

   _____

2. Which subcategory best reflects the E/M service provided? Explain your rationale.

   _____

   _____

   _____

3. Which level of service best reflects the E/M service provided? Explain your rationale.

   _____

   _____

   _____

Exercise 14.2 E/M Category, Subcategory, and Level for Fecal Impaction

Read the following medical documentation, and then answer the following questions.

Timmy, a 3-year-old, presents to the emergency room for significant abdominal and rectal pain. Patient's pain is identified in the lower abdomen but not focally identifiable. Patient states it hurts to poop. Father states after his son passed extremely hard, large stool, blood was noted on the toilet paper and in the toilet. Timmy is very agitated about pooping.

ROS: Prior to this episode, negative for bloody stools, dysuria, hematuria. Positive history for constipation. Timmy has recently been potty trained and has been postponing defecation. All other ROS pertaining to this problem are negative. Father states that Timmy's preschool went on a field trip to an apple orchard. When asked if Timmy likes apples, patient replies, "Not any more."

Past medical history: Negative history of small bowel obstruction or intussusception. No family history of abdominal problems.

Physical exam: T, 102.5. Timmy is calm but very uncomfortable. Abdomen is bloated. Palpation of abdomen reveals minimal guarding and pain, especially in quadrants. Patient reports little referring pain when asked to cough. No evidence of anal fissures, fistulas, or hemorrhoids noted during anal exam. Normal anal wink is noted. Presence of hard, dry stool is evident in rectal vault.

Diagnostic: WBC, 9,000; CRP, 150 mg/L. KUB significant stool in rectosigmoid and through descending colon.

Assessment: Fecal impaction. Recommend fecal disimpaction via oral cathartics. Due to Timmy's age, treatment would be most efficacious via enema or suppository application. Recommend education on healthy bowel habits.

Plan: Admit patient to observation status for fecal disimpaction and evacuation of bowels. Rehydration via oral fluids.

1. Which category best reflects the E/M service provided? Explain your rationale.

   _____

   _____

   _____

2. Which subcategory best reflects the E/M service provided? Explain your rationale.

   _____

   _____

   _____

3. Which level of service best reflects the E/M service provided? Explain your rationale.

   _____

   _____

   _____

Exercise 14.3 E/M Category, Subcategory, and Level for Joan's Severe Back Pain

Read the following medical documentation, and then answer the following questions.

Subjective: Joan was admitted to Five Wings Hospital yesterday for severe lower back pain. Pain well controlled with oxy-

codone. Patient more conversant and responsive. No bowel movement since admission. Remaining ROS: negative.

Objective: Head: normal, atraumatic. Eyes: PERRL, EOMI. Resp: clear sounds, good exchange. CV: RRR, normal sounds. GI: mild bloating, no guarding or rigidity.

continued

Exercise 14.3 *continued*

Assessment/Plan: Suspected vertebral fracture between T12 and L2 vertebrae of unknown severity.

1. Request consultation for vertebral fracture and spinal or nerve involvement.
2. Begin stool softener regimen.
3. Physical therapy ordered.

1. Which category best reflects the E/M service provided? Explain your rationale.

_____

_____

_____

2. Which subcategory best reflects the E/M service provided? Explain your rationale.

_____

_____

_____

3. Which level of service best reflects the E/M service provided? Explain your rationale.

_____

_____

_____

NURSING FACILITY SERVICES

skilled nursing facility facility that provides housing for chronically ill patients who require a variety of health-care services, including nursing care; physical, speech, or occupational therapy; rehabilitation; and other services of care

intermediate care facility transitional facility that provides rehabilitative care for patients who require care and services for a short period of time

long-term care facility facility that provides extended healthcare services for patients who require extensive or ongoing care, therapeutic support, or assistance with activities of daily living

convalescent care healthcare services provided for a patient who is recovering from an illness; also referred to as recuperative care

rehabilitative care healthcare services—such as therapy, education, and counseling—intended to enable a patient's return to good health in mind and body

The CPT manual utilizes the nursing facility services category to report E/M services provided to patients who have been admitted to nursing facilities commonly known as **skilled nursing facilities, intermediate care facilities**, or **long-term care facilities**. Nursing facilities provide services such as **convalescent care**, **rehabilitative care**, and long-term care. These nursing facilities are required to perform standardized assessments in a series of protocols to measure the functional capacity of each resident. Not only do these protocols and assessments indicate potential problems for the residents' health, but also they provide specific guidelines for any subsequent assessments, screenings, and protocols that are required. It is important that these measurements can be reproduced over time to ensure objective accuracy and quality patient care.

Physicians play a vital role in the promotion of these essential protocols and assessments, subsequent measurements, and the maintenance and provision of management options and medical plans for inpatient residents in nursing facilities. As a result, E/M services performed in a nursing facility setting require documentation of the mandatory assessments and protocols as well as the performance of the content of service and any pertinent contributing components. The category of nursing facility care lists four subcategories of services: initial nursing facility care, subsequent nursing facility care, nursing facility discharge, and other nursing facility services.

Initial Nursing Facility Care

The initial nursing facility care service reports the admission of the patient into the nursing facility. A distinction is not made between a new patient and an established patient, since each initial service reports a completely new admission into the nursing facility. Because any admission process may include certain complications and intricacies, each level of initial nursing facility care reports the E/M services provided on the date of admission into the nursing facility. As with the other initial services, the admission may be initiated during the course of a clinical encounter at a different site of service, such as a physician's clinic office, emergency department, or home care. In the event that the admission does commence during a clinical encounter at a different site of service, any E/M services related to the admission are considered part of the initial nursing facility care service and are considered when reviewing the content of service. Also, since admissions to nursing facilities can occur at anytime during the day or night, initial nursing facility care services are reported on a per diem basis. ■ TABLE 14.11 reflects the documentation requirements for the initial nursing facility care service.

As with each E/M category and subcategory, the specific guidelines listed in the CPT manual should be reviewed.

Subsequent Nursing Facility Care

Subsequent nursing facility care includes the E/M services provided each day of care, specifically in relation to the last assessment or protocol by the physician. These services may include review of records or the results of diagnostic testing, as well as identification of changes in the patient's health status according

■ TABLE 14.11   **INITIAL NURSING FACILITY CARE REQUIREMENTS**

NURSING FACILITY SERVICES: INITIAL NURSING FACILITY CARE	99304	99305	99306
History	Detailed or comprehensive	Comprehensive	Comprehensive
Physical Examination	Detailed or comprehensive	Comprehensive	Comprehensive
Medical Decision Making	Straightforward or low	Moderate	High
Intraservice Time	25 minutes of unit/floor time	35 minutes of unit/floor time	45 minutes of unit/floor time
Nature of Presenting Problem	Low severity	Moderate severity	High severity

■ TABLE 14.12   **SUBSEQUENT NURSING FACILITY CARE REQUIREMENTS**

NURSING FACILITY SERVICES: SUBSEQUENT NURSING FACILITY CARE	99307	99308	99309	99310
History	Problem-focused	Expanded problem-focused	Detailed	Comprehensive
Physical Examination	Problem-focused	Expanded problem-focused	Detailed	Comprehensive
Medical Decision Making	Straightforward	Low	Moderate	High
Intraservice Time	Although this is a per diem code, 10 minutes of unit/floor time is typical.	Although this is a per diem code, 15 minutes of unit/floor time is typical.	Although this is a per diem code, 25 minutes of unit/floor time is typical.	Although this is a per diem code, 35 minutes of unit/floor time is typical.
Nature of Presenting Problem	Severity is not defined, but generally the patient is stable, recovering, or improving.	Severity is not defined, but generally the patient is responding inadequately to therapy or has developed a minor complication.	Severity is not defined, but generally the patient has developed a significant complication or a significant new problem.	Severity is not defined, but the patient may be unstable or may have developed a significant new problem requiring immediate medical attention.

to the documented content of service. ■ TABLE 14.12 illustrates the documentation requirements for subsequent nursing facility care services.

Nursing Facility Discharge Services

The nursing facility discharge services are considered "day management" services because they report the total amount of time the performing physician spends discharging the patient from the nursing facility. For this reporting, specific durations of time are identified for the completion of the nursing facility discharge: 30 minutes or less spent by the physician or more than 30 minutes spent by the physician. These specific allotments of time may include a final physical examination of the patient, discussion with or counseling of the patient and/or family about care the patient received, prescriptions, care management, referrals, and preparation of discharge records.

Other Nursing Facility Services

Although this subcategory suggests a variety of services from which to choose, it specifically includes E/M services provided to an inpatient resident of the nursing facility in relation to the **annual nursing facility assessment**. This annual assessment provides the standardized measurement required for nursing facility services and requires the content of service and contributing components shown in ■ TABLE 14.13.

This nursing facility subcategory may not be reported on the same date as any other nursing facility care service.

annual nursing facility assessment the standardized protocols intended to assess and measure the patient's progress, ability, and function throughout the patient's stay in the nursing facility

■ TABLE 14.13 OTHER NURSING FACILITY SERVICES REQUIREMENTS

OTHER NURSING FACILITY SERVICES	99318
History	Detailed
Physical Examination	Comprehensive
Medical Decision Making	Low to moderate complexity
Intraservice Time	30 minutes of unit/floor time
Nature of Presenting Problem	Severity is not defined, but generally the patient is stable, recovering, or improving.

DOMICILIARY, REST HOME, OR CUSTODIAL CARE SERVICES

activities of daily living (ADLs) the activities necessary for an independent person to perform in order to live alone, including, but not limited to, grooming oneself, feeding oneself, cooking, and getting dressed

Domiciliary, rest home (e.g., boarding home), or custodial care services are provided in facilities that provide legal residence for patients—for example, room, board, and any other services that assist the personal function, ability, or mobility of the patient. Each of the components of this category represents a different aspect of these E/M services. Domiciliary services are provided in a patient's permanent or semi-permanent dwelling. A rest home is commonly a home in which elderly or frail patients reside and receive care. Custodial care services are E/M services provided for patients who are unable to perform **activities of daily living (ADLs)**, such as personal grooming, cooking, or dressing themselves. The E/M services provided in the domiciliary, rest home, or custodial care category include the medically necessary care for each of the subcategories: new patient and established patient.

New Patient

The new patient subcategory requires that the patient has not received professional, clinical, or medical services from the physician or group during 3 years prior to the domiciliary, rest home, or custodial care service in question. The documentation requirements for this subcategory are consistent with those for all new patients, as illustrated in ■ TABLE 14.14.

Established Patient

The established patient subcategory of domiciliary, rest home, or custodial care requires that the patient has received professional, clinical, or medical services from the physician or group during 3 years prior to this specific service date in question. As shown in ■ TABLE 14.15, the documentation requirements for the

■ TABLE 14.14 DOMICILIARY, REST HOME, OR CUSTODIAL CARE SERVICES: NEW PATIENT REQUIREMENTS

DOMICILIARY, REST HOME, OR CUSTODIAL CARE SERVICES: NEW PATIENT	99324	99325	99326	99327	99328
History	Problem-focused	Expanded problem-focused	Detailed	Comprehensive	Comprehensive
Physical Examination	Problem-focused	Expanded problem-focused	Detailed	Comprehensive	Comprehensive
Medical Decision Making	Straightforward	Low	Moderate	Moderate	High
Intraservice Time	20 minutes of face-to-face time with patient and/or family	30 minutes of face-to-face time with patient and/or family	45 minutes of face-to-face time with patient and/or family	60 minutes of face-to-face time with patient and/or family	75 minutes of face-to-face time with patient and/or family
Nature of Presenting Problem	Low severity	Moderate severity	Moderate to high severity	High severity	Severity is not defined, but the patient may be unstable or has developed a significant new problem requiring immediate physician attention.

■ TABLE 14.15   DOMICILIARY, REST HOME, OR CUSTODIAL CARE SERVICES: ESTABLISHED PATIENT REQUIREMENTS

DOMICILIARY, REST HOME, OR CUSTODIAL CARE SERVICES: ESTABLISHED PATIENT	99334	99335	99336	99337
History	Problem-focused	Expanded problem-focused	Detailed	Comprehensive
Physical Examination	Problem-focused	Expanded problem-focused	Detailed	Comprehensive
Medical Decision Making	Straightforward	Low	Moderate	Moderate
Intraservice Time	15 minutes time with patient and/or family or caregiver	25 minutes time with patient and/or family or caregiver	40 minutes time with patient and/or family or caregiver	60 minutes time with patient and/or family or caregiver
Nature of Presenting Problem	Self-limited or minor severity	Moderate severity	Moderate to high severity	Moderate to high severity; generally, the patient may be unstable or may have developed a significant new problem requiring immediate physician attention.

established domiciliary, rest home, or custodial care services follow the standards for all established patient services.

HOME SERVICES

E/M services provided for patients residing in a private residence are identified as home services. The content of service documents the E/M services performed for the patient, whereas the contributing components may also include the needs of the patient's family. The home service category lists two subcategories: new patient and established patient.

New Patient

For the new patient home services subcategory, the documentation requires that the patient has not received professional, clinical, or medical home services from the physician or group during 3 years prior to the home service in question. The documentation requirements for a new patient home service are consistent with those for all new patients, as shown in ■ TABLE 14.16.

■ TABLE 14.16   HOME SERVICES REQUIREMENTS: NEW PATIENT

HOME SERVICES: NEW PATIENT	99341	99342	99343	99344	99345
History	Problem-focused	Expanded problem-focused	Detailed	Comprehensive	Comprehensive
Physical Examination	Problem-focused	Expanded problem-focused	Detailed	Comprehensive	Comprehensive
Medical Decision Making	Straightforward	Low	Moderate	Moderate	High
Intraservice Time	20 minutes of face-to-face time with patient and/or family	30 minutes of face-to-face time with patient and/or family	45 minutes of face-to-face time with patient and/or family	60 minutes of face-to-face time with patient and/or family	75 minutes of face-to-face time with patient and/or family
Nature of Presenting Problem	Low severity	Moderate severity	Moderate to high severity	High severity	Severity is not defined, but the patient may be unstable or has developed a significant new problem requiring immediate medical attention.

■ TABLE 14.17   **HOME SERVICES REQUIREMENTS: ESTABLISHED PATIENT**

HOME SERVICES: ESTABLISHED PATIENT	99347	99348	99349	99350
History	Problem-focused	Expanded problem-focused	Detailed	Comprehensive
Physical Examination	Problem-focused	Expanded problem-focused	Detailed	Comprehensive
Medical Decision Making	Straightforward	Low	Moderate	Moderate to high
Intraservice Time	15 minutes time with patient and/or family	25 minutes time with patient and/or family	40 minutes time with patient and/or family	60 minutes time with patient and/or family
Nature of Presenting Problem	Self-limited or minor severity	Low to moderate severity	Moderate to high severity	Moderate to high severity, indicating that the patient may be unstable or has developed a significant new problem requiring immediate medical attention

Established Patient

The established patient subcategory requires that the patient has received medical, clinical, or professional home services from the physician or group during 3 years prior to the specific home service visit in question. ■ TABLE 14.17 illustrates the documentation requirements for the established patient home services.

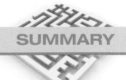

SUMMARY

- E/M services are divided into different categories. Each category reflects the site of service, the essential quality of service, or the manner of care provided for the patient. Nearly half of the E/M categories require specific documentation of the content of service as well as contributing components. These category-specific guidelines supply direction and instruction for identifying the most accurate service code. The directions may include references to different categories that may more appropriately reflect the performed and documented E/M service. Understanding the principle of each category of service is useful when reviewing the guidelines and identifying the most appropriate E/M service code. Each of the category guidelines included in this chapter require the documentation of content of service elements, as well as at least one of the contributing components.

- The term *outpatient* refers to any patient who does not reside at the healthcare facility or has not been admitted to the healthcare facility. The guidelines for E/M services provided in an outpatient setting require the documentation of the content of service elements and may include the contributing components. There are two subcategories for an E/M service: new and established patient. A new office or other outpatient E/M service requires the documentation of all three of the content of service elements. An established office or other outpatient E/M service requires the documentation of two of the three content of service elements. Intraservice time, coun-

seling, and coordination of care may be considered during the selection of the E/M service code; however, there must be documentation to support the inclusion of these contributing components.

- Hospital observation is a particular kind of service performed when the severity of the presenting problem precludes the patient's departure from the healthcare facility but is not severe enough to warrant admission into the healthcare facility. There are three different subcategories of hospital observation services: initial observation care, subsequent observation care, and observation care discharge services. The guidelines for the initial and subsequent observation care services require documentation of the content of service. The codes listed in these two subcategories are considered to be per diem codes, which consider any hospital observation services performed and documented throughout the day. Although the initial observation care codes are considered "per diem" codes, intraservice time has been included in the guidelines for only these initial observation care codes. Unlike the other hospital observation service subcategories, observation care discharge services do not require the content of service elements.

- A patient who has been formally admitted to a healthcare facility is considered an inpatient. Hospital inpatient services are provided for a patient who has been formally admitted to the hospital facility for treatment. Hospital inpatient services are considered per diem services. There are two subcategories of hospital inpatient services: initial hospital care and subsequent hospital care. Initial hospital care includes the actual admission of the patient into the hospital, whereas subsequent hospital care includes services provided for the patient on each consecutive day after admission. The E/M services provided during subsequent hospital care may be broken down into two different, more detailed subcategories: observation or inpatient care services (including admission and discharge services) and hospital discharge services. Observation or inpatient care services (including admission and discharge services) includes the observation or inpatient care services that have been provided to patients who have been admitted and discharged on the same date of service, whereas hospital discharge services include the care provided to a patient during discharge from the hospital.

- A consultation E/M service occurs when one physician performs an E/M service at the request of another physician for the sole purpose of providing a professional and clinical opinion about the patient's presenting problem. This request for consultation may come from a physician, physician assistant, nurse practitioner, insurance company, or other appropriate source. Consultations have three unique requirements: the requesting physician must provide a verbal or written request for consultation; the physician performing the consultation must render an opinion on the patient's presenting problem; the rendered opinion must be conveyed to the source of the consultation request. The two consultation subcategories reflect the settings in which a consultation can be performed: an outpatient setting or an inpatient setting. CMS eliminated payment for consultation services for any Medicare beneficiary in January 2010, although consultations are still listed in the numeric code set in the CPT manual.

- An emergency department is any section of a hospital facility that is specifically equipped to respond to and treat medical emergencies, staffed with medical professionals trained in emergency medical care, and remains open 24 hours a day. When a patient's presenting problem requires immediate medical attention and the patient presents to the emergency department, there is no distinction made between new and established patients.

- A nursing facility provides convalescent, rehabilitative, and long-term care for the patient. Nursing facilities have commonly been known as skilled nursing facilities, intermediate care facilities, and long-term care facilities. Because of the nature of care provided for patients, standardized assessments and protocols are required to provide accurate, inclusive measurements of the capability, function, and health of the patients. The content of service enhances and informs the documentation of the vital role the physician plays in nursing facility care. There are four subcategories of nursing facility care: initial nursing facility care, subsequent nursing facility care, nursing facility discharge services, and other nursing facility services.

- Domiciliary, rest home (e.g., boarding home), or custodial care E/M services occur in facilities designated as the patient's legal residence. These facilities provide the patient with room, board, and assistance with any necessary activities of daily living. There are two subcategories of services: new patient and established patient.

- When an E/M service is performed in the patient's private residence, it is known as a home service. There are two subcategories of home service: new patient and established patient.

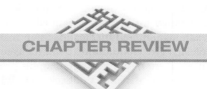

CHAPTER REVIEW

Multiple Choice

Choose the letter that best answers each question or completes each statement.

1. In the clinic office a pediatrician sees a 12-year-old girl for headache, dizziness, and neck pain. The previous night, she had been struck in the face with a ball while playing a game of dodge ball. Patient felt progressively worse as the night progressed. ROS pertinent to chief complaint: no nausea or vomiting, fever, or shortness of breath. All other ROS unremarkable. The patient's social history has not changed since her most recent annual physical. Physical exam: pupils equal, round, and reactive to light. Ocular nerves intact. Patient expresses significant pain upon palpation of shoulders and along cervical spine, but no dizziness upon palpation. Patient can stand on one foot with appropriate balance and displays good range of motion. Neck soft without lumps or tenderness. Cervical lymph nodes are normal. Plan: patient shows no sign of infection, cranial injury, or concussion. The physician discussed mother's concern regarding head injury,

instructed mother and patient regarding signs and symptoms of concern, and recommended ibuprofen or Tylenol for neck pain. Which of the following E/M codes best reflects the documented service?
   a. 99203
   b. 99213
   c. 99221
   d. 99219

2. A 24-year-old woman presents to the emergency department for severe abdominal pain. After collecting a detailed history, performing an expanded problem-focused physical examination, and medical decision making of moderate complexity, the supervising physician admits the patient to an observation status. Which of the following E/M service codes best reflects the documented service?
   a. 99221
   b. 99282
   c. 99224
   d. 99218

3. The medical documentation reports that an E/M service was provided for a frail 89-year-old woman where she resides, at Sunset Hills Rest Home. The clinician collected a brief HPI, a complete ROS, and a pertinent PFSH. Then the clinician performed a detailed physical examination and medical decision making of moderate complexity. The documentation states that a staff member prepared tea for the clinician and the patient since this was the patient's first visit from the clinician. Which of the following E/M service codes best reflects the documented service?

   a. 99336

   b. 99304

   c. 99235

   d. 99342

4. During a patient's recovery after a total knee replacement, the 68-year-old man presented to his primary care physician because he had not passed a bowel movement for 3 days, and the patient complained of significant lower abdominal pain. According to the patient's records, the patient had been taking oxycodone. During the expanded problem-focused physical examination performed by the primary care physician, the patient was found to be quite dehydrated, and when asked to get on the exam table, the patient experienced significant orthostatic hypotension and syncope. The primary care physician contacted the North Hills Nursing Home and requested an admission. During the course of the admission, which lasted a good portion of the day with several clinical encounters, the physician collected a comprehensive history, performed a detailed physical examination, and made medical decisions of moderate complexity. Which of the following E/M service codes best reflects the documented service?

   a. 99221

   b. 99305

   c. 99310

   d. 99215

5. An initial E/M service is provided in the private residence of an 83-year-old woman who has been discharged from a nursing home. The patient broke her fibula when she fell off a ladder. The clinician collects an extended HPI, a complete ROS, and a complete PFSH, making note of the number of family and friends who passed through the patient's home during the visit. Then the clinician performs a detailed physical examination and medical decision making of moderate complexity. The clinician documents that the patient is "a delightful older woman who laughs frequently and is quite alert, and even gregarious." Which of the following E/M service codes best reflects the documented service?

   a. 99343

   b. 99253

   c. 99349

   d. 99326

6. A 16-year-old boy is brought to the emergency department with a history of severe lower abdominal pain. The pain was severe enough to wake the boy from a deep sleep and has lasted for 24 hours. His pain has been persistent today, and he has complained of pain with urination. ROS is positive for mild nausea without fever, vomiting, or constipation. He has been healthy until this recent abdominal pain. Pain has kept patient from school, where he is a sophomore at East Orringtown High. Physical exam: no fever. Patient is breathing comfortably without signs of labor or any abnormal sounds. Abdomen is not distended but soft with no focal tenderness. No costovertebral tenderness noted upon palpation. Normal blood count and urinalysis. CT scan performed at hospital, and the radiologist report reveals mild dilation of the appendix, but no inflammation surrounding the appendix, as well as a large amount of stool in the recto-sigmoid. Plan: Due to the patient's asymptomatic status and normal physical examination, the patient is discharged home with his family. Which of the following E/M service codes best reflects the documented service?

   a. 99218

   b. 99221

   c. 99252

   d. 99283

7. According to the medical documentation, 2 days after presenting to the hospital after being pushed down the stairs by her boyfriend, the patient is beginning to eat and has slept through the night. During the course of the day, an expanded problem-focused physical examination is performed, as well as medical decision making of moderate complexity. Which of the following E/M service codes best reflects the documented service?

   a. 99221

   b. 99232

   c. 99218

   d. 99283

8. The medical documentation states that Dr. Goodtummy has requested the professional opinion of Dr. Longshanks regarding a patient's midback pain. Dr. Goodtummy sees the patient in the clinic office and documents the collection and performance of a detailed history, an expanded problem-focused physical examination, and medical decision making of moderate complexity. Dr. Goodtummy communicates to Dr. Longshanks in the form of a letter, detailing his professional opinion regarding the patient's midback pain. Which of the following E/M service codes best reflects the documented service?

   a. 99252

   b. 99214

   c. 99242

   d. 99202

9. Dr. Lingenbary has been Johnny's primary care physician for 3 years and has been unsuccessful in treating Johnny's irritating cough. Dr. Lingenbary requests that Dr. Hapilung accept the care of Johnny's irritating cough. Although Dr. Lingenbary will continue to provide primary care for Johnny in every other aspect of health, the care for Johnny's irritating cough will be provided by Dr. Hapilung. Which of the following E/M service categories best reflects the documented service?

   a. Observation care services

   b. Consultation services

   c. Transfer of care

   d. Office or other outpatient

10. The documentation reflects the patient's discharge from the hospital after a 2-day stay. The discharge process required 45 minutes to instruct the patient on the appropriate self-care, medications, and concerning signs and symptoms. Which of the following E/M service codes best reflects the documented service?

a. 99217
b. 99239
c. 99316
d. 99233

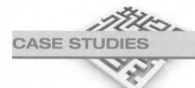

CASE STUDIES

Case Study 14-1

Read the following medical documentation, and then utilize all prior knowledge and your CPT manual to answer questions 1–5.

History: Suzie is a previously healthy 17-year-old girl who presents to the Children's Health Clinic of Metropolis Emergency Department with severe abdominal pain and mild vaginal bleeding lasting 10 days. Last night, patient felt especially ill with sharp cramping pain in her lower abdomen and nausea after passing a bowel movement. Three days ago, she missed her high school softball game, which her mother states is highly unusual as her daughter is an avid softball player. Today, her pain increased in severity to 7/10, and Suzie fainted at the dinner table. Her mother called 911, and Suzie was brought to the emergency department via ambulance.

Review of Systems: Patient has been healthy with no history of surgeries or major illnesses. Patient's last menstrual period was 7 weeks ago and was normal, although Suzie reports it was extremely heavy. Suzie's menstrual cycle is very erratic, and she averages between six and eight menses a year. She has experienced no dysuria or foul-smelling urine prior to onset of symptoms. Bowel movements have been daily with no pain or straining, and there has been no change of bowel habits prior to symptoms. No rashes were noted, and there has been no exposure to illness. No cough, chest pain, or joint pain reported in recent weeks; however, patient reports extreme dizziness over past week. As stated previously, patient is very active in her high school softball league. Suzie is doing well in Monterey High School, where she is in the 11th grade. Suzie is sexually active. She lives at home with mother, and father is currently serving in Afghanistan as a military chaplain. Mother has history of irritable bowel syndrome and also has a long history of oligoovulation, averaging between six and eight menses a year.

Exam: T, 100.76; weight, 138.6; heart rate, 76. She is very uncomfortable in the bed, and her face is significantly flushed. She appears very agitated that her sexual activity has been identified to her mother. Eyes clear. Neck soft without masses. Breast exam reveals very tender, swollen breasts. Lungs are clear of rattles, wheezes, and crackles. Heart sounds are clear of murmur with a regular heart rate and rhythm. No swelling of finger knuckles or ankles. Deep palpation of lower abdomen reveals mild tenderness; however, no tenderness, mass, or pain noted upon palpation of lower right abdomen.

Laboratory: WBC, normal. Pregnancy test is positive.

Assessment: Probable ectopic pregnancy requiring rule-out of internal bleeding. Admit patient to observation status to determine whether internal bleeding is present.

1. Which of the following best reflects the overall level of history for this medical documentation?
   a. Problem-focused
   b. Expanded problem-focused
   c. Detailed
   d. Comprehensive

2. Which of the following best reflects the physical examination according to the 1995 DGs?
   a. Problem-focused
   b. Expanded problem-focused
   c. Detailed
   d. Comprehensive

3. Which of the following best reflects the level of medical decision-making complexity?
   a. Straightforward
   b. Low
   c. Moderate
   d. High

4. Which of the following best reflects the E/M service category provided for Suzie?
   a. Hospital inpatient services
   b. Emergency department services
   c. Hospital observation services
   d. Consultation

5. Which of the following codes best reflects the E/M service provided?
   a. 99221
   b. 99283
   c. 99218
   d. 99252

Case Study 14-2

Using your CPT manual, identify the E/M category, subcategory, and numeric code for the following case study. Be sure to utilize all prior knowledge. Remember that Appendix D contains the full content of service worksheet.

Subjective: Franklin is doing well. Franklin recalls events of hospital admission and accident appropriately. Good recall of abdominal trauma, appropriate humor regarding tripping over the dog. No other voiced concerns. No bowel movement yet. Abdominal pain controlled. Remaining ROS: negative. Nursing notes reviewed by MD.

Objective: Temperature average (24 hrs), 100.25°F; minimum, 99.5; max, 101. Oxygen delivery: room air. One unit of blood transfused for patient in last 24 hours and IV fluids. Eyes clear, PERRL. Resp: good air entry, clear to auscultation bilaterally. CV: RRR, normal. GI: soft, supple, with minimal guarding. Neck is soft without masses. Auscultation of lungs reveals clear sounds without wheezes or rubs. Auscultation of heart reveals regular rate and rhythm with no abnormal sounds noted. Inflammation of upper left abdomen greatly reduced. Minimal tenderness upon palpation of upper left quadrant. Stool sample collected for occult blood test.

Assessment/Plan: 56-year-old man with confirmed grade 2 splenic laceration. Nonsurgical conservative management implemented with positive results.

1. Reduce physical examination to every 12 hours
2. Continue IV fluids
3. Repeat CT scan to identify internal bleeding
4. Instruction to patient for 7 days of strict bed rest

More than 50 percent of this 30-minute visit was spent coordinating care and counseling patient and family on grade 2 splenic injury.

1. Does this reflect a new patient or an established patient? __
   _____
2. What is the site of service? _____
3. Is the patient type applicable for this site of service?
   Yes/No: _____
4. Level of overall history: _____
   Supported by HPI level: _____
   ROS level: _____
   PFSH level: _____
5. Level of physical examination: _____
   Which physical examination guidelines were referenced to determine the type of physical examination? Please be sure to identify the overall findings.
   1995 body area/organ system (how many body areas and/or organ systems were documented?): _____
   General multisystem (how many elements identified by a bullet were documented?):_____
   Single organ system (which single organ system was referenced, and how many elements identified by a bullet, in both shaded and unshaded borders, were documented?):
   _____
6. Overall level of medical decision-making complexity:_____
   Supported by the following levels:
   Number of diagnoses and/or management options: _____
   Amount and/or complexity of data to be reviewed:_____
   Risk of complication, comorbidity, and/or mortality: _____
7. Category: _____ .
   Please explain your rationale for selecting this category.
   _____
8. Subcategory: _____
   Please explain your rationale for selecting this subcategory.
   _____
   _____
9. E/M service code: _____

Coding Challenge

Using your CPT manual, identify the E/M code that most appropriately reflects each of the following clinical scenarios.

1. New patient seen in a clinic office, comprehensive history, detailed physical examination, moderate medical decision making.
   CPT code: _____
2. Upon assessing the patient in the emergency room, the performing physician admits the patient to observation, documenting a detailed history, detailed physical examination, and moderate medical decision making.
   CPT code: _____
3. A patient is admitted to the hospital. The admitting physician documents a comprehensive history, a comprehensive examination, and moderate medical decision making.
   CPT code: _____
4. The primary care physician has requested that a general surgeon consult on a patient's condition. During the patient's visit in the general surgeon's clinic office, the surgeon documents a comprehensive history, an expanded problem-focused physical examination, and medical decision making of moderate complexity. The surgeon sends a letter to the primary care physician outlining his clinical opinion regarding the patient's condition.
   CPT code: _____
5. For a patient's 4-hour stay in the emergency department, the physician documents a detailed history, expanded problem-focused physical examination, and moderate medical decision making for a presenting problem of moderate severity.
   CPT code: _____
6. During the third day of the patient's admission in the nursing facility, the physician spends 45 minutes off the patient's unit/floor discussing the patient's pathology and radiology results. The physician records detailed documentation of the 25 minutes spent in counseling and coordination of care with the patient and the family of the patient regarding the patient's presenting problem.
   CPT code: _____
7. The patient is admitted to custodial care in a group home for the very first time, where the patient will receive help performing ADLs, maintaining correct medication schedules, and receiving occupational therapy. During the initial admission, the documentation reflects a comprehensive history, detailed physical examination, and medical decision making of moderate complexity during this 50-minute admission.
   CPT code: _____
8. Documentation of an expanded problem-focused history, detailed physical examination, and moderate medical decision making for a patient seen during an initial home service visit in the patient's private residence.
   CPT code: _____
9. Patient who has not sought any medical care for 6 years presents to family physician. Comprehensive history, detailed physical examination, low medical decision making.
   CPT code: _____
10. During the second day of observation status, the patient's condition has stabilized, as shown by the documented detailed history and detailed physical examination, as well as

the 45 minutes of intraservice time spent at the patient's bedside and on the patient's hospital floor or unit.

CPT code: _____

11. On the third day of admission in the hospital, an expanded problem-focused history, detailed physical examination, and moderate medical decision making are documented. No intraservice time is documented.

CPT code: _____

12. During a patient's admission in the hospital, the attending physician requests an oncologist's opinion regarding the patient's presenting problem and condition. The oncologist documents the following information in the patient's medical record: a detailed history, comprehensive physical examination, and moderate medical decision making, as well as her professional opinion regarding the patient's condition.

CPT code: _____

13. A patient is brought into the emergency department and requires urgent evaluation by the physician. During the 95-minute service, the physician documents that the patient's presenting problem has high severity but does not pose a significant threat to the patient's life. A comprehensive history, detailed physical examination, and moderate medical decision making are documented in the patient's medical record.

CPT code: _____

14. On the first day of the patient's admission in the nursing facility, a detailed history, a detailed physical examination, and medical decision making of low complexity are documented in the patient's nursing facility record.

CPT code: _____

15. A 97-year-old patient returns to a rest home after a 3-day hospital stay for pneumonia. Upon returning to the rest home, the physician spends 25 minutes with the patient documenting an expanded problem-focused history, detailed physical examination, and moderate medical decision making.

CPT code: _____

16. A patient is readmitted to home care for the second time in a year. Documentation of this visit reflects an expanded problem-focused history, expanded problem-focused physical examination, and medical decision making of moderate complexity.

CPT code: _____

17. Established patient seen in a physician's clinic, comprehensive history, expanded problem-focused physical examination, moderate medical decision making.

CPT code: _____

18. This new patient claims that her neighbor, dermatologist Dr. K, recommended she visit Dr. H, a gastroenterologist, for stomach pain. In the clinic office, the gastroenterologist documents a detailed history, expanded problem-focused physical examination, and low medical decision making.

CPT code: _____

19. On the third day of being admitted to observation status, the patient has improved enough to be discharged from observation care.

CPT code: _____

20. A patient presents to the emergency room at 6:30 a.m. and is admitted to inpatient care services for observation. By 4:00 p.m. that day, the patient's condition has improved enough to warrant discharge by the supervising physician. Documentation of the E/M services for this patient include a comprehensive history, detailed physical examination, and moderate medical decision making, with a documented presenting problem of low severity.

CPT code: _____

21. A nurse practitioner requests the professional opinion of a dermatologist about a patient's skin rash. The dermatologist documents an expanded problem-focused history, expanded problem-focused physical examination, and moderate medical decision making. The dermatologist dictates a response letter to the nurse practitioner outlining his professional opinion, resulting from his 45-minute face-to-face visit.

CPT code: _____

22. A 9-year-old boy is brought to the emergency department with suspected arm fracture. Documentation of a detailed history, expanded problem-focused physical examination, and low medical decision making indicates that the child's arm is only sprained, and the patient leaves the emergency room after a 3-hour stay.

CPT code: _____

23. An annual nursing facility assessment is performed for a patient in an inpatient nursing facility. Documentation reflects comprehensive history, physical examination, and medical decision making of moderate complexity.

CPT code: _____

24. This patient returns to a domiciliary care facility after a 4-year absence, during which the patient was living out of state with adult son. On the first day of admission in the domiciliary care facility, the physician documents a comprehensive history, a detailed physical examination, and moderate medical decision making during this 40-minute visit.

CPT code: _____

25. The patient is discharged from a nursing facility. The physician spends 15 minutes with the family and caregivers discussing the patient's stay in the nursing facility, but the physician is called away from the room. Upon returning to the patient and family, the physician spends another 25 minutes providing instructions regarding the patient's medication and care at home. The patient, family, and caregivers indicate clear understanding of everything discussed.

CPT code: _____

26. During the course of discharging the patient from a 4-day hospital admission, the physician spends 45 minutes performing a final examination of the patient, which includes extensive discussion with the patient and family about the care the patient received. Prescriptions are provided, and instructions are given to the family caregivers, as well as referrals for follow-up care.

CPT code: _____

27. On the second day of patient's inpatient visit, the attending physician requests a consultation by a general surgeon for the patient's presenting problem. General surgeon documents a comprehensive history, detailed physical examination, and moderate medical decision making. The patient's insurance carrier follows Medicare guidelines.

CPT code: _____

28. Documented problem-focused history, problem-focused physical examination, moderate medical decision making, and in-depth counseling and coordination of care provided during the 45 minutes the established patient was seen in a clinic office.

CPT code: _____

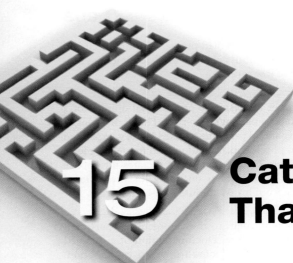

15 Categories Requiring More Than Content of Service

Learning Objectives

After completing this chapter, you should be able to do the following:

- Spell and define the key terms and abbreviations presented in this chapter
- Identify the requirements for care plan oversight services
- Recognize the requirements for domiciliary, rest home (e.g., assisted living facility), or home care plan oversight services
- Identify the requirements for case management services
- Understand the requirements for preventive medicine service
- Recognize requirements for non–face-to-face physician services
- Identify requirements for special E/M services

Key Terms

amphoric breath sound

anticoagulant

behavior change intervention services

bronchoscopy

care plan oversight

ceftriaxone

cerebrovascular accident

counseling risk factor reduction services

deep vein thrombosis

direct contact

domiciliary

gravida

home care agency

hospice care

human chorionic gonadotropin (hCG)

initial comprehensive preventive medicine services

internationalized normalized ratio (INR)

intramuscular

lactation

methotrexate

multidisciplinary nonphysician qualified healthcare professionals

myocardial infarction

non–face-to-face physician services

nonphysician qualified healthcare professional

nursing facility

para

periodic comprehensive preventive medicine services

placental abruption

postpartum

pulmonary embolism

CPT-4 codes in this chapter are from the CPT-4 2012 code set. CPT is a registered trademark of the American Medical Association.

qualified healthcare professionals

status post

stroke

verbal apraxia

Abbreviation

mIU/ml a unit of measurement for the amount of hCG hormone in a woman's body; represents a milli-international unit per milliliter in the bloodstream

INTRODUCTION

Each E/M service reflects variations on a theme: A physician utilizes his or her extensive education, skill, and expertise to promote the health and well-being of a patient. Although certain E/M services require the performance of the content of service to allow the physician to diagnose and treat the patient, other healthcare circumstances preclude the collection of content of service information because of the patient's need, the specific intent of the service, or the logistics of the situation. Some situations require an unusual or unexpected approach to the promotion of well-being. For instance, in the event that a variety of multi-disciplinary healthcare professionals are all providing care for one patient, a conference may be warranted to ensure the appropriate plan of care for the patient. In another case, a healthy patient may need to visit his or her primary care physician for an annual physical. Understanding the intent of the service is an important way of distinguishing among these E/M categories.

This chapter examines the categories that require something other than the content of service in reporting these unique services; the intent of these categories of service cannot be properly reflected with the content of service. The guidelines found in the CPT manual provide a foundation for the category requirements. However, further guidelines and regulations that are more explicit are maintained and updated by CMS and can be found on the official CMS website, www.cms.gov.

CARE PLAN OVERSIGHT SERVICES

In a healthcare setting, oversight is defined as the watchful management or supervision of a process or procedure to ensure the accurate, thorough completion of each necessary aspect of that process or procedure. A performing physician provides oversight whenever he or she supervises, providing watchful management over the care given to a patient. Such oversight can occur under varied circumstances, with different types of care, and in numerous settings. For example, a supervising physician may coordinate the efforts of different clinicians, other healthcare professionals, and even other physicians from a variety of healthcare disciplines who are all involved in providing hospice care for one patient. When one physician supervises the multifaceted or multidisciplinary treatment plan for a patient's healthcare, these E/M services are known as **care plan oversight**. Care plan oversight applies to three specific types of care: hospice care, the care provided by a home health agency, and the care provided by a nursing facility. Each of these types of care requires that one physician be solely responsible for overseeing the patient's care plan or provide a predominant percentage of that oversight.

Over the course of a 30-day period, or a calendar month, many different elements of care plan management and oversight may be performed, and the nature of the services provided explains why the patient need not be present during the provision of the services. For example, the patient does not need to be present when the supervising physician reviews diagnostic testing results, reviews follow-up or subsequent patient progress reports, or makes indicated adjustments in the care plan. Similarly, the patient does not need to be present when the supervising physician communicates with other health care professionals, family members, care providers, or legal guardians regarding the assessment of the care plan.

The CPT manual identifies care plan oversight services for three specific types of healthcare:

- Care provided by a home care agency for patients living in their own homes or domiciliary settings
- Hospice care
- Care provided by a nursing facility

A **home care agency** provides the coordinated services of different healthcare professionals and/or therapists—including nursing care; speech, physical, or occupational therapy; and even home aid workers who can provide assistance with light chores—for a patient who is residing in a private home or **domiciliary** residence. ■ TABLE 15.1 gives the specific service codes for care plan oversight services provided by a home health agency for a patient residing in a private home or domiciliary setting.

Hospice care is the provision of medical, emotional, psychological, and spiritual support by interdisciplinary healthcare and other skilled professionals, specifically for patients who are terminally ill. Hospice care is not limited to the home but may be provided in a variety of locations. ■ TABLE 15.2 gives the specific codes for care plan oversight services provided for a hospice patient.

care plan oversight the management and/or coordination of any multi-faceted or multidisciplinary treatment plans for a patient's healthcare; requires the participation of the supervising physician

home care agency the provider of the coordinated care of different healthcare professionals and/or therapists—including nursing care; speech, physical, and occupational therapy; and even home aid workers who can provide assistance with light chores—for a patient who is residing in a private home or domiciliary residence

domiciliary referring to the home or other dwelling in which a person lives and which is the person's legal place of residence; may be a multioccupant building or a private home

■ **TABLE 15.1   CARE PLAN OVERSIGHT SERVICES FOR PATIENT UNDER CARE OF HOME HEALTH AGENCY**

CPT CODE	TOTAL TIME OF PHYSICIAN SUPERVISION SERVICES DURING CALENDAR MONTH	TYPE OF CARE SUPERVISED AND/OR SETTING
99374	15–29 minutes	**Home health agency** care provided in home or domiciliary setting
99375	30 minutes or more	**Home health agency** care provided in home or domiciliary setting

■ **TABLE 15.2   CARE PLAN OVERSIGHT SERVICES FOR HOSPICE CARE PATIENT**

CPT CODE	TOTAL TIME OF PHYSICIAN SUPERVISION SERVICES DURING CALENDAR MONTH	TYPE OF CARE SUPERVISED AND/OR SETTING
99377	15–29 minutes	**Hospice care** for patient in any setting
99378	30 minutes or more	**Hospice care** for patient in any setting

hospice care the provision of medical, emotional, psychological, and spiritual support by interdisciplinary healthcare and other skilled professionals, specifically for patients who are terminally ill

nursing facility inpatient facility that provides various kinds of healthcare services for patients requiring care on a 24-hour basis

Nursing facilities are inpatient facilities that provide various kinds of healthcare services for patients requiring care on a 24-hour basis. Although specific codes report the initial visit, subsequent care on a per diem basis, and discharge, care plan oversight is a completely different kind of E/M service and must be represented by a different category. ■ TABLE 15.3 gives the specific codes for care plan oversight services that occur in a nursing facility.

The care plan oversight services performed by a physician provide watchful management and coordination of a patient's care, regardless of whether that care is provided by a home health agency, a hospice organization, or a nursing facility. Since these three different types of care address many differing medical needs, the presence and oversight of one supervising physician can be very important, even as the required allotment of time can vary according to individual circumstances. Two separate allotments of time identify the care plan oversight services performed during a 30-day period:

- 29 minutes or less
- 30 minutes or more

■ TABLE 15.4 summarizes the categories of care plan oversight services according to the time allotment and the type of care and/or setting in which the services occur.

■ **TABLE 15.3   CARE PLAN OVERSIGHT SERVICES FOR NURSING FACILITY PATIENT**

CPT CODE	TOTAL TIME OF PHYSICIAN SUPERVISION SERVICES DURING CALENDAR MONTH	TYPE OF CARE SUPERVISED AND/OR SETTING
99379	15–29 minutes	**Nursing facility** care
99380	30 minutes or more	**Nursing facility** care

■ **TABLE 15.4   SUMMARY OF CARE PLAN OVERSIGHT SERVICES**

CPT CODE	TOTAL TIME OF PHYSICIAN SUPERVISION SERVICES DURING CALENDAR MONTH	TYPE OF CARE SUPERVISED AND/OR SETTING
99374	15–29 minutes	**Home health agency** care provided in home or domiciliary setting
99375	30 minutes or more	**Home health agency** care provided in home or domiciliary setting
99377	15–29 minutes	**Hospice care** provided in any setting
99378	30 minutes or more	**Hospice care** provided in any setting
99379	15–29 minutes	**Nursing facility** care
99380	30 minutes or more	**Nursing facility** care

The guidelines listed in the CPT manual provide the foundation of the intent for this case management service and should be consulted. Furthermore, CMS maintains and updates specific regular guidelines for home care agencies, which it regulates, and these guidelines should be reviewed.

DOMICILIARY, REST HOME, OR HOME CARE PLAN OVERSIGHT SERVICES

The CPT manual further distinguishes care plan oversight services in a completely separate category of E/M services—domiciliary, rest home (e.g., assisted living facility), or home care plan oversight services—for patients who are not under the care of a home health agency, hospice organization, or nursing facility. This separate category of care plan oversight services includes a physician's supervision of care in a broad range of domiciliary facilities. For patients residing in domiciliary or assisted living facilities or receiving healthcare services in their own private residences, the participation of a supervising physician may be required to coordinate the plan of care and the management or treatment options for the patients. As in the earlier category of oversight services, this type of care plan oversight may require a supervising physician to revise a patient's current plan of care or to review subsequent records or documentation of follow-up visits, the review of the patient's status of health, or the patient's physical response to any prior treatment plans. Likewise, results of laboratory tests may need to be reviewed, as well as the report of any other diagnostic testing. Any one of these pieces of information may introduce new data or factors that need to be integrated into the patient's plan of care.

Similarly, the supervising physician may need to communicate with other healthcare professionals about the patient's care or the assessments required to measure the patient's progress. This communication may also extend to nonmedically trained persons, such as the following:

* Family members
* Legal guardians
* Surrogate decision makers
* Primary caregivers

This communication may occur in a variety of forms, including via telephone. As with the review of reports, results, or documentation, the supervising physician may receive new information during this communication that needs to be integrated into the care plan and may even necessitate an adjustment to one or more aspects of the patient's care.

These oversight services provided by the supervising physician, again, do not require the patient to be present when the physician is performing the services. Consequently, documentation of the content of service is not required for domiciliary, rest home, or home care plan oversight services, and classification of these services is determined by the allotment of time. From month to month, the amount of time necessary to provide care plan oversight can vary depending on the oversight performed. Therefore, the numeric codes for domiciliary, assisted living, or home care plan oversight identify two specific periods of time that the supervising physician spends in care plan oversight:

* 15–29 minutes
* 30 minutes or more

■ TABLE 15.5 clarifies the codes for care plan oversight services for these particular settings.

As with each category of E/M service, the guidelines listed in the CPT manual should be consulted. Likewise, CMS maintains and updates specific regular guidelines for domiciliary, rest home, or home care plan oversight services.

CASE MANAGEMENT SERVICES

Management is the control, organization, or administration of a process, event, or procedure. Case management services are a category of E/M care in which one physician facilitates the organization of, access to, and supervision of any healthcare services required by the patient. Under case management, a single physician or other qualified healthcare professional is solely responsible for the direct care of the patient,

■ **TABLE 15.5   DOMICILIARY, REST HOME, OR HOME CARE PLAN OVERSIGHT SERVICES**

CPT CODE	TOTAL TIME OF PHYSICIAN SUPERVISING SERVICES DURING CALENDAR MONTH	TYPE OF CARE SUPERVISED AND/OR SETTING
99339	15–29 minutes	Domiciliary residence, assisted living facility, or private home
99340	30 minutes or more	Domiciliary residence, assisted living facility, or private home

anticoagulant a category of pharmaceutical medication intended to reduce or prevent the abnormal or pathological clotting of blood

pulmonary embolism a medical emergency that involves a blockage of the main artery of the lung or one of the arterial branches within the lungs; caused by a substance or material called an embolus, which obstructs blood flow and increases pressure on the right ventricle of the heart; can cause difficulty breathing, painful and/or rapid breathing, and heart palpitations

myocardial infarction a medical emergency during which blood supply to the heart is interrupted, causing the cells of the affected part of the heart to die; more commonly known as a heart attack

stroke a medical emergency caused by an interruption or disturbance of the blood flow to and through a part of the brain; impairs or prevents the affected part of the brain from functioning; can be one of many types, each of which impacts and impairs the neurological function in different ways

deep vein thrombosis a medical emergency involving the formation of a clot in a vein deep within the body, most commonly a lower extremity; causes severe pain, redness, significant warmth and swelling of the affected area, engorgement of superficial veins of the affected limb, and can lead to a pulmonary embolism if the clot dislodges and travels to the lung

internationalized normalized ratio (INR) a measure of the coagulation tendency of the blood, used to monitor anticoagulant therapy; may also be called a prothrombin (PT) test

as well as for coordinating care for the patient, which may include managing the patient's access to care. This process may also include supervising any other healthcare services the patient may need and potentially initiating any specific treatment or therapy. Since E/M services that primarily involve case management can be very involved, CMS maintains and updates regulations and guidelines that provide clarification for the proper use and reporting of these services. There are two subcategories of case management services: anticoagulant management and medical team conferences.

Anticoagulant Management

An **anticoagulant** is a category of pharmaceutical medication intended to reduce or prevent the abnormal or pathological clotting of blood. Anticoagulants are used in the treatment and prevention of several pathologies and conditions, including these:

- **Pulmonary embolism**,
- **Myocardial infarction**, or **stroke**
- **Deep vein thrombosis**

Although these medications are very helpful, the patients must be carefully monitored to ensure proper dosages and prevent undesirable side effects, as well as adverse interactions with other medications. The prothrombin (PT) test, better known as the **internationalized normalized ratio (INR)**, identifies the coagulation tendency of the blood—that is, the rate at which the blood clots—and is the primary test utilized to monitor anticoagulant therapy. For a patient being treated with anticoagulant medication, an INR level that is too low can signal that the blood is clotting too quickly, which increases the risk of a blood clot, or embolism. On the other hand, a level that is too high indicates that the blood is taking too long to clot, which could lead to problems such as persistent nosebleeds, unusual bruising, blood in the urine, or hemorrhaging. Anticoagulant case management services are provided only in outpatient settings and, most importantly, should not be the basis of reporting an E/M service or time spent in care plan oversight. Reporting anticoagulant management is identified in blocks of 90 days: the initial 90 days of anticoagulant therapy, which includes a minimum of eight measurements of the patient's INR, and each subsequent 90 days of therapy, which must include a minimum of three INR measurements. ■ TABLE 15.6 presents a visual aid for the determination of the anticoagulant management subcategory of case management services.

Certain inpatient services—such as hospital care, hospital observation, nursing facility, and critical care services—require anticoagulant management as an inherent part of the patient's care. As a result, it would be inappropriate to report anticoagulant management services separately in these circumstances. Because of the complexity involved in outpatient anticoagulant therapy, the guidelines for anticoagulant case management services provide exhaustive directions for correctly reporting these services.

Medical Team Conferences

A conference in this context is a meeting of various professionals who have gathered to exchange ideas about and discuss a plan of action. The category of medical team conference represents a special kind of E/M service that involves an interdisciplinary team of at least three healthcare professionals who have each provided face-to-face healthcare services for a specific patient within 60 days prior to the medical team conference. It is important to note a distinction between qualified healthcare professionals and nonphysician qualified healthcare professionals. **Qualified healthcare professionals** have gained the education, experience, and expertise to legally practice medicine—for example, physicians; nurses; physical, occupational, and speech therapists; nutritionists; and many more. A **nonphysician qualified healthcare professional** refers to those healthcare professionals who are not physicians.

■ TABLE 15.6   CASE MANAGEMENT SERVICES: ANTICOAGULANT MANAGEMENT

CPT CODE	CASE MANAGEMENT SERVICES DURING 90-DAY PERIOD	TYPE OF CARE MANAGED AND/OR SETTING
99363	First 90 days of therapy—a minimum of 8 INR measurements	Anticoagulant therapy for a patient in an outpatient setting
99364	Each subsequent 90 days of therapy—a minimum of 3 INR measurements	Anticoagulant therapy for a patient in an outpatient setting

Note: Anticoagulant management services may not be reported with certain inpatient or critical care services, since anticoagulant therapy may be an inherent and necessary part of the patient's care in these settings.

When at least three qualified healthcare professionals from different specialties and disciplines gather to exchange plans, therapies, and management options regarding the provision of care for a specific patient, for whom each has provided face-to-face healthcare services, each professional brings important and valuable knowledge to the conference. Together, they may participate in the meeting with or without any of the following:

- Patient
- Patient's family members
- Any community agency
- Any social service agency Legal guardians or other surrogate decision makers
- Caregivers

Everyone who participates in the medical team conference plays an important role in any development and/or performance of healthcare services for the patient, as well as in any changes made to those services and coordination of the different specialties or disciplines. Even though more than one healthcare professional from the same discipline or specialty may participate in the medical team conference, no more than one individual from the same discipline or specialty may simultaneously report that participation. In other words, if two physical therapists, three occupational therapists, and two social workers are all present at a medical team conference, a report may be submitted from only one physical therapist, one occupational therapist, and one social worker.

Nonphysician Medical Team Conference with Direct Contact with Patient and/or Family

Coordination of a medical team conference and the appropriate reporting of this service involve a variety of exclusions and requirements, which the CPT manual lists in detail. The two most important aspects of medical team conferences are whether the patient (or patient's family) and/or the physician is present in the medical conference. When the medical team conference of an interdisciplinary team of healthcare professionals includes the patient and/or the patient's family, this is referred to as **direct contact**, or face-to-face contact. In the event that such a conference involves *only* nonphysician qualified healthcare professionals and lasts 30 minutes or more, it may be reported with a specific numeric code (see ■ TABLE 15.7).

It is important to note that when the patient and/or patient's family participates in the medical team conference, it may be reported with this code if *only* nonphysician qualified healthcare professionals are participating. Once a physician participates in the medical team conference in direct contact with the patient and/or family, then the nature of the visit has changed to a service during which the physician is providing direct care to the patient. In such a case, that medical team conference should be reported according to intraservice time, which includes the physician's counseling and/or coordination of care for the patient.

Medical Team Conference without Direct Contact with Patient and/or Family

Certain clinical circumstances require a medical team conference that consists of physician and nonphysician qualified healthcare professionals *without* direct contact with the patient and/or patient's family. Such a conference still represents the active participation of all parties in the development and performance of healthcare services for the patient, as well as in any changes to those services or in the coordination of the different specialties or disciplines.

As previously mentioned, a physician's participation in a medical team conference of **multidisciplinary nonphysician qualified healthcare professionals** is represented differently than a medical team conference composed entirely of nonphysician qualified healthcare professionals. Regardless of the physician's involvement, each of these two kinds of medical team conferences represents the assembly of qualified healthcare professionals with no direct contact with the patient and/or patient's family. ■ TABLE 15.8 charts the medical team conference without patient and/or family contact.

■ TABLE 15.9 shows the various configurations of medical team conferences.

Since both kinds of medical team conferences represent the complicated participation of qualified healthcare professionals involved in the patient's care, CMS maintains and updates regulations specifically

qualified healthcare professionals healthcare professionals who have education, experience, and expertise to legally practice medicine; includes a wide range of professionals, such as physicians; nurses; physical, occupational, or speech therapists; nutritionists; and more

nonphysician qualified healthcare professional any healthcare professional who is not a physician

direct contact the presence of the patient (or the patient's family) with the performing physician or in the team conference during the E/M service

multidisciplinary nonphysician qualified healthcare professionals clinicians from different disciplines such as physical therapy, occupational therapy, speech therapy, psychology, other specialties, and nursing

■ TABLE 15.7 CASE MANAGEMENT SERVICES: MEDICAL TEAM CONFERENCE WITH DIRECT PATIENT AND/OR FAMILY CONTACT

CPT CODE	PROFESSIONAL PARTICIPATION	PATIENT AND/OR FAMILY REPRESENTATION	DURATION OF TIME
99366	Nonphysician qualified healthcare professionals	Patient and/or family	30 minutes or more

■ TABLE 15.8 CASE MANAGEMENT SERVICES: MEDICAL TEAM CONFERENCE WITHOUT DIRECT PATIENT AND/OR FAMILY CONTACT

CPT CODE	PROFESSIONAL PARTICIPATION	PATIENT AND/OR FAMILY REPRESENTATION	DURATION OF TIME
99367	Physician and nonphysician qualified healthcare professionals	None	30 minutes or more
99368	Nonphysician qualified health care professionals	None	30 minutes or more

■ TABLE 15.9 CASE MANAGEMENT SERVICES: MEDICAL TEAM CONFERENCES

CPT CODE	PROFESSIONAL PARTICIPATION	PATIENT AND/OR FAMILY REPRESENTATION	DURATION OF TIME
99366	Nonphysician qualified healthcare professionals	Patient and/or family	30 minutes or more
99367	Physician and nonphysician qualified healthcare professionals	None	30 minutes or more
99368	Nonphysician qualified healthcare professionals	None	30 minutes or more

Note: Medical team conferences of less than 30 minutes should not be reported separately.

related to the accurate reporting of medical team conferences. These should be reviewed for the most up-to-date revisions to the guidelines.

PREVENTIVE MEDICINE SERVICES

Prevention is any action intended to forestall a potentially abnormal or undesired outcome or occurrence. In healthcare, preventive services are precautionary services utilized to forestall undesired or unpleasant pathology. Preventive medicine services are E/M services intended to promote and ensure a patient's good health and identify the status of the patient's health. Performed in office or outpatient settings, these services are provided for any patient regardless of age.

Preventive medicine services are not intended to provide treatment or management of a presenting problem, associated condition, or underlying disease; preventive services are precautionary and are intended to provide guidance for a patient's continued health. Therefore, if one or more significant abnormalities are identified by the performing physician during the preventive medicine service *and* the identified abnormalities require the physician to collect and/or perform elements of the content of service, then the appropriate office or outpatient E/M service should be reported in addition to the preventive medicine service. As healthcare has evolved and questions about insurance have become more complex, further extensive regulations have been introduced and updated to help ensure proper reporting and identification of E/M services that provide preventive medicine for patients. CMS maintains and updates these regulations, which should be consulted when preparing to report preventive medicine services.

There are three subcategories of preventive medicine services:

- New preventive medicine
- Established preventive medicine
- Counseling risk factor reduction and behavior change intervention

New and Established Preventive Medicine Services

initial comprehensive preventive medicine services the first preventive medicine service performed for a patient by the physician

periodic comprehensive preventive medicine services any preventive medicine services that occur after the first comprehensive preventive medicine service that is performed for a patient by the physician

New preventive medicine services are known as **initial comprehensive preventive medicine services**, whereas any preventive services performed for established patients are referred to as **periodic comprehensive preventive medicine services**. During preventive medicine services, the performing physician collects a thorough, appropriate history and performs an appropriate physical examination to provide a baseline for future comparison. These activities are referred to as *comprehensive* preventive medicine services. However, this use of *comprehensive* is not the same as its use with content of service elements and key components, such as history, physical examination, or medical decision making. ■ TABLE 15.10 gives the different codes for preventive medicine services for new patients and for established patients.

■ TABLE 15.10 PREVENTIVE MEDICINE SERVICES: NEW PATIENT AND ESTABLISHED PATIENT BY AGE GROUP

	LESS THAN 1 YEAR (INFANT)	AGES 1–4 YEARS (EARLY CHILDHOOD)	AGES 5–11 YEARS (LATE CHILDHOOD	AGES 12–17 YEARS (ADOLESCENCE)	AGES 18–39 YEARS	AGES 40–64 YEARS	AGES 65 YEARS OR OLDER
New Patient	99381	99382	99383	99384	99385	99386	99387
Established Patient	99391	99392	99393	99394	99395	99396	99397

Note: Preventive medicine services are intended to identify the status of the patient's health at the time of the visit. If an abnormality or presenting problem is addressed during the preventive medicine service and the documented content of service supports at least a problem-focused level, then the appropriate office or other outpatient service should be reported.

Again, there may be an occasion during a preventive medicine service when the performing physician identifies a presenting problem or abnormality that is significant enough for the physician to address during the course of the preventive medicine visit *and* that requires a problem-oriented E/M service, the appropriate office or outpatient service level should be reported in addition to the preventive medicine service. CMS identifies extensive requirements for properly reporting preventive medicine services. These requirements are maintained and updated often and should be reviewed when reporting preventive medicine services.

Counseling Risk Factor Reduction

Counseling risk factor reduction services are provided to a patient by a physician or other qualified healthcare professional in face-to-face contact with the patient; they are intended to promote health and prevent illness or injury. These services address issues such as problems in the family, use of substances, injury prevention, dental health, sexual practices, and more. These services are identified by the specific amounts of time spent in counseling the prevention of risk factors or intervening for the change of a specific behavior. ■ TABLE 15.11 identifies the specific codes for preventive medicine services that address counseling risk factor reduction.

Counseling for the reduction of risk factors targets the intended avoidance of disease or conditions associated with high-risk factors. Once again, if the performing physician identifies a presenting problem that requires the documentation of content of service elements or components and that calls for at least a problem-oriented E/M service, the appropriate office or outpatient service level should be reported in addition to the preventive medicine service.

counseling risk factor reduction services E/M services intended to encourage an intentional avoidance of disease or conditions associated with high-risk factors

Behavior Change Interventions

Behavior change intervention services are provided for patients engaging in a behavior or condition that can itself be considered an illness, such as obesity or the abuse of or addiction to tobacco, alcohol, or illicit substances. These interventions are reported according to the intensity of the service provided, as well as the amount of time involved in the provision of the care. ■ TABLE 15.12 shows two reportable behavior change interventions.

behavior change intervention services services intended to promote change in a behavior that could be considered an illness, such as obesity, use of or addiction to tobacco, alcohol use or abuse

■ TABLE 15.11 PREVENTIVE MEDICINE SERVICES: COUNSELING RISK FACTOR REDUCTION BY TIME SPENT

Counseling Risk Factor Reduction Service	99401	99402	99403	99404
Individual Counseling	15 minutes	30 minutes	45 minutes	60 minutes

■ TABLE 15.12 PREVENTIVE MEDICINE SERVICES: INDIVIDUAL BEHAVIOR CHANGE INTERVENTIONS BY TIME SPENT AND INTENSITY

INDIVIDUAL BEHAVIOR CHANGE INTERVENTION	INTERMEDIATE INTENSITY	HIGH INTENSITY	EXCLUSIONS
Smoking and Tobacco Cessation Counseling	99406 3–10 minutes	99407 More than 10 minutes	99406 cannot be listed in conjunction with 99407
Alcohol and/or Substance Abuse Screening and Intervention	99408 15–30 minutes	99409 More than 30 minutes	99408 cannot be listed in conjunction with 99409

■ **TABLE 15.13** **PREVENTIVE MEDICINE SERVICES: GROUP BEHAVIOR CHANGE INTERVENTION BY TIME SPENT**

GROUP BEHAVIOR CHANGE INTERVENTION	99411	99412
Counseling provided to individuals in a group setting	Approximately 30 minutes	Approximately 60 minutes

These services are intended to promote behavior change and may be reported when the service is performed as an inherent part of the treatment of a condition or pathology that is intricately related to, or worsened by, this specific behavior. For example, if, during the treatment of a condition related to tobacco addiction, the performing physician counsels the patient regarding the cessation of smoking, a behavior change intervention service may be reported. Likewise, if, during the treatment of a condition or pathology that is potentially related to alcohol or substance abuse, the performing physician screens the patient for alcohol and/or substance abuse and engages in an intervention regarding this behavior, a specific behavior change intervention service may be reported.

Behavior change services may also be reported in the context of group counseling. ■ TABLE 15.13 shows the codes for counseling patients in a group setting.

Each behavior change intervention service targets the avoidance of disease or conditions associated with high-risk factors or behaviors. As with each of the other preventive medicine services, if the performing physician identifies a presenting problem that requires the documentation of content of service elements or components and calls for at least a problem-oriented E/M service, the appropriate office or outpatient service level should be reported in addition to the preventive medicine service.

NON–FACE-TO-FACE PHYSICIAN SERVICES

non–face-to-face physician services services between a physician and an established patient that, unlike any other E/M service, may occur over the phone or via the Internet

Non–face-to-face physician services represent E/M services between a physician and an established patient that have been initiated by this established patient and stand apart from any other E/M service. CMS updates additional guidelines for non–face-to-face services, since identifying and reporting these interactions may present challenges.

Telephone Services

If the non–face-to-face service between a physician and an established patient results in a decision to see this physician within 24 hours, then that specific non–face-to-face physician service is considered to be part of the subsequent E/M service. Likewise, if the non–face-to-face physician service relates to a presenting problem for which the patient received E/M service within 7 days prior to the non–face-to-face physician service, the non–face-to-face physician service is considered part of the previous E/M service visit. ■ TABLE 15.14 provides the specific E/M codes for non–face-to-face physician telephone services of varying duration.

Online Medical Evaluation

An online medical evaluation is a non–face-to-face physician service that uses Internet communications resources to provide responses to a patient's inquiry. This non–face-to-face medical evaluation must not

■ **TABLE 15.14** **NON–FACE-TO-FACE PHYSICIAN SERVICES: TELEPHONE SERVICES**

	99441	99442	99443
Telephone Time Spent in Medical Discussion	5–10 minutes	11–20 minutes	21–30 minutes

Notes: (1) Telephone services may not originate from a related E/M service within 7 days prior to the telephone service.

(2) Telephone services may not directly lead to an E/M service within the 24 hours following the telephone service.

(3) Telephone services should be carefully separated from case management services.

■ **TABLE 15.15   NON–FACE-TO-FACE PHYSICIAN SERVICES: ONLINE MEDICAL EVALUATION**

Provision of online evaluation and management services to established patient, guardian, or healthcare provider	99444

Notes: (1) Online medical evaluation may not originate from a related E/M service within 7 days prior to the online medical evaluation.
(2) Online medical evaluation should be carefully separated from case management services.

originate from any related E/M service provided during the previous 7 days. ■ TABLE 15.15 gives the code for online medical evaluation.

SPECIAL E/M SERVICES

Special E/M services involve identifying baseline clinical data for two different reasons: issuance of basic life insurance or disability insurance policies and identification of medical or work-related disability. These services may be provided in an office setting, and no distinction is made between new or established patients. Specific criteria that must be identified during the provision of these services are identified by the AMA and listed in the CPT manual. ■ TABLES 15.16 and 15.17 identify the differences between the two special services: basic life insurance and/or disability insurance evaluation services and work or medical disability evaluation services.

These criteria should be clearly documented in the special E/M service. Since these services relate specifically to insurance and disability policies, regulations exist not only for the proper documentation of these services, but also for the setting, the provider, and sometimes even the forms on which these services must be documented. CMS should be consulted for regulation updates, and the specific agency providing the insurance policy or disability certification should be consulted as well.

■ **TABLE 15.16   SPECIAL E/M SERVICES: BASIC LIFE INSURANCE AND/OR DISABILITY INSURANCE EVALUATION**

99450 BASIC LIFE INSURANCE AND/OR DISABILITY INSURANCE EVALUATION
Measurement of vital signs, including height, weight, blood pressure
Collection of history as directed
Collection of fluids, including blood or urine sample, according to protocols
Completion of all required documentation

■ **TABLE 15.17   SPECIAL E/M SERVICES: WORK-RELATED OR MEDICAL DISABILITY EVALUATION**

99455 EXAMINATION THAT MUST BE PERFORMED BY THE PHYSICIAN WHO TREATS THE PATIENT	99456 EXAMINATION THAT MUST BE PERFORMED BY A PHYSICIAN *OTHER THAN THE PHYSICIAN WHO TREATS THE PATIENT*
Collection of medical history	Collection of medical history
Performance of physical examination	Performance of physical examination
Determination of a diagnosis as well as the patient's capabilities	Determination of a diagnosis as well as the patient's capabilities
Calculation of the extent of impairment	Calculation of the extent of impairment
Development of plan of care or treatment	Development of plan of care or treatment
Completion of all required documentation	Completion of all required documentation

Exercise 15.1   E/M Category Identification

Read the following medical documentation, and then answer the questions that follow.

Joanie Smith presents for her annual physical. She has completely recovered from her sinus infection. She identifies no problems or complaints. Physician reviews her history. Joanie has changed jobs and is working as an elementary school administrator. She reports that she has been experiencing heartburn and feels very anxious during the day with difficulty sleeping at night.

Comprehensive physical examination is performed, including neck, cardiovascular, respiratory, neurologic, musculoskeletal, and gastrointestinal. Examination of breasts performed; however, a pap smear is deferred since a pap smear was performed 3 months ago when Joanie wished to begin using oral contraceptives. Ear exam is normal. Dark staining of teeth noted, which Joanie reported is related to the five to six cups of coffee she drinks a day.

Visit concluded with counseling Joanie regarding the dangers of excessive caffeine intake and the impact of caffeine on stress levels, dehydration, insomnia, and stomach upset. Recommend weaning caffeine intake down to two cups a day before noon during the next month and drinking decaffeinated coffee for the rest of the day.

1. Which category best reflects the E/M service provided?

_____

2. Why has this category been selected?

_____

3. Does this category necessitate identification of the patient as new or established?

_____

4. Identify the factors that are most important when considering this category of E/M service.

_____

_____

Exercise 15.2   E/M Category Identification

Read the following medical documentation, and then answer the questions that follow.

Medical team conference regarding Janet Tomas, a 34-year-old-woman **para 1 gravida** 1 who experienced a class 3 **placental abruption** at 37 weeks gestation, followed by significant blood loss and maternal coagulopathy. Janet required transfusion of three units during surgery. Recovery delayed due to **verbal apraxia**, which raised concern regarding risk of stroke during placental abruption. Neurology consulted regarding possibility of **cerebrovascular accident**. No evidence of CVA identified, and therapies included physical, occupational, speech. Janet is currently 2 weeks **postpartum** and ready to discharge home under the care of home health agency.

Coordination of occupational therapy to build strength and coordination for carrying her baby; goal for occupational therapy is to carry 10-pound bag of flour in one arm while performing basic ADLs. **Lactation** consultation has been involved in Janet's care as Janet has expressed a desire to breastfeed baby Francis. Lactation consultation will continue at home in coordination with occupational therapy visits. Physical therapy coordinates with occupational therapy for muscle strengthening and coordination up and down the flight of stairs in the house. Per physical therapy, flight of stairs consists of two flights of 10 stairs each connected by a 4-foot-square landing. Per Janet's husband, who is present for medical team conference, a bed has been arranged on the ground floor until physical and occupational therapy considers Janet capable of safely ascending and descending stairs. Sleeping space pending approval by home health nurse and occupational therapy. Speech therapy reports that Janet's facial muscles have recovered strength and coordination, and verbal apraxia has dissipated. Speech therapy will ensure good swallowing capabilities at home and during performed ADLs.

SafeHouse Home health agency to coordinate nursing and therapy visits with Janet and her husband. Janet expresses excitement about going home with baby Francis and is looking forward to being strong enough to carry baby Francis alone. 45 minutes of counseling and coordination of care was performed in this medical team conference with Janet, her husband, and baby Francis.

1. Which category best reflects the E/M service provided?

_____

2. Why has this category been selected?

_____

3. Does this category necessitate identification of the patient as new or established?

_____

4. Identify the factors that are most important when considering this category of E/M service.

_____

_____

Exercise 15.3 **E/M Category Identification**

Read the following medical documentation, and then answer the questions that follow.

John Bigbute has a history of one CVA and one deep vein thrombosis. John has been taking 2.5 milligrams of Coumadin for 2 months with weekly checks for the last 3 weeks. INR, 1.7. No report of rash, but John reports one nosebleed last night before bed. John admits that he took an ibuprofen pain reliever for a headache yesterday morning. No report of weakness or dizziness. No swelling identified in toes, fingers, or ankles. Coumadin dose increased to 3 milligrams, and recommended John return for INR tomorrow. Counseling provided for warning signs, including unusual bruising, bleeding from gums when he brushes his teeth, black bowel movements, or a recurrent headache.

1. Which category best reflects the E/M service provided?

_____

_____

2. Why has this category been selected?

_____

_____

3. Does this category necessitate identification of the patient as new or established?

_____

4. Identify the factors that are most important when considering this category of E/M service.

_____

_____

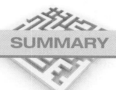

SUMMARY

- When a single physician provides a supervisory role for the management and/or coordination of a patient's multidisciplinary treatment plans, this is known as care plan oversight. This requires that the supervising physician be solely responsible for, or responsible for a significant percentage of, the oversight of the plan of care, management, and treatment for the patient, who may or may not be present during the provision of these services. This E/M service provides oversight for a patient receiving one of three types of care: hospice care, home care by agency, or nursing facility care. Care plan oversight services are reported in blocks of time during a calendar month, reflecting the effort involved in coordination of the multidisciplinary teams, which are intended to facilitate the management and/or treatment of the patient's condition(s) and needs. The guidelines identified in the CPT manual provide the foundation for understanding care plan oversight services, and CMS maintains and updates more detailed and explicit regulations for the proper reporting of these services.

- When the care plan oversight service involves a patient residing in a private home, assisted living facility, or other domiciliary residence, the nature of the E/M service changes a little bit. The change in setting affects the role of the supervising physician because of the difference in the care available to the patient. As with every other E/M service that does not require content of service, the CPT guidelines provide a foundational understanding of these care plan oversight services. CMS maintains and updates explicit regulations for the reporting of

domiciliary, rest home, or home care plan oversight services and should be consulted regularly.

- Case management services involve a single physician or other qualified healthcare professional who is solely responsible for the direct care of the patient—that is, who supervises any healthcare services the patient may require, which includes coordinating care for the patient, as well as managing the patient's access to care and/or initiating any specific treatment or therapy. Case management services include two subcategories: anticoagulant management and medical team conferences. Anticoagulant management services monitor the INR for patients undergoing anticoagulant therapy; services are defined in terms of a minimum number of INR measurements within a set period of time in an outpatient setting. Medical team conferences represent an assembly of at least three qualified healthcare professionals of varied disciplines who have each provided face-to-face healthcare services for a single patient within 60 days prior to the medical team conference. These qualified healthcare professionals may include both physicians and nonphysicians, although there is a distinction made when reporting these case management conferences in which a physician participates. Medical team conferences may include the patient and/or family. However, any conference involving the physician *and* the patient and/or family should be reported using the documented content of service. Regulations that are more specific are maintained by CMS and should be reviewed when reporting case management services.

- Preventive medicine services represent healthcare services intended to promote the continuation of the patient's good health. These services are not intended to provide treatment or management of a patient's presenting problem, associated condition, or underlying disease. The prior relationship between the physician and the patient affects how the preventive medicine service is reported, so new and established patients are recognized as subcategories and are reported according to the age of the patient. A separate subcategory of preventive medicine services includes counseling in the reduction of risky behavior, as well as interventions intended to change harmful behavior. In-depth regulations for reporting preventive medicine services are maintained and updated by CMS and should be reviewed when reporting any preventive medicine services.

- Certain clinical circumstances require the patient and the physician to engage in non–face-to-face services. These non–face-to-face E/M services must be performed by a physician and may be provided via telephone or online communication resource. A non–face-to-face E/M service cannot occur within 7 days of a related E/M service and cannot lead to a related E/M service within 24 hours after the non–face-to-face service. CMS maintains and updates regulations specific to non–face-to-face services, which should be reviewed when reporting a non–face-to-face E/M service.

- In order to identify a baseline of clinical information before the issuance of a basic life insurance and/or disability insurance policy or the identification of a medical or work-related disability, special E/M services may be performed and reported. The CPT manual clearly identifies the foundational guidelines for the performance, documentation, and reporting of these services; however, specific and explicit regulations maintained and updated by CMS should be reviewed, as well as any pertinent regulations provided by the specific agency requiring this healthcare service.

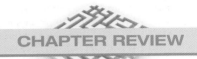

CHAPTER REVIEW

Multiple Choice

Choose the letter that best answers each question or completes each statement.

1. When a physician or other qualified healthcare professional performs an INR in an outpatient setting, which of the following E/M services has been performed?
   a. Preventive medicine service: new patient
   b. Case management service: anticoagulant management
   c. Care plan oversight: nursing facility
   d. Special E/M service

2. When a physician or other qualified healthcare professional performs counseling for the reduction of one or more risk factors, which of the following categories of service is being performed?
   a. Care plan oversight services
   b. Case management services
   c. Preventive medicine services
   d. Non–face-to-face physician services

3. A physician supervises the coordination and management of care for a 68-year-old established patient diagnosed with acute exacerbation of COPD. Involved in the care of the patient are three disciplines of a home health agency: physical therapy, home health nurse, and occupational therapy. The physician documents review of documentation, diagnostic reports, coordination of home health agency involvement, and communication with the patient's adult children, who each provide daily care and assistance with ADLs. Which of the following best reflects this E/M service?
   a. Domiciliary, rest home (e.g., assisted living facility), or home care plan oversight services
   b. Case management services

   c. Non–face-to-face physician services
   d. Care plan oversight services

4. A 17-year-old man presents to his regular pediatrician for an annual physical. During the course of the visit, the physician notices an **amphoric breath sound**. Further collection of history reveals that the patient has had a persistent and productive cough that began last week. Patient remembers eating pistachio nuts while playing video games with friends and distinctly remembers choking. After recovering from the episode, video game play resumed, and he thought nothing of it. Physical examination: Reveals distinct amphoric breath sounds accompanied by right-sided wheezes. Assessment: Probable foreign-body airway obstruction of right bronchi. Plan: Recommend **bronchoscopy** to identify and, if necessary, remove foreign body. Physician documents a detailed history, expanded problem-focused physical examination, and moderate medical decision making. Other than this presenting problem, physician performs an age and gender appropriate history, physical examination, and risk factor counseling pertinent to a young man—specifically, good driving habits, safe sexual practices or abstinence, and identification of alcohol or drug use. Which of the following best reflects the service(s) provided?
   a. One code: office or other outpatient service, new patient, level 3
   b. One code: preventive medicine, established patient
   c. Two separate codes: (1) preventive medicine, established patient, and (2) office or other outpatient; established patient, level 4
   d. Two separate codes: (1) preventive medicine, new patient, and (2) office or other outpatient service, new patient, level 3

5. Four healthcare professionals participate in a face-to-face conference at the hospital regarding a 59-year-old man 4 days

status post right-foot amputation due to severe ulceration of the foot secondary to type I diabetes. Patient is recovering from surgery well and will remain at the hospital for 3 more days before being transferred to ActiveWay Rehabilitation for follow-up rehab. Participating in medical conference is physical therapy, occupational therapy, physician, and patient's wife. 40 minutes spent in conference coordinating the active participation of each discipline in patient's rehabilitation. Patient's wife has been educated on postsurgical rehabilitation, as well as her coordination with physical and occupational therapy during her husband's recovery and rehabilitation. Which of the following best reflects the service(s) provided?

   a. Case management services: medical team conference, direct contact with patient and/or family

   b. Care plan oversight service

   c. Hospital inpatient services: subsequent hospital care

   d. Domiciliary, rest home (e.g., assisted living facility), or home care plan oversight

6. Jamie, a 10-year-old child, is recovering from a case of late-stage Lyme disease and requires IV **ceftriaxone**. Jamie's pediatrician supervises and coordinates medical team conferences by phone with the epidemiologist, home health nurse, and school nurse to ensure that Jamie's education will not be adversely effected by her extended absence from school. Over the course of the month during which Jamie has received the IV ceftriaxone, more than 40 minutes have been spent in reviewing records, coordinating, and implementing Jamie's healthcare plan. Which of the following best reflects the service(s) provided?

   a. Case management services: medical team conference without direct contact with patient

   b. Care plan oversight services

   c. Domiciliary, rest home, or home care plan oversight services

   d. Office or outpatient services: established patient, level 4

7. A 34-year-old woman is seen by her primary care physician for an examination as part of her work-related disability. One week ago, she was struck by a car while she was collecting shopping carts for her job at the Pinch-a-Penny shopping mall and was knocked to the ground, striking her head on a car bumper as she landed. She reports loss of consciousness for 40 minutes after the accident, although she recalls nothing from that entire day and night. She was treated emergently but remembers nothing of the care she received or how long she remained at the hospital. Records have been received and reviewed. She has suffered dizziness, severe headaches, and numbness in her fingertips and toes since her accident. The physician documents a medical history and physical examination, which are both proportionate to the patient's presenting problem. The physician's diagnosis is a moderate traumatic brain injury as rated on the Glasgow Coma Scale; recommendation for neurologic consultation. Physician strongly recommends the patient is unable to work until she receives full consultation and complete care from neurologist. Physician educates patient on the risk of further brain injury, recommending she wear head protection at all times. All necessary documentation required by the employer's insurance company, the driver's

insurance company, and the medical disability agency has been completed in full. Which of the following best reflects the service(s) provided?

   a. Office or outpatient services, established patient, level 2

   b. Special E/M services: work-related or medical disability evaluation services

   c. Care plan oversight services

   d. Case management services: medical team conference with direct contact with patient

8. A pediatrician returns a call placed by the mother of his 11-month-old established patient. Pediatrician informs the mother that her child's blood culture was positive for the pertussis antibody. The blood test was drawn 10 days ago during an office visit at the pediatrician's office. The physician prescribes antibiotics for the child and recommends the mother get screened for the pertussis antibody as well. The physician spends 15 minutes on the call, providing counseling for the mother regarding the antibiotic course, home care for the patient, and education about pertussis. Which of the following best reflects the service(s) provided?

   a. Care plan oversight services

   b. Non–face-to-face physician services

   c. Case management services

   d. Service that cannot be reported

9. A physician supervises the care of a 79-year-old woman who is receiving several different therapies at home. The patient is recovering from a fall from a kitchen stool, resulting in a broken ulna and sprained wrist. The physician coordinates the involvement and participation of a private physical therapist and the patient's adult daughter, the patient's power of attorney, and the private home aide who provides assistance with the patient's ADLs. According to the patient's daughter, the patient will not leave her home but received adequate care from the home aide, with positive results from the physical therapy. Over the course of 1 calendar month, the physician spends 35 minutes in supervision of documented physical therapy records, laboratory results, and telephone conference with the patient's adult daughter and home aide. Which of the following best reflects the service(s) provided?

   a. Non–face-to-face physician services

   b. Care plan oversight services

   c. Case management services

   d. Domiciliary, rest home (e.g., assisted living facility), or home care plan oversight services

10. The condition of a 95-year-old woman with lung and liver cancer has deteriorated. The physician supervised the coordination of hospice services during the patient's final month of life. During this month, the physician spent 45 minutes coordinating and revising the care plans and communicating with the hospice chaplain, hospice nurse, and psychologist. Which of the following best reflects the service(s) provided?

   a. Care plan oversight services

   b. Case management services

   c. Domiciliary, rest home (e.g., assisted living facility), or home care plan oversight services

   d. Non–face-to-face physician services

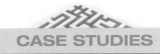

CASE STUDIES

Case Study 15-1

Read the following medical documentation, and then answer the questions that follow.

Suzie initiated a telephone call regarding concern about abdominal cramping. Patient 28 days status post hospital discharge for medical intervention of ectopic pregnancy at 37 days gestation. Initial **intramuscular methotrexate** injection was well tolerated by patient with **human chorionic gonadotropin (hCG)** levels dropping from 2150 mlU/ml to 1828 mlU/ml within the first 24 hours, with subsequent intrasmuscular methotrexate injection at 36 hours leading to a subsequent hCG level of 1462 mlU/ml at 48 hours. Suzie experienced significant abdominal cramping during the first 3 days after methotrexate injection, which improved with exercise, heat application, and positioning. Patient was seen in my office 10 days ago for follow-up with hCG level of 0.4 mlU/ml. Pregnancy test negative at that visit.

Suzie says she forgot about the recommendation to avoid ibuprofen and took 400 mg of ibuprofen this morning for a headache. After school, when she was preparing to take another 400 mg of ibuprofen for abdominal cramping, her mother reminded her about the potential adverse effect of ibuprofen and methotrexate. Suzie is now concerned about an adverse interaction.

Per verbal interview, patient denies any rashes, itching, or hives. No tightness in chest, tingling of lips or face. Bowel movements normal without black or red indicators, and no nausea or vomiting. No visual auras noted by patient.

Counseled patient that hormonal changes of body may lead to early menses rather than her usual oligoovulation. Recommend to Suzie that her body may be preparing for another menses; recommended expectant waiting. Suzie noted that she feels better in the evening. Recommended rest, increased fluid. Suzie will schedule an appointment next week if abdominal cramping increases in severity or frequency. Suzie displayed appropriate good humor when she commented that she has discontinued any sexual activity for the future. Suzie in good spirits at end of the 17-minute medical discussion.

1. Which of the following best reflects the service(s) provided?
   a. Non–face-to-face physician services
   b. Preventive medicine services
   c. Case management services
   d. Service that should not be reported

2. What do these words mean in relation to the performed service: "Patient was seen in my office 10 days ago for follow-up with hCG level of 0.4 mlU/ml. Pregnancy test negative at that visit"?
   a. This service should not be reported since the patient was seen within 10 days of the telephone contact.
   b. This service is actually part of the case management medical team conference since the physician had no direct contact with the patient.
   c. The physician provided risk reduction counseling and behavior change intervention, which supports preventive medicine services.

d. The telephone call was not the result of an E/M service within the previous 7 days, which supports a non–face-to-face physician service.

3. What does the following excerpt mean in relation to the service provided: "Suzie will schedule an appointment next week if abdominal cramping increases in severity or frequency. Suzie displayed appropriate good humor when she commented that she has discontinued any sexual activity for the future"?
   a. This service is actually part of the case management medical team conference since the physician had no direct contact with the patient.
   b. The physician provided risk reduction counseling and behavior change intervention because the patient said she wouldn't engage in risky sexual activity anymore, which supports preventive medicine services.
   c. The telephone call did not result in an E/M service within the following 24 hours, which supports a non–face-to-face physician service.
   d. This service should not be reported since the patient will be seen within the next week after the telephone contact.

Case Study 15-2

Identify the E/M category, subcategory, and criteria for the following case study. Be sure to utilize all prior knowledge. Remember that Appendix D contains the full content of service worksheet.

Franklin had received home care services from Georges Valley Home Health agency—specifically, physical therapy, occupational therapy, and home nursing. Franklin's primary care physician supervised the coordination and provision of all home health care through Georges Valley Home Health agency, including one physical therapy visit, one occupational therapy visit, and two home health nursing visits.

Franklin, a 59-year-old established patient, then called his primary care physician regarding abdominal pain. Franklin's abdominal pain had increased over the previous 24–36 hours, and Franklin wanted to know what pain relievers he could safely take. He did not want any more narcotic pain relievers. Franklin's abdominal pain began after he and his wife moved patio furniture into the garage. Physician recommended continued rest with minimal physical activity. Franklin educated about warning signs and symptoms, especially worsening abdominal pain or swelling, chest pain or difficulty breathing, fever over 101°F. Physician recommended NSAIDs such as ibuprofen, Motrin, Advil. Ten minutes were spent in telephone conference with Franklin.

1. Is content of service documented in this case study?

_____

2. Is direct contact with the patient and/or family documented in this E/M service?

_____

3. Is time a factor in this E/M service?

_____

4. Which E/M service category best reflects this documented case study?

_____

5. Which E/M service code best reflects this documented case study?

_____

Coding Challenge

Using your CPT manual, identify the E/M code that most appropriately reflects each of the following clinical scenarios.

1. On the 5th day of the patient's stay in the hospital, the physician, occupational therapist, physical therapist, and speech therapist meet in a face-to-face conference to review treatment plans, outcomes, and future coordination of the patient's care. Total time of conference is 35 minutes.
   CPT code: _____

2. Documentation reflects 13 minutes spent educating about and counseling tobacco cessation for a healthy 14-year-old girl who has been smoking cigarettes for the past 10 months.
   CPT code: _____

3. Patient Q is terminally ill and receiving hospice care. Dr. K supervises all of the care provided to patient Q and his family members during the final month of life, including review of patient status and nursing notes, as well as communication with and counseling of the patient's family. A total of 65 minutes of supervisory care for patient Q is documented by Dr. K, during which time patient Q was not present.
   CPT code: _____

4. Pediatrician G documents a 16-minute telephone conference with mother of 14-year-old girl who is experiencing abdominal pain and fever. Patient is well-known to pediatrician G. Most recent clinical visit was 2 weeks prior to phone conference. Pediatrician documents a comprehensive history and recommends the mother bring her daughter into the clinic the following morning if her daughter's fever does not respond to Tylenol. Patient presents to pediatrician G's clinic the following morning, where pediatrician G documents an expanded problem-focused history, expanded problem-focused physical exam, and moderate medical decision making for this established patient. Rapid strep test is positive for strep throat. Pediatrician prescribes antibiotics.
   CPT code: _____

5. Medical record documents physician review and interpretation of 15 separate INR tests during the first 90 days of a patient's anticoagulant therapy.
   CPT code: _____

6. A 46-year-old woman has transferred all her care to a new physician, and her first visit with her new physician is a comprehensive annual physical exam with comprehensive history and low medical decision making. No abnormalities are documented.
   CPT code: _____

7. Physician documents 48 minutes spent performing individual supervision of the care provided for a patient residing in a domiciliary setting; the time involved communication and coordination with physical and occupational therapy care plans.

Documentation clearly states patient was not present during the independent supervision of the individual patient care.
   CPT code: _____

8. The physician provides counseling for a healthy 18-year-old male patient who has experienced interest in becoming sexually active with his girlfriend. Safe-sex practices and abstinence are discussed during this 10-minute visit.
   CPT code: _____

9. Patient O was a resident of Oceanside Nursing Residence, which is an inpatient facility, from February 12 to March 11. Medical documentation indicates that Dr. W provided 25 minutes of supervision for the care provided to patient O, including independent review of clinical laboratory results, review of nursing notes and patient status, and telephone communication with other physicians and family members.
   CPT code: _____

10. Physician documents a 10-minute telephone conference with a patient whom he has not seen in 10 days. MD evaluates the presenting problem, gathers a comprehensive history, and recommends an OTC analgesic. Patient expresses understanding. Telephone call does not lead to an E/M visit.
    CPT code: _____

11. Documentation reflects a 45-minute face-to-face conference with an occupational therapist, physical therapist, speech therapist, and patient's family on the 10th day of the patient's stay in the hospital. The clinician reviewed the patient's condition, treatment, and plan of care and answered the family's questions.
    CPT code: _____

12. Documentation reflects a 10-year-old boy who presents to the pediatrician for his first annual physical exam after moving to the area. Comprehensive history, detailed physical exam, low medical decision making, and 10 minutes spent counseling the patient about healthy nutritional habits. All findings are within normal limits for a 10-year-old male.
    CPT code: _____

13. During the month of January, Dr. X personally supervises care provided for patient G, a resident of Sunny Home's assisted living center. Dr. X documents reviews and revision of the care plans, personal review of laboratory results, and communication of patient G's status with her family. A total of 20 minutes of Dr. X's independent, individual supervision took place without the presence of patient G.
    CPT code: _____

14. Documentation reflects a comprehensive annual evaluation for a 58-year-old man with well-controlled hypertension. Comprehensive history, detailed physical exam, and moderate medical decision making, including counseling regarding appropriate dietary and exercise guidelines, are documented, and routine labs are ordered.
    CPT code: _____

15. Patient has taken a health hazard appraisal. The physician interprets the appraisal for the patient and documents the findings in the patient's medical record.
    CPT code: _____

16. Pediatrician G documents an email conversation with the mother of a 14-year-old girl who is experiencing abdominal pain. Patient is well-known to pediatrician G, but pediatrician

G has not seen patient for over 2 weeks, when the patient was treated for strep throat. Pediatrician G collects a comprehensive history and performs low medical decision making, recommending a liquid diet to settle the patient's stomach. Mother expresses understanding. No clinic visit is recommended by pediatrician G or requested by the mother.

CPT code: _____

17. Patient presents to physician for physical assessment during the process of applying for a life insurance policy. Physician performs a comprehensive physical examination and documents appropriate history and findings on the forms provided by the life insurance provider.

CPT code: _____

18. Pediatrician G documents an email conversation with the mother of a 14-year-old girl who is experiencing abdominal pain. Patient is well-known to pediatrician G as most recent visit was 3 days previous, when pediatrician G treated the patient for strep throat with antibiotics. Pediatrician G collects detailed history and performs low medical decision making, recommending that the patient take the antibiotics with food rather than on an empty stomach. No follow-up visit in the clinic is recommended.

CPT code: _____

19. Patient who has been treated for a football-related back injury presents to family physician for assessment prior to resuming regular duties at work as a shipping and receiving manager. Physician documents a detailed history and examination that are specifically related to the back injury. Medical decision making includes prevention of future recurrence. Physician completes all necessary paperwork required by employer before patient can return to work.

CPT code: _____

20. During the month of January, Dr. A documents 50 minutes of supervision for the care provided for patient M, who is under care of South District Home Care. Dr. A documents his personal review of diagnostic testing results; performs coordination of physical therapists, occupational therapists, and home care RNs; and communicates any change of care or treatment to the family members of patient M. Documentation clearly indicates that patient M was not present during any of Dr. A's supervision.

CPT code: _____

21. A physician, occupational therapist, physical therapist, and speech therapist spent 45 minutes in face-to-face conference with the patient and family on the 10th day of the patient's stay in the hospital. During the conference, the clinicians review the patient's condition, treatment, and plan of care. Documentation reflects a problem-focused history and low medical decision making.

CPT code: _____

22. The physician documents a comprehensive annual evaluation for a 16-year-old boy who is physically active with no health complaints.

CPT code: _____

---

para a woman who has delivered at least one live birth; often used with a number to indicate how many live births the woman has delivered

gravida a woman's state of pregnancy; often used with a number to indicate how many pregnancies the woman has experienced

verbal apraxia a neurological condition that causes an inability of the muscles of the face and mouth to form words

placental abruption an abnormal separation of the placenta from the wall of the uterus prior to the birth of a baby; can lead to severe, uncontrollable uterine bleeding

cerebrovascular accident also known as a stroke; an occlusion or blockage of vessels in the brain caused by an embolus, thrombus, or other pathology that can cause lack of blood flow in the tissues of the brain

postpartum after birth

lactation the production of milk in the mammary glands in females

amphoric breath sound an abnormal hollow, blowing sound heard during auscultation of the lungs; can be indicative of an abnormal opening into the bronchus or pneumothorax or an obstruction of the bronchus

bronchoscopy the act of inserting a cylindrical fiber optic tube with a video function into the airway; allows direct visualization of the mucosal tissues of the airways for diagnostic purposes

status post a term indicating that a person has recently had a significant procedure or experienced a medical event; often preceded by a time designation and followed by a medical procedure, as in "4 days status post appendectomy" to indicate that this individual had an appendectomy 4 days prior

ceftriaxone an antibiotic

intramuscular within a muscle; for example, describing an injection into the muscle tissue

methotrexate an antineoplastic antimetabolite that acts as a folic acid antagonist as well as an immunosuppressive agent for autoimmune diseases such as rheumatoid arthritis; also used in the medical treatment of ectopic pregnancies

human chorionic gonadotropin (hCG) also known as the "pregnancy hormone"; measured to identify the gestation stage of pregnancies

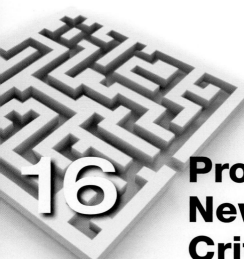

16

Prolonged Services, Newborn Care, and Critical Care

Learning Objectives

After completing this chapter, you should be able to do the following:

- Spell and define the key terms and abbreviations presented in this chapter
- Understand prolonged services
- Identify services for newborn care
- Identify critical care
- Recognize services for inpatient neonatal care, as well as pediatric and neonatal critical care
- Recognize the unlisted E/M services

Key Terms

add-on service codes

Apgar assessments

birthing room

broviac catheter

cardiopulmonary function

cardiothoracic surgeon

central nervous system failure

chest compressions

colostomy

critical care

delivery room

diaphragmatic rupture

dilated intestinal loops

emergency medical technician (EMT)

extrauterine

fetus

general surgeon

heart failure

heart failure with acute pulmonary edema

HELLP syndrome

homeostasis

indomethacin

infant

intensive care

intrauterine

labored breathing

Legionnaire's disease

low birth weight

malrotation

moxifloxan

neonatal medicine

newborn

oxygenation

CPT codes in this chapter are from the CPT 2012 code set. CPT is a registered trademark of the American Medical Association.

patent ductus arteriosus

pediatric medicine

perineal

persistent cyanosis

pneumatosis intestinalis

positive pressure ventilation

prolonged services

rales

respiratory failure

resuscitation

shock

testicular

unlisted E/M service

very low birth weight

vital organ system failure

INTRODUCTION

Every category of E/M service identifies a specific kind of clinical interaction between a physician and a patient. There are times when the nature of the patient's presenting problem requires the performance of an E/M service that exceeds what could be documented in the content of service. Some of these services address pathologies that require significant and extreme measures of treatment and management. Other categories of E/M service represent a specific stage of the patient's life. This chapter examines some of the most complicated categories of E/M services: prolonged service, newborn care, critical care, inpatient neonatal and pediatric critical care, and unlisted E/M services.

PROLONGED SERVICES

When the word *prolonged* is used in reference to an event, it suggests that the time during which an event should have occurred has extended beyond the typical, or expected, length. When an E/M service is prolonged, the provision of the service takes longer than the service would typically require. This lengthy service cannot be reported through the documentation of the history, physical examination, or medical decision making, since these elements identify the content of service and the extended intraservice time may involve the collection of the content of service *or* the contributing components. By definition, **prolonged services** require a longer amount of time to perform than the intraservice time typically allows and may occur in an outpatient or an inpatient setting. Prolonged services report the total amount of intraservice time the physician or other qualified healthcare professional has spent providing care for an individual patient on a specific date, even if the total intraservice on that specific date has been interrupted. The specific prolonged service codes should be reported in addition to the code that best reflects the performed E/M service.

prolonged services
services requiring a longer amount of time to perform than the intraservice time typically allows; may occur in an outpatient or an inpatient setting

The three subcategories of prolonged services reflect the different circumstances that may require an unusually lengthy E/M service. The subcategories are prolonged service with direct patient contact, prolonged service without direct patient contact, and physician standby services.

Prolonged Services with Direct Patient Contact

In the context of prolonged services, specific nuances must be identified when defining the term *direct patient contact*. The phrase refers to the face-to-face time the physician or other qualified healthcare professional spends with the patient but also includes any additional non–face-to-face services provided on the patient's floor or unit in the hospital or nursing facility during the same session. Therefore, prolonged services involving face-to-face contact with a patient are considered prolonged services with direct patient contact. In each case, the physician or other qualified healthcare professional must document content of service appropriate to the setting and patient type.

These prolonged services with direct patient contact report the total length of time spent by the physician or other qualified healthcare professional on a particular date of service, regardless of whether this time is continuous or interrupted. Therefore, each of these services may be reported only once per date.

Prolonged services with direct patient contact may occur in an outpatient or an inpatient setting. Since these services require the collection, performance, and documentation of content of service, they may be reported only with certain categories of E/M services.

Prolonged Services with Direct Patient Contact in an Outpatient Setting Prolonged services involving direct patient contact may be reported with outpatient E/M services that require

content of service. Specifically, prolonged services may be reported in conjunction with the following categories:

- Office or outpatient services
- Outpatient consultations
- Domiciliary, rest home (e.g., boarding home), or custodial care services
- Home services

Each of these E/M categories specifically requires content of service or lists typical intraservice times.

The subcategory of prolonged service with direct patient contact identifies two different allotments of time—the first hour of additional time (which the CPT manual defines as 30–74 minutes) and each additional 30 minutes beyond that first hour—and assigns the two periods separate E/M service codes. Both of these individual codes are considered to be **add-on service codes**, identified by a "+," which means they represent E/M services that may be reported only in conjunction with a different E/M service and may never be listed independently.

Prolonged services with direct patient contact require an extensive length of time over and above that of the E/M service. This prolonged service should be listed with the highest level of the appropriate category. The CPT guidelines state that prolonged services involving direct patient care in an outpatient setting provide an additional hour beyond the typical intraservice time, including both face-to-face and non–face-to-face services. However, the manual goes further to state that any prolonged service consisting of less than 30 minutes should *not* be reported in addition to the appropriate outpatient E/M service. Since this can become confusing, it is worthwhile to consider the appropriate reporting of prolonged service with direct patient contact in an outpatient setting as a three-part conditional statement:

> *If …*
>
> a physician or other qualified healthcare professional performs an E/M service for an established patient in an outpatient setting
>
> > *and*
>
> the duration of the visit exceeds the required intraservice time by at least 30 minutes
>
> > *and*
>
> the service involves direct patient contact,
>
> > > *then*
> >
> > a prolonged physician service with direct patient contact may be reported in addition to the highest level of office or outpatient service for an established patient.

add-on service codes numeric codes representing E/M services that may be reported only in conjunction with a different E/M service and may never be listed independently; identified with the symbol "+"

The CPT manual identifies guidelines and recommendations for the appropriate identification and reporting of prolonged services. Since the individual category of prolonged service does not require content of service on its own but instead must be linked to a separate E/M outpatient service, the guidelines for this category are lengthy. As it does for every other category of E/M service that does not individually require the content of service, CMS maintains and updates additional guidelines and requirements for prolonged services with direct patient contact in an outpatient setting, which should be consulted whenever considering these prolonged physician services. ■ TABLE 16.1 gives the codes for prolonged service with direct patient contact in an outpatient setting.

Prolonged Services with Direct Patient Contact in an Inpatient Setting The inpatient E/M services that may be listed in conjunction with prolonged services involving direct patient contact are hospital inpatient services, inpatient consultations, and nursing facility services. These services each require the collection, performance, and documentation of the content of service and/or the contributing components, including typical intraservice time. The prolonged services with direct patient

■ TABLE 16.1 PROLONGED SERVICE WITH DIRECT PATIENT CONTACT IN AN OUTPATIENT SETTING

CPT CODE	SETTING	DURATION OF PROLONGED SERVICE
+99354	Office or other outpatient setting	First hour (30–74 minutes)
+99355	Office or other outpatient setting	Each additional 30 minutes

■ **TABLE 16.2** **PROLONGED SERVICE WITH DIRECT PATIENT CONTACT IN AN INPATIENT SETTING**

CPT CODE	SETTING	DURATION OF PROLONGED SERVICE
+99356	Inpatient setting, requiring unit/floor time	First hour (30–74 minutes)
+99357	Inpatient setting, requiring unit/floor time	Each additional 30 minutes

contact must be provided while the physician is on the patient's unit/floor in the hospital or nursing facility *and* must be performed on the same date as the hospital inpatient service, inpatient consultation, or nursing facility service. ■ TABLE 16.2 provides the codes for the inpatient prolonged services with direct patient contact.

Both of these codes are identified as add-on codes, which require that any reported prolonged service with direct patient contact identify the specific inpatient setting with the appropriate inpatient E/M service code. The following example reveals the coding of inpatient prolonged services with direct patient contact in conjunction with a subsequent hospital care service.

During the second day of a 45-year-old man's inpatient stay in the hospital for complaints of excruciating upper abdominal pain and nausea, the documented content of service supports the highest level of subsequent hospital care with 95 minutes of documented intraservice time.

E/M service with documented content of service	99223	35 minutes intraservice time
Prolonged service with direct patient contact	+99356	First additional hour (30–74 minutes) of prolonged service

Even though the three inpatient E/M service categories that may identify prolonged service with direct patient contact require documentation of content of service, the specific prolonged service subcategory does not require content of service. CMS identifies and maintains specific guidelines for the correct reporting of any prolonged service with direct patient contact performed in an inpatient setting.

Prolonged Service without Direct Patient Contact

Sometimes the care provided by a physician or other qualified healthcare professional occurs without direct contact with the patient. When such professional services relate directly to an E/M service for this specific patient, any prolonged services may be considered a prolonged service without direct patient contact. Examples of prolonged service without direct patient contact include an extensive review of patient records, research into a patient's condition, extensive review of diagnostic results, and more. As these examples suggest, prolonged service without direct patient contact should be reported only when this service relates directly to one specific E/M service that did involve direct contact between the patient and the physician or other qualified healthcare professional. In this way, these prolonged services without direct patient contact support the physician's effective provision of care of the patient. However, this prolonged service may not be listed for the physician's time spent in case management services, non–face-to-face services, or care plan oversight services. Beyond these exclusions, the CPT manual lists no specific categories with which prolonged service without direct patient contact may be reported.

The prolonged service without direct patient contact is reported in blocks of time—the first hour beyond the typical intraservice time and each additional 30 minutes. Unlike the prolonged service that involves direct patient contact, this prolonged service without patient contact may be listed independently and on a different date from that of the E/M service visit.

Example: Documentation of Prolonged Service

On February 15, a 9-year-old girl was seen by her pediatrician for abdominal pain in a 40-minute established outpatient visit. A barium swallow and CT scan were ordered to determine the nature of the patient's anatomy. The imaging reports, results, and scans were sent to the pediatrician for review on February 17, and the pediatrician spent 55 minutes examining the patient's previous medical records, imaging results, scans, and laboratory results.

| E/M service with documented content of service | 99215 | 40 minutes intraservice time | Date of service: February 15 |
| Prolonged service without direct patient contact | +99358 | First additional hour (30–74 minutes) of prolonged service | Date of service: February 17 |

rales an abnormal sound in the lungs, identified by auscultation; characterized by crackles and caused by accumulation of fluid within the trachea, bronchi, or lungs

However, the additional 30 minutes of prolonged service time *is* an add-on code that must be listed, when applicable, along with the initial hour of prolonged service without direct patient contact.

Exercise 16.1   Respiratory Illness and Rule-Out Pertussis

Read the following medical documentation, and then answer the questions that follow.

Ruby, a 10-month-old girl, is well-known to me and presents for severe cough, lethargy, and high fever. Patient appears haggard and weak with thick, green mucus draining from both nares and a severe, rough cough that leaves her breathless. Ruby's mother states the patient has not slept more than an hour straight over the past 2 days because of her persistent cough, has very poor appetite, and has coughed so much she vomited last night. Ruby's cough is significantly worse at night and was severe enough her mother was concerned she had stopped breathing.

Physical Exam: Vital signs: T, 103.1°F; Wt, 28 lbs; pulse, 120. Ruby is very pale, and skin is hot to touch with no notation of spots, nodules, or rash. She is alert and responsive during exam but prefers to be in mother's arms. Neck: palpation causes significant discomfort due to swollen lymph nodes. Eyes: red and irritated bilaterally with no identified discharge. EOMI. ENT/M: significant clear fluid identified behind right tympanic membrane; serous fluid behind left tympanic membrane with minimal pressure identified. Nares red and inflamed bilaterally. Oropharynx red, inflamed, with significant green phlegm and white exudates apparent throughout, occluding the tonsils. Patient is clearly in significant pain during mouth and throat exam. Auscultation reveals sonorous rhonchus, fine **rales**, and pleural friction rub identified. Soft, nontender abdomen with no identified masses.

Laboratory and Assessment: Sputum gram stain and culture positive for Streptococcus pneumonia. Due to lung auscultation, chest X-ray ordered. Independent visualization of chest X-ray reveals significant inflammation of pleural lining as well as the bronchi. Recommend blood test for pertussis.

Diagnosis: Streptococcal pneumonia, pleurisy, and bronchitis. Rule out pertussis.

Plan: Prescribed cefotaxime antibiotic for Streptococcus pneumonia. Indomethacin prescribed to reduce inflammation of pleural lining. Hydrocodone cough suppressant prescribed for reduction of cough. More than 95 minutes of direct contact were spent providing counseling for Ruby's mother, reviewing chest X-ray film with Ruby's mother, coordinating care at the hospital for the pertussis test, as well as providing care for Ruby.

1. Which category best reflects the E/M service provided?
   _____

   Why has this category been selected? _____
   _____
   _____

2. Does this category necessitate identification of the patient as new or established? _____

3. Identify the factors that are most important when considering this category of E/M service. _____
   _____
   _____

4. Which code(s) best reflect the E/M service provided?
   _____
   _____

Physician Standby Services

Consider the **general surgeon** Dr. A, who is preparing to perform a stage 3 splenectomy for an adult patient. Because the radiology scans show the possibility of **diaphragmatic rupture**, Dr. A requests that Dr. C, a **cardiothoracic surgeon**, stand by in case Dr. A needs the additional assistance that Dr. C could provide. The period of time that Dr. C is standing by, waiting to provide assistance if needed, is categorized as physician standby services. This duration of time is identified in blocks of 30 minutes and may be reported only if Dr. C is waiting, standing by, and not providing care for any other patients. Physician standby services may also be reported with newborn care E/M services.

As with every other category of E/M service that does not require content of service, CMS identifies and maintains specific guidelines for reporting physician standby services, which should be reviewed whenever considering a physician standby service.

general surgeon a physician specially trained to investigate and repair the internal structure and function of abdominal organs, as well as treating disease and injury through manual manipulation

diaphragmatic rupture a tear or created abnormality of the muscle that aids inspiration and separates the thoracic cavity and the abdominal cavity

Janet Tomas's Postpartum Care

Read the following medical documentation, and then answer the questions that follow.

Janet Tomas presents to her primary care physician 4 months after her discharge from a home health agency. Currently 6 months postpartum, she is feeling well, physically. During the visit, Janet becomes tearful and expresses concern regarding her state of mind, especially given that her menstrual cycle has begun again.

A detailed history is collected, a detailed physical examination performed, and medical decision making of moderate complexity. Extensive time during this 95-minute visit is spent in discussion with Janet about methods of contraception, as well as self-care during the transition.

1. Which category best reflects the E/M service provided?

   _____

   Why has this category been selected? _____

   _____

2. Does this category necessitate identification of the patient as new or established? _____

3. Identify the factors that are most important when considering this category of E/M service. _____

   _____

   _____

4. Which code best reflects the E/M service provided? ____

   _____

cardiothoracic surgeon a physician specially trained to investigate and repair the internal structure and function of the organs of the chest, including, but not limited to, the lungs, heart, mediastinum, and pleura

infant a child from birth to approximately 1 year of age, or about the time the infant learns to walk

newborn an infant from birth to 28 days of life

NEWBORN CARE SERVICES

An **infant** is a child from birth to approximately 1 year of age, or about the time a young child learns to walk. The term **newborn** refers to an infant from birth to 28 days of life. Newborn care services are provided to newborns in a variety of settings: delivery rooms, birthing centers, and hospitals. These E/M services include the initial care provided for newborns after birth and before the newborn's trip home from the hospital. This initial care includes the collection of history (which may include the mother's history and the prenatal history of the newborn), performance of the newborn's first physical examination, and the ordering of any initial diagnostic procedures. In addition, if the physician needs to meet with the family, this meeting is included in the newborn care service.

Newborn care services are per diem services and identify the E/M care for a normal newborn. These services are distinguished by two different factors: where the newborn care service is provided and whether the newborn care service is an initial or subsequent service. The locations in which newborn care services can be provided are hospitals, birthing centers, and any other settings that are not hospitals or birthing centers. Since the newborn care services are per diem codes, the initial newborn care service reflects the E/M services provided during the entire day for the newborn after birth. Subsequent newborn care services include the E/M services provided for the newborn after the initial newborn care service but before the newborn is discharged from the hospital. ■ TABLE 16.3 presents each of the newborn care codes with appropriate, simplified examples for normal newborn infants.

However, if the newborn care service reveals an abnormality that requires treatment, this E/M service should be reported using the appropriate hospital inpatient service level *and* the appropriate neonatal intensive and critical care service.

■ TABLE 16.3 NEWBORN CARE SERVICES

CPT CODE (PER DIEM)	SETTING	SERVICE
99460	Hospital or birthing center	Initial care provided for newborn baby (e.g., Sue is born in a hospital)
99461	Other than hospital or birthing center	Initial care provided for newborn baby (e.g., Sam is born at home and admitted to the hospital 3 hours after birth)
99462	Hospital	Subsequent care provided for newborn baby (e.g., either Sue or Sam)
99463	Hospital or birthing center	Initial care provided for newborn baby born and discharged on the same date (e.g., Sarah is born in a birthing center and goes home with parents that same day)

■ **TABLE 16.4** NEWBORN CARE SERVICES: DELIVERY/BIRTHING ROOM ATTENDANCE AND RESUSCITATION SERVICES

CPT CODE	SERVICE	EXAMPLE
99464	Performing physician's attendance at delivery of newborn and initial stabilization of newborn	Dr. G is delivering newborn baby Sarah and requests Dr. K's attendance at delivery for initial stabilization of the newborn while Dr. G provides care for the mother directly after this complicated birth. Dr. K reports his attendance.
99465	Resuscitation of newborn, positive pressure ventilation, and/or chest compressions	Immediately after the delivery of newborn baby Sarah, Dr. K provides resuscitation in the birthing room. Dr. K reports the resuscitation service.

Delivery/Birthing Room Attendance and Resuscitation Services

Since newborn care services represent E/M services provided for an infant 28 days old or younger, these services also include any E/M services provided during the birth—in the **delivery room** or the **birthing room**.

The birth process marks the transition from **intrauterine** life within the uterus to **extrauterine** life as a newborn infant. During this transition, the newborn infant must take initial, spontaneous breaths to clear its lungs of fluid. Specific cardiopulmonary changes must also occur to ensure the proper **oxygenation** of the newborn, as well as the proper body temperature. **Apgar assessments** evaluate the newborn's heart rate, breathing, and muscle tone, as well as its reflexive response to the suctioning of the nasal and oral cavities. Skin color indicates the oxygenation level of the newborn, reflecting **cardiopulmonary function**. The results of these assessments indicate any need for **resuscitation**.

In the event that resuscitation is required because of **labored breathing**, gasping, or **persistent cyanosis**, **positive pressure ventilation** may be initiated. This is the process of forcing oxygenated air into the lungs through mechanical means and, for newborns, can pose clinical complications requiring specific equipment and skill. Similarly, if **chest compressions** are required in the event that the newborn's heart rate is less than desired, such compressions require skill and expertise because of the typical size of a newborn. ■ TABLE 16.4 gives the codes and examples of these services.

The delivery and/or birthing room attendance and resuscitation services may be reported in conjunction with an initial hospital or birthing center care service or with initial inpatient neonatal critical care.

CRITICAL CARE

A **critical care** service is the provision of personalized, continuous care for one specific patient whose health has been abruptly damaged by an illness, injury, or disease that simultaneously poses a significant and definite threat to the patient's life. The provision of critical care services requires extensive training and expertise, as well as specialized equipment required to provide the appropriate care. Critical care requires time to assess the presentation of the critical illness and to identify the any injury, illness, or disease process that is contributing to or causing the **vital organ system failure**. Critical care services require a greater amount of time to perform than the typical intraservice time allows.

The human body is composed of many different organ systems, some of which provide vitally important functions that ensure the continued health and life of the person and are known as vital organ systems. The cardiovascular and respiratory organ systems are only two examples. All of these vital organ systems function together to maintain **homeostasis**, which occurs when the systems not only function within normal limits, but also ensure the normal physiology of the person. Certain illnesses or injuries disrupt this homeostasis, causing one or more of the vital organ systems to deteriorate or even fail. When one vital organ system fails, there is an increased risk of failure of additional vital organ systems. Therefore, when a patient experiences the failure of one or more vital organ systems, he or she must receive critical care services from a physician.

The provision of critical care services requires several important skills: very complex medical decision making, the ability to assess a clinical situation quickly and identify any diagnostic results, and the capacity to rapidly adjust treatment plans and management options in order to prevent single or multiple vital organ system failure. Some examples of vital organ system failure are **shock**, **heart failure**, **respiratory failure**, **heart failure with acute pulmonary edema**, and **central nervous system failure**.

delivery room a designated room or area specially equipped to deal with the delivery and care of newborns

birthing room one designated room or area specially equipped to deal with the delivery and care of newborns

intrauterine within the uterus

extrauterine outside the womb

oxygenation the normal flow of oxygen to the tissues

Apgar assessments five different assessments at the time of birth that determine the patient's blood flow, heart rate, respiratory function, and neurologic function

cardiopulmonary function the heartbeat that pumps the blood to the lungs during respiration

resuscitation manual establishment of the functions of heart and lungs after a sudden cessation of normal cardiac or respiratory function

labored breathing mechanical function of respiration due to disease or injury

persistent cyanosis a symptom of decreased flow of oxygen to the tissues, most often presenting as a bluish coloration of the skin

positive pressure ventilation process of forcing oxygenated air into the lungs through mechanical means

chest compressions the manual compression of the chest for the purpose of restoring heart function; most often associated with cardiopulmonary resuscitation

critical care personalized, continuous care provided for one specific patient whose health has been abruptly damaged by an illness, injury, or disease that simultaneously poses a significant and definite threat to the patient's life

vital organ system failure the interruption or cessation of normal physiological function of one of the important organ systems that is vital to the normal function of the human body

homeostasis the physical state when vital organ systems not only function within normal limits, but function together to ensure the normal physiology of a patient

shock one of several life-threatening conditions that lead to the inadequate flow of blood to the body and a decrease of oxygen in the tissues; can lead to a buildup of toxins in tissues and quickly to brain damage and death; includes distributive shock, hypovolemic shock, and carcinogenic shock

heart failure the failure of the heart to pump blood

respiratory failure the failure of the lungs to function

heart failure with acute pulmonary edema the failure of the heart to pump blood, combined with the collection of fluid within the pulmonary tissues, leading to intense difficulty breathing

central nervous system failure the breakdown of the human central nervous system through pathology, illness, disease, or injury

The purpose of critical care is to treat the single or multiple organ system failure and prevent any further deterioration of the patient's condition. Critical care can be provided on a number of consecutive days, regardless of whether the life-threatening condition changes. Even though critical care is often provided in a specially designated area of a healthcare facility, such as an intensive care unit or a cardiac care unit, critical care services are not required to occur in a designated unit or ward.

The time spent by the physician providing critical care should be recorded in the patient's medical record. The requirements for this time are similar to the requirements for unit/floor intraservice time; that is, the time spent on the unit or floor providing critical care services may be reported as critical care time because critical care services require the physician's quick access to the patient. These services include reviewing records and diagnostic results and discussing the patient's critical illness or injury with other qualified healthcare professionals, services that may not occur at the patient's bedside or in the presence of the patient's family. As with unit/floor intraservice time, any activities performed or time spent by the physician away from the unit or off the floor may not be counted as critical care time.

Because of the intensity of the critical care services and the emergent nature of the patient's pathology, it is important that the performing physician provide care to no other patient than the patient experiencing the critical illness, injury, or disease. Critical care services require that all services must directly relate to the diagnosis, management, and treatment of this one patient's critical illness, disease, or injury. The duration of time spent by the physician providing critical care services is reported in 29-minute segments of time. However, if the physician provides critical care services to the patient for less than 30 minutes, then the appropriate E/M service category and level are reported. For example, if 25 minutes of critical care services are provided to a patient during a subsequent inpatient visit, the critical care services should be reported as a level 2 established hospital inpatient service, based on the unit/floor intraservice time with appropriate documentation. But if 30 minutes or more have been spent providing critical care services to a patient, critical care services can be reported. Consideration of critical care can be thought of as a four-part conditional statement:

> *If* ...
>
> the physician spends at least 30 minutes providing critical care services for a patient
>
> > *and*
> >
> > the physician's assessment of the critical injury or illness requires a high level of decision making
> >
> > > *and*
> > >
> > > the management or treatment of the critical injury or illness involves a comprehensive evaluation of the vital organ systems
> > >
> > > > *and*
> > > >
> > > > a very significant amount of support and care goes into preventing further deterioration of the patient's vital organ system(s),
> > > >
> > > > > *then*
> > > > >
> > > > > critical care services may be reported.

The CPT manual makes clear in the guidelines for critical care services that all of the listed criteria must be met in order to report critical care services.

Critical care services are reported according to the total amount of time spent by the physician providing critical care for one specific patient. This total amount of time does not need to be consecutive or uninterrupted time. The first 30 to 74 minutes of critical care services are identified by one specific numeric code as the first block of critical care time. ■ TABLE 16.5 shows the essential components of this one code.

■ TABLE 16.5   CRITICAL CARE GUIDELINES FOR 99291

If . . .	at least 30–74 minutes are spent . . .	providing critical care
and . . .	physician assessment of critical injury or illness requires . . .	high-level medical decision making
and . . .	management or treatment of critical injury or illness requires . . .	comprehensive evaluation of vital organ systems
and . . .	significant amount of clinical support and care is given to . . .	preventing further deterioration of vital organ systems
then	critical care code **99291** may be reported.	

■ TABLE 16.6   CRITICAL CARE GUIDELINES FOR ADD-ON CODE +99292

If . . .	at least an additional 30 minutes beyond the initial 30–74 minutes is spent	providing critical care
and . . .	physician assessment of critical injury or illness requires . . .	high-level medical decision making
and . . .	management or treatment of critical injury or illness requires . . .	comprehensive evaluation of vital organ systems
and . . .	significant amount of clinical support and care is given to . . .	preventing further deterioration of vital organ systems
then the add-on critical care code **+99292** may be reported in addition to 99291.		

Any additional time spent providing critical care after the initial 74 minutes is identified in periods of up to 30 minutes. ■ TABLE 16.6 shows the components of this critical care add-on code.

The total amount of time may be reflected in something resembling an equation, depending on the total amount of time involved.

Example: Documentation of Critical Care

A physician spends a total of 2 hours and 45 minutes providing critical care services for a patient suffering from penetrating abdominal trauma with multiple organ system failure. All of the necessary criteria for critical care services are met. Therefore, the critical care services are reported as follows:

99291 × 1 (representing the first 74 minutes of critical care) and +99292 × 3 (representing each additional period of 30 minutes each)

The CPT manual provides extensive guidelines for the services that may not be listed separately from critical care services because these other services are commonly performed during critical care and are therefore considered a part of codes 99291 and 99292. The services that may not be listed separately include, but are not limited to, cardiac output measurements, gastric intubation, and vascular access procedures. As with all E/M services that require elements other than content of service, CMS maintains and updates extensive guidelines, requirements, and recommendations for the correct reporting of critical care services, and these should be referenced when considering critical care services.

INPATIENT NEONATAL CARE AND PEDIATRIC AND NEONATAL CRITICAL CARE SERVICES

When a critical healthcare situation occurs in a pediatric patient or a neonate patient, critical care or intensive care may be required. Although the phrases "critical care" and "intensive care" are often used interchangeably, there is a subtle difference between the two. Critical care represents personalized, continuous care provided by one specially trained healthcare professional for one specific patient whose disease process, injury, or condition poses a critical and imminent threat to the patient's life. **Intensive care** reflects a team of healthcare professionals trained in critical care and operating on a unit dedicated to the critical care of patients. Regardless of the nuances of the phrases, both intensive care and critical care reflect healthcare services provided for a patient whose life is threatened by a critical injury, illness, or disease. This category—inpatient neonatal intensive care services and pediatric and neonatal critical care services—identifies the E/M services dedicated to the provision of critical care and intensive care for newborn infants, as well as older infants, children, and adolescents. Although the requisite criteria for these critical care services are consistent with those of critical care services provided for any other patients, the age requirements identified by the CPT manual are isolated to the pediatric and neonate population.

The CPT guidelines define the age parameters for the terms *pediatric* and *neonate*. **Neonatal medicine** refers specifically to healthcare services provided to a newborn infant from birth up to 28 days of age. **Pediatric medicine** refers to any healthcare services provided to infants at least 29 days old but no more than 71 months, or approximately 5 years and 11 months. The two groups differ greatly because of the unique physiological and anatomical maturity of each group. For instance, it is not uncommon for a neonate patient to lose as much as 10 percent of his or her body weight in water loss during the first 3 to 5 days after birth. However, it is equally common for this neonate patient to *regain* this weight by 7 to 10 days after

intensive care the critical care provided by a team of healthcare professionals operating on a unit that is dedicated to the critical care of patients

neonatal medicine healthcare services provided to a newborn infant from birth up to 28 days of age

pediatric medicine any healthcare services provided to infants older than 29 days but younger than 71 months

birth, an important measurement and health marker for the development of this neonate. In contrast, if a 5-year-old pediatric patient experienced this kind of fluctuation in weight over such a short period of time, this could pose an imminent health risk to the child and be a cause for serious concern. Because of such differences, the age parameters become very important in the provision and reporting of critical care services and intensive care services. Nonetheless, all critical care services identify and require the same criteria to be met in order to report critical care services.

Pediatric Critical Care Patient Transport

Consider an 8-month-old patient who presents to the physician's office because of lethargy, clammy skin, back pain, and fever. During the collection of history, the physician learns the pediatric patient has not produced urine for 2 days. Through complex medical decision making, the physician assesses that the patient is at risk of renal failure, a critical illness. The physician determines the patient must be admitted to the hospital immediately, requests an ambulance to transport the pediatric patient to the hospital, and rides in the ambulance with the patient, providing critical care for this patient. This physician has provided face-to-face critical care to this pediatric patient during the transportation to the inpatient facility, thereby supporting the pediatric critical care patient transport subcategory.

The CPT manual places distinct age requirements on this subcategory, pediatric critical care transport—specifically, that the patient must be no older than 24 months of age. Although the manual does not explain its rationale, important developmental changes occur in many children at about 24 months of age. For example, it is common for the language capacity of a toddler to grow exponentially between 18 and 24 months, potentially increasing from 50 words to close to 300 words. Regardless of the rationale, however, the age requirement must be followed.

Because this subcategory deals with the transportation of a pediatric patient who is receiving critical care services, the basic rules of critical care still apply: one physician must provide critical care services that relate directly to the diagnosis, management, and/or treatment of the critical illness, disease, or injury during the interfacility transport of this one patient who is no older than 24 months of age. Although the method of transportation is not specified, the greatest emphasis is placed on the continual presence of the physician who is providing the critical care services and who must remain present with the pediatric patient during the entire critical care transport.

Pediatric critical care patient transport is reported according to two different blocks of time. The first block includes the first 30 to 74 minutes of hands-on care during the transport of the critically ill or injured pediatric patient. Each additional 30 minutes of hands-on care provided during the transport is reported with an add-on code that must be used in conjunction with the first pediatric critical care patient transport code. ■ TABLE 16.7 shows the guidelines for these two pediatric critical care patient transport codes.

If the performing physician had not provided hands-on care during the transport of the patient—but perhaps had directed the **emergency medical technicians (EMTs)** with a two-way radio, telephone, or other form of voice communication—this service would be reported as "other emergency services." This subcategory of emergency department services includes physician direction of EMTs, which would also apply to advanced life support.

Inpatient Neonatal and Pediatric Critical Care

Since the physiology of a newborn infant or young child differs from that of an older child, adolescent, or grown adult, the provision of neonatal intensive care services, neonatal critical care services, and pediatric critical care services stand apart from any other critical care services. For example, as the **fetus** transitions from intrauterine to extrauterine life, the health of the transitioning fetus is closely monitored. At birth, identifying measurements are made to ensure the health and development of the newborn infant. If an abnormality is discovered during the birth that requires critical care services, neonatal inpatient critical care may be required. Similarly, critical injuries or illnesses among pediatric patients pose a unique set of

emergency medical technician (EMT) a specially trained medical professional capable of performing medical services such as resuscitation, cardiac monitoring, and other services

fetus the term that identifies an unborn human young from the 8th week of gestation up to birth

■ TABLE 16.7   PEDIATRIC CRITICAL CARE PATIENT TRANSPORT SERVICES

CPT CODE	INTRASERVICE TIME	SERVICES DELIVERED BY PHYSICIAN	AGE OF PATIENT
99466	First 30–74 minutes	Face-to-face and hands-on care of critically ill or injured patient	24 months of age or younger
+99467	Each additional 30 minutes	Face-to-face and hands-on care of critically ill or injured patient	24 months of age or younger

■ TABLE 16.8   INPATIENT NEONATAL CRITICAL CARE SERVICES

CPT CODE	AGE OF PATIENT	SERVICES
99468	Neonate (28 days or younger)	Initial neonatal critical care per day
99469	Neonate (28 days or younger)	Subsequent neonatal critical care per day

■ TABLE 16.9   INPATIENT PEDIATRIC CRITICAL CARE SERVICES (AGES 29 DAYS THROUGH 24 MONTHS)

CPT CODE	AGE OF PATIENT	SERVICES
99471	Pediatric (29 days through 24 months)	Initial pediatric critical care per day
99472	Pediatric (29 days through 24 months)	Subsequent pediatric critical care per day

healthcare needs and requirements to assess, manage, stabilize, or treat the problem. Both inpatient neonatal and pediatric critical care services are per diem codes and are divided according to patient age.

Inpatient Neonatal Critical Care   Two codes identify the initial inpatient neonatal critical care service and the subsequent inpatient neonatal critical care service for a neonate patient from birth through 28 days of age. ■ TABLE 16.8 gives the guidelines for these neonatal critical care codes.

Time is not a factor when reporting these services, because these inpatient neonatal critical care codes are considered per diem services.

Inpatient Pediatric Critical Care (Ages 29 Days through 24 Months)   Upon the 29th day of life, the patient's status changes from neonatal to pediatric, reflecting the changes in the anatomy and physiology of the patient. ■ TABLE 16.9 gives the codes for initial and subsequent inpatient pediatric critical care services for this patient population.

Again, since these services address critical care services provided during an entire day, time is not a factor for these per diem services.

Inpatient Pediatric Critical Care (Ages 2 Years through 5 Years)   Between the ages of 2 years and 5 years, the patient is still considered a pediatric patient; however, the changes in the patient's anatomy and physiology require a different identification for critical care services. ■ TABLE 16.10 gives the codes for both initial and subsequent inpatient pediatric critical care services provided for a patient aged 2 years through 5 years.

These services are per diem services and include all critical care services provided for the pediatric patient regardless of the amount of time spent in the provision of these services.

The CPT manual provides extensive guidelines and requirements for the correct reporting of critical care services for neonatal and pediatric patients. Since there may be countless different clinical circumstances requiring such services, the guidelines indicate wide variations on the possible ways of reporting neonatal and pediatric critical care services. As with each E/M service that requires something more than the content of service, CMS maintains and updates guidelines for accurately reporting critical care services. These updated guidelines should be reviewed whenever inpatient neonatal and pediatric critical care services are considered.

Initial and Continuing Intensive Care Services

Even though some pathologies do not pose an imminent threat to the patient's life, they may still require continued intensive observation to prevent any deterioration of the patient's condition and ensure that the

■ TABLE 16.10   INPATIENT PEDIATRIC CRITICAL CARE SERVICES (AGES 2 YEARS THROUGH 5 YEARS)

CPT CODE	AGE OF PATIENT	SERVICES
99475	Pediatric (2 years to 5 years)	Initial pediatric critical care per day
99476	Pediatric (2 years to 5 years)	Subsequent pediatric critical care per day

■ **TABLE 16.11** **INITIAL AND SUBSEQUENT INTENSIVE CARE SERVICES**

CPT CODE	SERVICE	AGE OF PATIENT	WEIGHT OF PATIENT
99477	Initial intensive observation, intervention, or care per day	28 days or younger	N/A
99478	Subsequent intensive care per day	Not a factor	Present bodyweight less than 3.3 lbs (1500 gms)
99479	Subsequent intensive care per day	Not a factor	Present body weight of 3.3–5.5 lbs (1500–2500 gms)
99480	Subsequent intensive care per day	Not a factor	Present body weight of 5.51–11.02 lbs (2501–5000 gms)

low birth weight weight of a newborn baby that is between 3.3 pounds and 5.5 pounds, or 1500 grams to 2500 grams, at the time of birth

very low birth weight weight of a newborn baby that is less than 3.3 pounds, or 1500 grams, at birth

patient's condition continues to improve. Such services may be required for neonate and pediatric patients of **low birth weight** or **very low birth weight**. *Birth weight* defines the neonate's actual weight at the time of birth.

- The average birth weight in the United States is between 5.5 pounds and 11.02 pounds, or 2501 grams and 5000 grams.
- A low birth weight is between 3.3 pounds and 5.5 pounds, or 1500 grams to 2500 grams.
- A very low birth weight is any weight less than 3.3 pounds, or 1500 grams.

Low birth weight, or very low birth weight, causes complications for the neonate's body temperature regulation and can lead to respiratory complications, feeding difficulties, or an imbalance in fluids, electrolytes, and glycogen, as well as many other potential complications. This confluence of physiology, anatomy, and potential pathologies increases the necessity for intensive observation care.

Only one performing physician may report these services, and only one of these services may be reported for one patient on any given day. The initial intensive observation service provided in the hospital for a neonate is reported for the first intensive observation and care, regardless of the weight of the neonate. Subsequent intensive care services are identified according to the birth weight of the infant. It is important to note that, although the subsequent intensive care services listed in the CPT manual denote the patient as an infant rather than a neonate, a neonate with a birth weight of 500 grams may continue to receive continuing intensive care services long after 28 days of age. Therefore, the subsequent intensive care codes identify the patient as an infant. Also, the subsequent intensive care services identify the patient's weight at the time of the service, *not* the patient's weight at birth. Subsequent intensive care services are categorized as follows:

- Infants recovering from very low birth weights with a present body weight of less than 3.3 pounds, or 1500 grams
- Infants recovering from low birth weights with present body weight between 3.3 pounds and 5.5 pounds, or between 1500 grams and 2500 grams
- Infants recovering from low birth weights with present body weight between 5.51 pounds and 11.02 pounds, or between 2501 grams and 5000 grams

■ TABLE 16.11 charts the guidelines and codes for initial and subsequent intensive care services.

Exercise 16.3 Critical and Intensive Care Services

Read the following medical documentation, and then answer the questions that follow.

Continuing Intensive Care Services for Baby Francis

Day One: Baby girl, a 2400 gram neonate, born full term. Umbilical cord wrapped twice around infant's neck, delayed cry, but no respiratory resuscitation required. Apgar scores are 7 and 9, respectively. Identified two lateral scratches along eyebrow, with evidence leading to facial scratching during birth transition.

Day Two: Baby Francis slept through the night. Voided 2cc/kg/hr after 36-hour mark. Facial scratches closed appropriately. Francis showed little interest in breastfeeding.

1. Which category best reflects the E/M service provided?

_____

Why has this category been selected? _____

_____

_____

Exercise 16.3 *continued*

2. Does this category necessitate identification of the patient as new or established? _____

3. Identify the factors that are most important when considering this category of E/M service. _____

4. Which code best reflects the E/M service provided? ____

_____

_____

UNLISTED E/M SERVICES

When the E/M service performed by the physician does not meet any of the categories or subcategories listed in the CPT manual, the category "other evaluation and management service" may be considered. However, an **unlisted E/M service** may be considered and reported only if no other E/M service reflects, reports, or identifies the performed service. The E/M services listed in the CPT manual identify two unlisted services: unlisted preventive medicine service and unlisted E/M service. In this way, the AMA has attempted to include any possible scenario in which an E/M service can be performed.

unlisted E/M service the E/M service code that can be used to report a performed service that no other service reflects, reports, or identifies

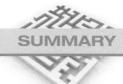

SUMMARY

- Occasionally, the severity of the presenting problem requires an unusually prolonged E/M service. Prolonged service codes may be used to report the unusual effort and time expended by the performing physician during a specific E/M service, in the event that the content of service and typical intraservice time cannot provide a sufficient reflection. Prolonged service codes are add-on codes, which means they must be used in conjunction with an inpatient or outpatient E/M service that utilizes the content of service. Therefore, prolonged service codes may not be reported separately.

- Newborn care services identify E/M services performed for a newborn after birth. These services include the initial service as well as any subsequent services performed before the discharge of the newborn.

- Critical care services indicate intense, personalized care provided by one physician to a patient who is critically ill or who has been critically injured. The criteria for reporting critical care services identify the patient's severe, life-threatening condition; the physician's complex assessment and intense management of the critical illness or injury; and the significant amount of support and time required by the patient's critical condition. Critical care services are reported in terms of the amount of time spent performing the services. The CPT manual lists extensive guidelines, requirements, and criteria for the reporting of critical care services.

- The critical care of a neonate or pediatric patient requires unique skill and expertise. Intensive care demands quick,

comprehensive assessment and complex medical decision making to treat or prevent further deterioration of the patient's condition. This category includes pediatric critical care transport, which reports the performing physician's intensive care provided to a pediatric patient during emergency transport to a qualified critical care unit. Inpatient neonatal and pediatric critical care services include the management and treatment of vital organ system failure in patients younger than 6 years of age. Inpatient continuing intensive care services include any intensive observation or treatment of pediatric or neonatal patients. Initial hospital care services provide inpatient care of a neonate who is not critically ill but who requires intensive or frequent observation. Subsequent intensive care services are specifically reported according to the current weight of the patient. Content of service is not required to report these services, but the guidelines should be reviewed.

- Occasionally, a physician must perform an E/M service that departs from any reported service. In the event that no category, subcategory, or code listed in the CPT manual accurately reflects the performed E/M service, an unlisted service may be reported. However, the medical documentation for this unlisted E/M service should clearly show the unusual set of circumstances and the medical necessity for the physician's performed service. There are two unlisted E/M service codes: unlisted preventive medicine service and unlisted E/M service.

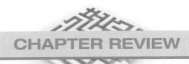

CHAPTER REVIEW

Multiple Choice

Choose the letter that best answers each question or completes each statement.

1. Patient is 26-year-old pregnant woman who has been admitted to the Well-Health Critical Care ward for management and treatment of diagnosed **HELLP syndrome** at 28 weeks gestation. On the second day of admission, patient complained of right upper quadrant pain and developed pitting edema and neck pain associated with right upper quadrant pain. Patient began expressing difficulty breathing and then developed adult respiratory distress with concomitant decrease in fetal movements. Obstetrics noted decreased fetal heart rate. A detailed history was collected, detailed physical examination performed, and complexity of medical decision making was high during this subsequent inpatient visit. Emergency C-section recommended. Total time of visit—including review of diagnostic results, discussion of case and symptoms with patient and husband, discussion with neonatology and obstetrics—was 100 minutes. Which of the following best represents the service provided?

   a. Critical care services

   b. Subsequent hospital care, level 3, and inpatient prolonged service with direct patient contact

   c. Intensive neonatal and pediatric critical care

   d. Physician standby services

2. A general pediatric surgeon requests a cardiopulmonary surgeon to be on standby during the repair of a diaphragmatic hernia, in the event of significant respiratory complications. Cardiopulmonary surgeon services are not required. 35 minutes spent on standby. Which of the following best reflects the service provided?

   a. Prolonged physician service without direct patient contact

   b. Critical care services with direct patient contact

   c. Newborn care

   d. Physician standby services

3. An E/M service is provided for a 2-day-old newborn. Expanded problem-focused maternal history collected, as well as a detailed physical examination of neonate and a low level of medical decision making performed. No abnormalities noted. Which of the following best reflects the E/M service provided?

   a. Newborn care services

   b. Initial and continuing intensive care services

   c. Subsequent hospital care, level 2

   d. Prolonged service

4. A 6-day-old full-term neonate is brought into the rural pediatric office for abdominal bloating, bloody diapers, and vomiting. Radiographic results demonstrate **dilated intestinal loops** indicating **pneumatosis intestinalis** resulting from **malrotation** or intussusception. Pediatrician requests immediate transport to trauma 1 hospital for immediate surgical and medical intervention. Pediatrician places **Broviac catheter** for fluids and accompanies neonate during transport to provide medical support and prevent further deterioration of fragile neonate. Which of the following best reflects the provided E/M service?

   a. Newborn care services

   b. Inpatient neonatal and pediatric critical care

   c. Pediatric critical care patient transport

   d. Initial and continuing neonatal intensive care services

5. This 45-year-old woman was admitted to the critical care ward of Healthy Hospital with **Legionnaire's disease**. Patient has not responded to intravenous **moxifloxan**, and cardiopulmonary function has decreased, followed by a sudden decrease in the oxygen level of the blood. Respiratory failure is diagnosed. 110 minutes are spent in extensive measures to prevent acute kidney failure and septic shock. Which of the following best reflects the E/M services provided?

   a. Prolonged care with direct patient contact

   b. Critical care: first 30–74 minutes, and one additional 30-minute block of time

   c. Critical care: first 30–74 minutes

   d. Physician standby services

6. Patient is a 12-year-old boy who is 4 months status post colorectal repair after sustaining massive rectal, **perineal**, and **testicular** wounds from falling backwards onto the silverware basket of an open dishwasher. Injuries included traumatic puncture wounds caused by forks, as well as penetrating injuries caused by both table knives and steak knives. Colorectal repair included **colostomy**. Patient's mother has requested an office visit tomorrow to ensure the patient's complete understanding of the care and precautions required. Mother also wishes to ensure the continued recovery of the patient, since the patient wishes to return to soccer practice. More than 60 minutes are spent in extensive review of radiograph images and discussion with pediatrician cardiology and gastroenterology surgeons in preparation for tomorrow's visit in my clinic. Which of the following best reflects the E/M service provided?

   a. Physician standby services

   b. Prolonged physician service without direct patient contact

   c. Prolonged physician service with direct patient contact

   d. Critical care

7. A 3-day-old neonate undergoes intensive observation during **indomethacin** IV therapy for **patent ductus arteriosus**. Patient's present weight is 3900 grams. Two days of intensive neonatal observation are reported. Which of the following best reflects the services provided?

   a. Inpatient neonatal and pediatric critical care

   b. Critical care

   c. Initial and continuing intensive care services

   d. Newborn care services

8. Which of the following is NOT a criterion for critical care services?

a. Management or treatment of the critical illness or injury involves a comprehensive evaluation of vital organ systems.

b. The physician's assessment of the critical injury or illness requires a high level of decision-making complexity.

c. A substantial amount of support and care go into preventing further deterioration of the patient's vital organ system(s).

d. The amount of time spent by the physician is not relevant to the reporting of critical care services.

9. The AMA defines the age of a neonate as

a. birth to 10 days.

b. birth to 15 days.

c. birth to 28 days.

d. birth to 2 months.

10. The AMA defines the age for inpatient pediatric critical care services as

a. birth to 28 days.

b. 29 days to 18 years.

c. birth to 71 months.

d. 29 days to 71 months.

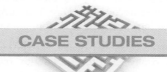

CASE STUDIES

Case Study 16-1

Read the following medical documentation, and then answer the questions that follow.

On the second day of life, E/M services were provided for a 2500-gram neonate. The following content of service was documented: a detailed history was collected, a moderate physical examination was performed, and medical decision making was of moderate complexity. No abnormalities were identified. More than half of this 45-minute visit was spent in providing counseling for the mother and father regarding neonatal care and lactation, since the mother wished to breastfeed.

1. Which of the following best reflects the documented E/M service?

a. Newborn care services

b. Pediatric critical care patient

c. Inpatient neonatal and pediatric critical care

d. Initial and continuing intensive care services

2. Which of the following best reflects the purpose of this visit?

a. Subsequent inpatient neonatal critical care for neonate younger than 28 days

b. Care provided for critically ill newborn under 24 months of age

c. Subsequent hospital care of healthy newborn, per diem

d. Subsequent intensive care of infant younger than 28 days

3. Provide the rationale for the category of E/M service.

_____

_____

Case Study 16-2

Identify the E/M category, subcategory, and criteria for the following case study. Be sure to utilize all prior knowledge. Remember that Appendix D contains the full content of service worksheet.

Presenting Problem: A 29-year-old man has been admitted to critical care with very sharp pain in shoulders, neck, and chest. He has vomited repeatedly today and has had two episodes of emesis in ER, as well as citing a nearly constant urge to urinate. He also has a quarter-sized puncture hole on the lateral edge of his right foot. Patient is an insulin-dependent diabetic.

History: Patient has been living in a transitional shelter for 3 weeks after losing his job and being evicted from his apartment. He had been working at Bob's Best Bell Shop in South Chicago as line worker, where he stood on his feet for his entire 8-hour shift. He has had many problems with his feet and decreased circulation due to diabetes. Patient states when he requested a stool to sit on, he was fired from his job. Shortly after his termination, he was evicted from his apartment when the bank foreclosed on the property. With the help of his church, he moved into Helping Hands Transitional Shelter, where he currently resides. He has no living family although he does record his church as an emergency contact.

Review of Systems: Patient has reported minor weight loss with significant fatigue associated with joint pain and muscle weakness; he complains of feeling weak "like a sick baby." He wears no glasses, although he reports blurred vision over the last month. He has had several nosebleeds over past 4 weeks, which he thought were due to the cold weather. He does report a recent development of canker sores along his lower lip, which have inhibited his appetite. He testifies to a feeling of heaviness in his chest prior to this most acute episode, and he describes experiencing a panic attack when he could not breathe and his chest hurt; however, his chest pain was different from this most recent episode. He admits it has been difficult for him to track his blood sugars since he moved into the shelter, and he has not been eating well, especially since his appetite has been extremely erratic. He reports that he has been bruising easily, which has caused him problems because it makes others at the shelter nervous. The shelter has only one bathroom, which has caused significant problems for him during the past 24+ hours when he describes feeling overwhelmed with the need to urinate. One week ago he cut his right foot on a broken tile in the shelter shower room, but he felt too embarrassed to ask for any Neosporin or bandage. Remainder of system review is positive for dizziness, although no loss of consciousness reported; negative for abdominal pain, although he has described significant pain prior to urinating.

Physical Exam: WBC, 23,000; T, 100.6°F; pulse, 87. Patient is not sure what day it is and cannot remember the name of the person who brought him to the hospital, even though this person is sitting in the exam room. Patient is very pale with clammy skin. He is clearly exerting great effort during respiration; thoracic musculoskeletal structures clearly visible when breathing. Lungs clear, although significant rubbings can be heard. Neck tense with no identifiable masses or lumps. Thyroid slightly enlarged. Heart sounds clear, although patient continues to report sharp chest pain. Right ankle and foot edematous, and skin tinged purple around toes and around lateral foot wound. Patient cannot assess toe pinch on right foot at all. Patient can minimally identify toe pinch on left foot. The soles of his feet are heavily callused and cracked with large white areas between the cracks.

Laboratory: Pertinent blood results: plasma glucose level, 275 mg/dl; serum bicarbonate, 10 mEq/L; blood ketones, 1.5mmol/l.

Assessment: Diabetic ketoacidosis with right foot diabetic wound.

Plan: IV fluids with potassium to reduce dehydration and dilute glucose and acid level. Admission to intensive care with immediate request for endocrinologist consultation for insulin dosage to prevent further ketone formation. Immediate consultation requested from neurologist and wound care NP for the right foot wound.

More than half of this 120-minute visit was spent in review of patient records and diagnostic results, interview of patient and collection of patient information, counseling patient, and performing critical services for the patient's care.

1. Is content of service documented in this case study?_____
2. Is direct contact with the patient and/or family documented in this E/M service? _____
3. Is time a factor in this E/M service?_____
4. Which E/M service code best reflects this documented case study? _____

Coding Challenge

Using your CPT manual, identify the E/M code that most appropriately reflects each of the following clinical scenarios.

1. Due to the onset of maternal distress during the birth process, the obstetrician requested the presence of Dr. Z for the initial stabilization and evaluation of the newborn. Directly after birth, the stabilization and evaluation of Baby Judy revealed a healthy newborn girl with no abnormalities.
   CPT code: _____

2. Patient is admitted to hospital for treatment after being struck by a vehicle. Significant thoracoabdominal injuries and degloving of lower left extremity have caused severe blood loss. Compartment syndrome is identified in lower right extremity. 120 minutes of critical care is provided in order to stabilize patient and prepare for surgery.
   CPT code(s):_____

3. On the second day of hospital admission, Dr. G sees the patient in relation to a significant upper left abdominal contusion. Dr. G documents 100 minutes of direct patient care, including review of current abdominal imaging, discussion of traumatic injury with the parents of the patient, review of laboratory results, a detailed physical examination, and identification of the need for emergency major splenorrhaphy.
   CPT code(s):_____

4. Four-year-old Suzie is admitted Tuesday night to hospital for treatment of head injury sustained in a fall in the bathroom. Patient has not regained consciousness. A nondisplaced basilar skull fracture is suspected due to the bleeding from nose and ears, as well as identification of cerebrospinal fluid via the nares. Patient is under constant supervision and intensive care, with 45 minutes of critical care provided from Tuesday night through Wednesday morning.
   CPT code: _____

5. Xavier is a 1200-gram infant undergoing intensive supportive care for necrotizing enterocolitis. Day 3 of supportive care reveals recordable improvement of abdominal integrity.
   CPT code: _____

6. The patient presents to physician for a follow-up regarding lower left abdominal pain and nausea. The most recent laboratory results and diagnostic imaging have been provided for the physician's review prior to the patient's visit. Documentation reflects a comprehensive history, comprehensive physical examination, and high level of medical decision making, as well as extensive counseling regarding the laboratory results and diagnostic imaging, the patient's stress management, and family history of Crohn's disease and colon cancer. More than 100 minutes of direct patient contact are documented.
   CPT code(s):_____

7. On the first day of life, Baby Drake is evaluated, with all findings identified as within normal limits.
   CPT code: _____

8. Damon is a 4500-gram infant admitted for pneumocystis pneumonia. Patient is currently on day 5 of pentamidine therapy. Day 5 reveals substantial improvement of patient's condition. Documentation includes discussion with foster family regarding future care of Damon and prevention of recurrent lung infection.
   CPT code: _____

9. On the second day of life, Baby Jane's condition rapidly deteriorates with rapid breathing, significant drop in blood pressure, and one documented paroxysmal seizure. During 40 minutes of critical care, catheterization releases amber urine. Patient eventually stabilized and rushed for exploratory abdominal surgery.
   CPT code: _____

10. On the second day of life, Baby Ruby has stabilized with stronger oxygen levels. Ruby has passed meconium and has initialized feeding. Facial lacerations due to self-inflicted fingernail scratching during transition show no sign of infection.
    CPT code: _____

11. In Friendly Family Pediatrics, Dr. X sees a new young child who complains of persistent joint pain, abdominal swelling, and low-grade fever. Dr. X documents at least 115 minutes during which a comprehensive history, detailed physical examination, and moderate medical decision making are performed, as well as extensive counseling of patient and parents. Dr. X

also documents 65 minutes of time spent in review of laboratory data and results, diagnostic imaging, and discussion of case with colleagues on the day following the patient's visit.

CPT code(s):_____

12. Patient has been admitted to the hospital for treatment of anaphylaxis due to exposure to peanuts. Symptoms rapidly progress from angioedema to wheezing and significant stridor, blue lips, followed by a rapid drop in blood pressure. The patient is identified as entering circulatory shock. 40 minutes of critical care is provided before patient's blood pressure, oxygen levels, and edema begin to subside.

CPT code: _____

13. Baby June is an 800-gram neonate who develops apnea, bradycardia, and abdominal swelling. Critical care is initiated in an attempt to stabilize patient; however, blood pressure begins to fall rapidly. Radiographic scans reveal pneumatosis intestinalis. Critical care provided for 35 minutes prior to emergent abdominal surgery for suspected necrotizing enterocolitis.

CPT code: _____

14. Georgie has been admitted to the hospital for treatment of a serious adverse event after ingestion of alkali causative agent, or dishwasher powder. On day 3 of admission, patient's temperature rapidly increases, blood pressure drops, patient passes bloody stool and becomes very short of breath. 50 minutes of critical care is provided to stabilize patient, during which time radiographic imaging reveals hemoperitoneum of unknown origin.

CPT code: _____

15. While on vacation in Yellowstone National Park in September, Dr. O is stranded in the rangers' station at the northeast entrance. While there, one of the rangers complains of right wrist and arm pain, and Dr. O performs a clinical visit in the ranger station of Yellowstone National Park. Through the evaluation and management, Dr. O identifies a sprained left wrist and recommends ice therapy and splinting.

CPT code: _____

HELLP syndrome a life-threatening condition occurring during pregnancy that is often associated with preeclampsia; characterized by destruction of red blood cells, elevated liver enzymes, and low platelet count

dilated intestinal loops the swelling and bulging of the intestines caused by a buildup of gases or fluid produced by infection and/or obstruction within the intestines

pneumatosis intestinalis the presence of air within the intestines, usually indicative of a life-threatening infection, necrosis, or abscess within the intestines

malrotation an emergent condition in which the bowels become twisted; can cause ischemia of the bowels and necrotic bowel

broviac catheter a small, flexible, tubular instrument threaded into a large vein and inserted into one of the large chambers of the heart; used to deliver medication or nutrition to the central venous system

Legionnaire's disease a potentially life-threatening infection caused by an aerobic bacterium, which often causes a virulent form of pneumonia

moxifloxan an antibacterial medication used in the treatment of respiratory infections, anthrax, intra-abdominal infections, and other high-risk diseases

perineal pertaining to the skin and tissue at the base of the torso; in males, the tissue space between the scrotum and the anus; in females, the tissue between the vaginal opening and the anus

testicular referring to the testicles

colostomy an abnormal opening that is surgically created to allow the release of feces from the body via an opening other than the anus

indomethacin an NSAID used to reduce fever, pain, swelling, and stiffness; used in the treatment of various conditions, including rheumatoid arthritis and patent ductus arteriosus

patent ductus arteriosus a congenital abnormality in which the opening between the aorta and the pulmonary artery, which normally closes at birth, remains open

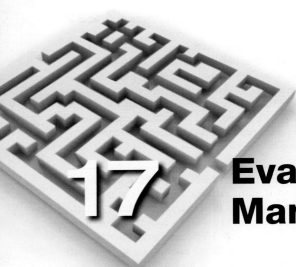

17 Evaluation and Management Modifiers

Key Terms

emergent surgery

excised

explored

gastrostomy tube

global period of surgery

gluteal crest

infraorbital

laparotomy

mandated

nail matrix

open procedure

pilonidal abscess

pilonidal cyst

repaired

same physician

semi-elective surgery

thoracotomy

transplanted

urgent surgery

INTRODUCTION

Each E/M service code represents a clinical interaction between a patient and a qualified healthcare professional. Regardless of where these E/M services occur, each service code reflects the documented content of service, the setting in which the service was performed, and the intent of the performed service.

However, certain E/M circumstances require an additional identification to indicate the precise nature of the performed service. For instance, if an E/M service is provided for a patient 5 days after surgery, how can the E/M service code clearly identify whether or not this service was related to the surgery?

The word *modify* means to adjust or change the meaning of something. In E/M services, modifiers are used to identify an adjustment to the intent of the performed E/M service. The CPT manual identifies four modifiers that provide additional information about and insight into the performed service. This chapter examines these four E/M service modifiers: modifiers 32, 24, 25, and 57. They adjust the meaning of a performed E/M service to reflect that the specific E/M service is mandated or to identify a decision for immediate surgery, an E/M service performed during a postoperative period, or an unrelated E/M service performed on the same day as a completely separate procedure. Each of these modifiers provides additional nuance to the service performed by the physician and can help to ensure proper payment.

MODIFIER 32

Although a patient's presenting problem generally instigates the E/M service, occasionally the service is **mandated** to occur. When an E/M service is mandated, it is required to occur and cannot be postponed or ignored. Specific agencies, organizations, or companies that are unrelated to the physician performing the service may order these mandated services. The CPT manual identifies several examples of companies, organizations, or agencies that mandate an E/M service, including an insurance company, a government agency, and regulatory agencies. If an agency, company, or organization mandates the performance of an E/M service, modifier 32 should be appended to the service to indicate that the patient did not initiate it, nor did the patient's family or another physician. The following example illustrates the proper use of modifier 32.

mandated ordered to occur at the request of another organization, agency, or company

> **Example: Modifier 32**
>
> Judy was involved in a car accident 3 days ago. Her car was broadsided when the other driver was making an illegal U-turn. During the police report, Judy experienced dizziness and nausea. The police officer recommended that Judy include her symptoms in her automobile insurance claim. After the submission of her claim to both her automobile insurance agency and the insurance agency of the other driver, the insurance adjuster mandated Judy to submit to a full physical by her primary care physician. Specific forms were sent to Judy from her insurance company, which she was instructed to take to her primary care physician. During the E/M service visit, Judy's physician collected a comprehensive history, performed a comprehensive physical examination, and identified medical decision making of moderate complexity. Judy's physician documented the E/M service in her medical record and completed the required paperwork before returning it to Judy's insurance company in the envelope provided.

It is important to note that modifier 32 cannot be reported if the E/M service is the result of the patient's care or is performed at the request of the patient's family. For example, if Judy's husband became concerned about her dizziness and she went to the physician at his request, modifier 32 could not be appended to the E/M service. Modifier 32 can be utilized only when the service has been performed at the request or direction of an outside organization, agency, or company unrelated to the performing physician.

GLOBAL PERIOD OF SURGERY

The term *global* refers to a comprehensive inclusion of any issue or factor relating to a specific topic. When used in reference to a surgical procedure, the **global period of surgery** refers to the time, services, and actions required not only to prepare for and perform the surgery, but also to ensure the complete recovery of the patient. Depending on the complexity and intensity of the surgical procedure, this global period of surgery may represent no days required for a complete recovery, 10 days required for a complete recovery, or 90 days required for a complete recovery.

Although surgery includes a very broad field of medicine, there are two generalized types of surgical procedures: major surgery and minor surgery. Because these two types of procedures represent very

global period of surgery the period of time recognized for a patient's full recovery after surgery; accounts for the materials, services, and procedures that are required for the performance of and recovery from a surgical procedure

different levels of complexity, the global period of surgery is very different for each. The global period of surgery for major surgical procedures is 90 days, otherwise known as 090, whereas the global period of surgery for minor surgical procedures is either 0 or 10 days, otherwise known as 000 or 010, respectively.

Global Period for Major Surgery

A major surgery is, by definition, a big deal. Generally, major surgeries require incisions and dissection to allow the surgeon access to the organs, tissues, or structures within the human body. Major surgery is not considered lightly because, regardless of the benefit a major surgery can provide, this intervention inevitably causes a substantial impact on the physiology and health of the patient. Major surgery is considered because the complexity of the patient's presenting problem requires an equally complex management option, which carries a higher risk. Because of the significant, occasionally extreme nature of major surgery, general anesthesia is nearly always required.

Although the spectrum of major surgeries is extremely broad with a wide variety of methods, rationales, and treatments, this chapter will consider major surgeries according to the level of invasiveness and complexity. Therefore, major surgery will be referred to as "open" or "minimally invasive" procedures. An **open procedure** refers to the creation of an opening in the human body. This type of major surgery is performed by creating a large incision to access a specific cavity, organ, or structure to be **explored, excised, repaired, or transplanted**. Two examples of open procedures are a **laparotomy** and a **thoracotomy**. A laparotomy is performed by creating a large incision along the abdominal cavity to explore, repair, remove, or transplant organs or tissues between the diaphragm and the pelvis. A thoracotomy requires an incision in the chest wall, retraction of the ribs, and dissection of the pleural cavity to gain access to the heart, lungs, mediastinum, esophagus, trachea, or other organs, tissues, or structures within the chest cavity. Given the complexity of these open procedures and the necessary care required to ensure the complete recovery of the patient during the postoperative period, a global period of 90 days is attached to the major open procedures.

Minimally invasive procedures are, by definition, less invasive than open procedures. Minimally invasive surgical procedures are performed by creating small incisions in the skin and inserting a thin tube-like camera to inspect the contents of a body cavity or structure within the patient. The broad spectrum of minimally invasive surgical procedures may be performed for a variety of pathologies and anatomic structures, such as the abdomen, joints, and chest cavity. A laparoscopic procedure is performed on the abdomen by creating small incisions in the skin and insufflating, or inflating, the abdominal cavity to allow the surgeon to thoroughly inspect the internal organs and structures with a small camera. With this visual assistance and additional devices, the surgeon is able to perform a surgical procedure within the abdominal cavity. A thoracosopic procedure is performed by creating small incisions in the skin and between the ribs and inserting a specialized, small, flexible camera into the thoracic cavity. With this visual assistance and additional surgical devices, the surgeon is able to perform a surgical procedure within the thoracic cavity. As these descriptions suggest, these surgeries still present risk to the patient and require an extensive amount of time for the patient's complete recovery.

CMS recognizes that the 90-day global period of surgery includes the day before the surgery as well as the following 89 days after the surgery, along with any necessary preoperative, intraoperative, and postoperative care or services required to ensure the complete recovery of the patient. This period includes any services or treatments related to the surgery or the condition for which the surgery was performed. CMS maintains and updates the global period of surgery for every service listed in the CPT manual in the Physician Fee Schedule, which can be viewed on the CMS website, www.cms.gov.

Global Period for Minor Surgery

Other surgical procedures present even less risk to the patient. Surgical procedures such as suturing a laceration, performing a skin biopsy, or percutaneously obtaining a biopsy of the liver via a needle present less risk and require less time for the patient's complete recovery. Endoscopic procedures are surgical or diagnostic procedures that introduce a flexible tube into a passage or structure of the body to inspect or perform a surgical procedure on that specific part of the body. Endoscopic procedures can be performed on a variety of anatomical parts of the body, such as the digestive tract, respiratory system, and reproductive or urinary systems.

CMS recognizes the global period of surgery for minor surgical procedures as 0 days and 10 days. A 10-day global period of surgery includes the day before the surgery as well as the following 9 days after the surgery, along with any necessary preoperative, intraoperative, and postoperative care or services required to ensure the complete recovery of the patient. A 0-day global period of surgery includes only the day the surgery is performed. It also includes any services or treatments related to the surgery or the condition for which the surgery was performed. CMS maintains and updates the global period of surgery for every service listed in the CPT manual in the Physician Fee Schedule, which may be viewed on the CMS website, www.cms.gov.

---

open procedure an invasive surgical procedure that requires incision through the exterior of the body to access internal organs, structures, or cavities

explored surgically investigated (e.g., a specific portion of the human anatomy)

excised surgically removed (e.g., a specific part of the human anatomy)

repaired surgically restored or reconstructed (e.g., a specific part of the human anatomy)

transplanted surgically transferred (e.g., a portion of the human anatomy) from one section of the body to another section of the body or from one body to a different but compatible body

laparotomy the major, invasive surgical procedure that creates a large incision along the abdominal cavity to explore, repair, remove, or transplant organs or tissues between the diaphragm and the pelvis

thoracotomy the major, invasive surgical procedure that creates an incision in the chest wall, retracts the ribs, and dissects the pleural cavity to gain access to the heart, lungs, mediastinum, esophagus, trachea, or other organs, tissues, or structures within the chest cavity

What Does the "Same Physician" Mean?

In the modern world, one physician practice office may include several different physicians of the same specialty. For instance, consider the family practice clinic Well-Health Physicians in Someplace, America, which includes four different internists. Over the years that Patient Jill has been a patient at Well-Health Physicians, more than one physician within the practice has seen Jill and provided care for her. However, each of the physicians practicing at the clinic is considered the "**same physician**" because each of them practices the same specialty in the same clinic.

In the CPT manual, the phrase "same physician" is used to identify the individual physician who has performed the service or procedure or another physician of the same specialty within the practice. In the context of an E/M service, the term "same physician" is used in the determination of an established patient. In the context of the global period of surgery, the term "same physician" refers to not only the physician who performed the surgical procedure, but also to any physician of similar specialty within the performing physician's group practice. This means that when Dr. G of the Well-Health Physicians performs an intermediate repair of a wound on Jill's forearm, the 10-day global period of surgery applies not only to Dr. G, but also to the other three physicians practicing at Well-Health Physicians. Therefore, if Jill receives care or services related to the wound or surgical repair of her forearm, these are considered part of the global surgical package for this repair.

same physician the individual physician who has performed the service or procedure in question, or another physician of the same specialty within the practice who has also performed the E/M service

MODIFIER 24

In an ideal world, a person would experience only one health issue at any given time. However, there are occasions when a patient may experience two or more health problems simultaneously. Further, a patient may occasionally experience one or more presenting problems that are completely unrelated to one another. In the context of surgery, it would be ideal if the patient experienced no other health problems during the postoperative recovery. However, there are times when an unrelated presenting problem requires evaluation and management to ensure the continued health of the patient. If, during the postoperative period, the physician who performed the surgery then provides an E/M service that is unrelated to the surgery, modifier 24 identifies the unique nature of this service.

> **Example: Modifier 24**
>
> Consider the patient Jill, who has undergone an intermediate surgical repair of a wound on her forearm. This surgical repair carries a 10-day global period, during which time professional services related to the wound repair are considered part of the postoperative care. However, if Jill returns to Well-Health Physicians because of a sinus infection, the simple care and service she receives related to her sinus infection have nothing to do with the wound repair and, as a result, are separate from the postoperative care.

In order to identify that Jill's sinus infection is a presenting problem and is unrelated to the surgery and that the performed service is unrelated to the wound repair, modifier 24 is appended to the E/M service code.

infraorbital referring to the area below the orbital cavity of the eye

---

Exercise 17.1 **E/M Modifier: Julian's Sore Face**

Read the following medical documentation, and then answer the questions related to modifier usage.

Julian is a 12-year-old boy well-known to me who sustained accidental rectal and perineal wounds and testicular bruising after falling backwards onto the silverware basket of an open dishwasher. My partner, Dr. H of Well-Health Physicians, performed the colorectal repair and colostomy. Julian is 5 weeks status post colorectal repair. Colostomy and colorectal recovery have been progressing nicely.

Julian presents today for a sore neck and recurrent headaches, which have bothered him for the past 5 days. He complains of pain when swallowing, a hot face, and aching in his teeth. His mother describes him as "glassy eyed" and dazed for the past 2 days, and she noted an elevated temperature of 99.2 this morning. Julian reports that he has been coughing a little at night but that his primary complaint is of nasal congestion and a sore throat. He reports coughing up greenish sputum in the morning. No complaints of chest pain or shortness of breath. Julian denies painful urination, and colostomy production has not changed significantly over the past week.

Palpation of face reveals significant tenderness of the **infraorbital** areas bilaterally, as well as the frontal sinus area of forehead. Suppurative serous fluid apparent behind tympanic membrane upon inspection. Neck is normal with the exception

continued

Exercise 17.1 *continued*

of minimal swelling in lymph nodes. Conjunctivae mildly red. Oropharynx red and inflamed, but no exudates noted. Lungs clear to auscultation. Heart rate normal without murmur.

It is my impression that Julian has a mild sinus infection exacerbated by the change of seasons. Recommend increased fluid intake combined with a humidifying practice such as steam inhalation or hot showers to facilitate decongestion. Recommend ibuprofen for pain and rest. Recheck of sinus infection in 3 days.

1. In order to reflect the documented E/M service, is a modifier required?_____

2. If a modifier is required, which modifier would best reflect the nature and intent of the E/M service—modifier 24, 32, 25, or 57?_____

3. Explain why this modifier best reflects the nature and intent of the E/M service._____

_____

4. If a modifier is required, does this modifier relate to the global period of surgery? _____

5. If content of service for an E/M service has been documented, identify the appropriate category, subcategory, and level of service._____

_____

6. If an E/M service has been identified, include your rationale supporting the identified category, subcategory, and level of service._____

_____

MODIFIER 25

Modifier 25 is very different from modifier 24. Modifier 25 reflects a distinct E/M service performed on the same day as another procedure or service. Modifier 25 is reported in conjunction with the E/M service performed by a physician who also performs a completely distinct, independent, noteworthy service or procedure on the same day. These distinct, noteworthy services or procedures may include a minor surgical procedure with a global period of 0 days, such as percutaneously changing a **gastrostomy tube**, or a minor surgical procedure with a global period of 10 days, such as the excision of a **pilonidal cyst**. In the event that a minor surgical procedure is performed on the same day as a significantly distinct E/M service, modifier 25 should be appended to the service code. The following example can help illustrate modifier 25.

gastrostomy tube a tube that is inserted directly into the stomach through the abdominal wall; introduces nutrients to patients who are unable to take nourishment through the mouth

pilonidal cyst literally, "nest of hair"; a collection of hair that has become infected, although it may be asymptomatic; most commonly occurs on the gluteal cleft near the sacrum, or near the base of the back

nail matrix the structure from which toenails and fingernails grow

> **Example: Modifier 25**
>
> Jack presents to Well-Health Physicians for a nasty, barking, productive cough. Dr. G collects a detailed history, performs an expanded problem-focused physical examination, and makes medical decisions of moderate complexity. During the visit, Dr. G comments on Jack's limp and identifies that Jack's left big toe has a severely ingrown toenail. Dr. G performs a partial excision of the nail and **nail matrix**, which is a minor surgical procedure with a global period of 10 days.

Since this partial excision of the nail and nail matrix was completely separate from the E/M service, modifier 25 should be added to the service code to identify that each of these services was necessary, separate, and noteworthy.

One of the most important aspects of modifier 25 is the intent of the procedure or service. In this last example, Jack presented to Dr. G's office because of his barking cough, and the problem of the ingrown toenail was separately identified during the visit. Therefore, the intent of this visit was to address Jack's barking cough, not to excise his ingrown toenail. This scenario meets the criteria for modifier 25 because Dr. G performed a separate, identifiable E/M service addressing Jack's barking cough on the same day and at the same time as Dr. G performed the surgical excision of the ingrown toenail. In considering the use of modifier 25, the intent of the procedure or service must be identified. The intent of the E/M service must be separately identifiable from the performed procedure. If Jack had presented to Dr. G because of his ingrown toenail, then the intent of the visit would have been to evaluate and manage the ingrown toenail, and the excision of the nail matrix would be the surgical management of Jack's presenting problem, which would not meet the criteria for modifier 25. The criteria for modifier 25 can be viewed as a five-part conditional statement:

If ...

content of service has been documented for the E/M service

and

this content of service supports at least a problem-focused (or level 1) E/M service

and

the E/M service was performed for an identifiably different reason from that of the other performed service or procedure

and

the E/M service has been performed by the same physician who performed the other service or procedure

and

the E/M service occurred on the same day as the other performed service or procedure,

then

modifier 25 may be appended to the appropriate E/M service code to reflect the separately identifiable E/M service performed by the same physician on the same day.

However, modifier 25 does not relate only to E/M services performed on the same day as a minor surgical procedure performed by the same physician. During a patient's story of health, it may be necessary for the physician providing care to perform one or more services during a specific episode of care. For example, consider a preventive medicine service, otherwise known as an annual physical exam. The underlying paradigm of preventive medicine services is the assessment of the patient's health and the prevention of illness, not the evaluation and/or management of identified abnormalities or specific presenting problems. Therefore, if the physician identifies a significant abnormality or presenting problem during the preventive medicine service and this abnormality or presenting problem requires the documentation of content of service, then a separately identifiable, unrelated E/M service has been performed on the same day by the same physician as the preventive medicine service. The following example presents this additional aspect of modifier 25.

Example: Modifier 25

Tony, a 45-year-old man, presents to Dr. M's office for his annual physical examination. During Tony's preventive medicine service, Dr. M identifies a skin rash that is significant enough that evaluation and management of this rash are required. Since Tony must drive 65 miles to reach Dr. M's office, Dr. M provides a separately identifiable E/M service to address the skin rash. Thus, Dr. M performs a comprehensive preventive medicine service for Tony. Dr. M also collects an expanded problem-focused history and performs a problem-focused physical examination. Medical decision making is low in complexity.

In this scenario, the preventive medicine service is considered the primary E/M service, since this is the reason Tony has presented to Dr. M's office, whereas the E/M service addressing the skin rash is a separately identifiable service performed by Dr. M that happens to be provided on the same day as the preventive medicine service. To fully represent this episode of care, the preventive medicine service code reports the annual physical exam, whereas modifier 25 is appended to the office or other outpatient E/M service to reflect the distinct, noteworthy service that was provided on the same day by the same physician.

Exercise 17.2 E/M Modifier: Joanie's Annual Physical

Read the following medical documentation, and then answer the questions related to modifier usage.

Joanie Smith presents for her annual physical. She has completely recovered from her sinus infection. She identifies no problems or complaints. Physician reviews her history. Joanie has changed jobs and is working as an elementary school administrator, reports that she has been experiencing heartburn, and feels very anxious during the day with difficulty sleeping at night.

Comprehensive physical examination is performed, including neck, cardiovascular, respiratory, neurologic, musculoskeletal, and gastrointestinal. Examination of breasts performed; however, a pap smear is deferred since a pap smear was performed 3 months ago when Joanie wished to begin using oral contraceptives. Ear exam is normal. Dark staining of teeth noted, which Joanie reports is related to the five to six cups of coffee she drinks a day.

Visit concludes with counseling Joanie regarding the dangers of excessive caffeine intake and the impact of caffeine on stress levels, dehydration, insomnia, and stomach upset. Recommend weaning caffeine intake down to two cups a day before noon during the next month and drinking decaffeinated coffee for the rest of the day.

1. In order to reflect the documented E/M service, is a modifier required?_____

2. If a modifier is required, which modifier would best reflect the nature and intent of the E/M service—modifier 24, 32, 25, or 57?_____

3. Explain why this modifier best reflects the nature and intent of the E/M service._____
_____

4. If a modifier is required, does this modifier relate to the global period of surgery?_____
_____

5. If content of service for an E/M service has been documented, identify the appropriate category, subcategory, and level of service._____
_____

6. If an E/M service has been identified, include your rationale supporting the identified category, subcategory, and level of service._____
_____

MODIFIER 57

A major surgical procedure represents a moderate or high level of risk to the patient. Every surgical procedure with a 90-day global period of surgery is considered major surgery because of the amount of time required for the patient's preoperative and postoperative care and recovery. Although there are many different types of major surgery, modifier 57 addresses a physician's medical decision that immediate major surgery is the most appropriate management option for a patient's presenting problem. Modifier 57 is appended to an E/M service to identify that the decision for major surgery has been made less than 24 hours before the actual surgery is performed. The presence of modifier 57 also recognizes that the associated E/M service that led to the decision for surgery was the first identification that major surgery was required. In addition, modifier 57 establishes that the E/M service should be acknowledged as separately reportable during the 90-day global period of surgery, which includes the day before surgery and the 89 days after surgery as part of the 90-day global period.

Modifier 57 does not apply to elective surgery, because elective surgery can be scheduled in advance, according to the availability of the physician and the patient. Modifier 57 pertains to the decision for **emergent surgery**, which must be performed at the earliest opportunity to address a life-threatening illness, condition, or injury. Modifier 57 also pertains to the decision for a **semi-elective surgery** or an **urgent surgery**, as long as the decision for surgery was made less than 24 hours before the performed surgery and the E/M service was the first identification of the need for this performed surgery. The following example illustrates the use of modifier 57.

emergent surgery a surgical procedure that is essential in order to save the life of the patient

semi-elective surgery an important surgical procedure that may be postponed for a limited number of days but must be performed to prevent further deterioration of the patient's condition

urgent surgery a surgical procedure that is very important for the patient's health

> **Example: Modifier 57**
>
> Joshua is brought into the emergency department after falling off his bicycle. He suffered massive blunt abdominal trauma and is having difficulty breathing. Dr. K suspects massive splenic injury and possible diaphragmatic trauma with possible eventration of abdominal contents into thoracic cavity. Emergency surgery is scheduled with Surgeon Q of ThoracoAbdomio Specialties to identify extent of diaphragmatic injury, with ensuing repair or excision as necessary. Joshua is prepped for emergency surgery.

Even though Dr. K does not know the exact major surgery that will be performed for Joshua, the ensuing surgery will definitely carry a 90-day global period. Since Dr. K's E/M service was the first identification of the need for surgery, modifier 57 should be appended to the E/M service to clearly identify Dr. K's decision for this major surgery.

Exercise 17.3 **E/M Modifier: Jane's Stuffy Head**

Read the following medical documentation, and then answer the questions related to modifier usage.

Jane is a 42-year-old woman who is well-known to me. Jane is 7 weeks postoperative after the closed treatment of a left Hume fracture. Cast was removed 8 days ago with no complications. Jane presents with complaints of chest congestion, headache, and nasal discharge. An expanded problem-focused history is documented, as well as an expanded problem-focused physical examination. Medical decision making is of low complexity due to negative strep test and negative lab results indicating any bacterial or viral infection. OTC pain reliever recommended, as well as increased rest. Follow-up recommended if symptoms do not improve within 10 days.

1. In order to reflect the documented E/M service, is a modifier required? _____

2. If a modifier is required, which modifier would best reflect the nature and intent of the E/M service—modifier 24, 32, 25, or 57? _____
_____

3. Explain why this modifier best reflects the nature and intent of the E/M service. _____
_____

4. If a modifier is required, does this modifier relate to the global period of surgery? _____
_____

5. If content of service for an E/M service has been documented, identify the appropriate category, subcategory, and level of service. _____
_____

6. If an E/M service has been identified, include your rationale supporting the identified category, subcategory, and level of service. _____
_____
_____

SUMMARY

- Modifier 32 applies in situations when a company, organization, or agency mandates the performance of an E/M service. In such a case, modifier 32 should be appended to the E/M service. Modifier 32 indicates that neither the patient nor the patient's family initiated the performed service. Modifier 32 should not be used when another physician has coordinated the performed E/M service as part of the patient's continuing care.

- Major and minor surgeries affect the human body in different ways. To reflect the postoperative care required after a major or minor surgery, global periods of surgery indicate the number of days generally required for the patient to return to health. Major surgeries have a global period of surgery of 90 days, whereas minor surgeries have a global period of surgery of 10 days or 0 days. The CPT manual defines the term "same physician" as the same individual physician or another physician of the same specialty within the performing physician's group practice.

- Modifier 24 reflects a physician's performance, during a postoperative period, of an E/M service for a presenting problem that is unrelated to the surgery performed by that same physician. The documentation must support content of service and clearly identify that the presenting problem is unrelated to the original procedure.

- Modifier 25 reflects a distinct E/M service performed on the same day as another procedure or service. In order to support the use of modifier 25, four specific criteria must be met: Content of service must be documented for the E/M service and must support at least a problem-focused (or level 1) service. Further, the E/M service must be performed for an identifiably different reason from that of the other service or procedure. Also, the same physician must perform both services. Lastly, the services must occur on the same day. If all four of the criteria have been met, modifier 25 may be appended to the appropriate E/M service.

- Modifier 57 identifies a physician's decision for immediate major surgery on the same day or the day after the performed E/M service. Modifier 57 should be appended to the E/M service to indicate that the decision for major surgery was made less than 24 hours before the actual surgery was performed. The very nature of this clinical situation precludes elective surgery, which can be scheduled at the convenience of the surgeon and the patient.

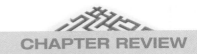

CHAPTER REVIEW

Multiple Choice

Choose the letter that best answers each question or completes each statement.

1. Physician W performs major surgery for a patient. Ten days later, this same patient presents to Physician W for a presenting problem that is unrelated to the surgery. Which of the following modifiers should be appended to the E/M service during a postoperative period?
   a. Modifier 25
   b. Modifier 32
   c. Modifier 24
   d. Modifier 57

2. Before being accepted into a state university's international student exchange program, Patient X is required by the program to submit to a comprehensive physical examination. Patient X presents to Physician Q for the E/M service. Physician Q performs the service and completes the necessary paperwork required by the exchange program. Which of the following modifiers should be appended to the E/M service?
   a. Modifier 57
   b. Modifier 25
   c. Modifier 32
   d. Modifier 24

3. During a preventive medicine service for a 38-year-old new patient, Dr. F identifies a significant abnormality and documents the collection of an expanded problem-focused history, performance of a problem-focused physical examination, and straightforward medical decision making, in addition to the initial comprehensive preventive medicine service. Which of the following modifiers should be appended to the E/M service?
   a. Modifier 24
   b. Modifier 25
   c. Modifier 32
   d. Modifier 57

4. Gina is a 10-year-old girl brought into the emergency department after she was attacked by a neighborhood dog, resulting in minor wounds to her back, buttocks, and thigh. After the wounds were cleaned in the emergency room, Gina was admitted to the hospital, where subsequent evaluation and management identified the need for exploratory surgery that evening to assess the extent of the damage and minimize complications with the injuries. Which of the following modifiers should be appended to the E/M service?
   a. Modifier 57
   b. Modifier 32
   c. Modifier 25
   d. Modifier 24

5. James Roberts is a well-known patient who returns for a postoperative follow-up 2 weeks after an abdominal exploration and splenorrhaphy. Seventeen days ago, James fell in his bathroom after stepping out of the shower and slipping on the wet tile floor, sustaining a grade 3 splenic laceration. Subsequent abdominal exploration and splenic repair was performed. Recovery has proceeded as expected, with appropriate healing of abdominal wound, no signs of infection or dehiscence; however, James is very concerned that the continued bruising that has remained on his abdomen and across his back is a symptom of a complication. Physician collects an expanded problem-focused history, performs an expanded problem-focused physical examination, and makes medical decisions of low complexity. The physician assures James that the bruising is a normal part of the healing process. The physician documents that more than half of the visit was spent in counseling the patient and his wife on postoperative care. An abdominal exploration and splenorrhaphy have a 90-day global period of surgery. Which of the following best reflects this E/M service?
   a. Office or other outpatient service, established patient, level 3, and modifier 32 because this service has been mandated by an outside organization
   b. Office or other outpatient service, established patient, level 3, and modifier 24 because this service occurred during the postoperative period and the intent of the service is unrelated to the surgery
   c. Office or other outpatient service, established patient, level 3, and modifier 57 because the physician decided surgery needed to occur
   d. No E/M service reportable because the intent of this service is related to the abdominal surgery and splenorrhaphy and is therefore part of the postoperative service

6. Sally Panther, who is applying to be a foster parent, is an established patient who presents to her primary care physician because of headaches she's been experiencing and debilitating muscle spasms in her shoulders and neck. Sally is sure that her symptoms are related to the stress surrounding her foster parent application, and more than half of the 45-minute visit is spent in counseling Sally regarding stress reduction techniques and in coordinating care for the reduction of the muscle spasms. During the visit, Sally shows her doctor the state-ordered paperwork that her caseworker has required her to fill out. Sally's primary care physician documents a detailed history, performs a detailed physical examination, and documents the medical decision making of low complexity, as well as the subjects addressed during the counseling and coordination of care. Which of the following best reflects the performed E/M service and modifier usage?
   a. Office or other outpatient service, established patient, level 4, with modifier 32
   b. Office or other outpatient service, established patient, level 4, with no modifier
   c. Office or other outpatient service, new patient, level 2, with modifier 32
   d. Office or other outpatient service, established patient, level 3, with no modifier

7. Joe Black is an established patient for whom I performed an inguinal hernia repair 3 weeks ago. The hernia repair has a 90-day global period of surgery. His hernia was caused by heavy lifting during a move to his new apartment. Today, Joe presents because of severe headaches, upper left abdominal pain, and heartburn, and he is concerned that he is experiencing a complication from the surgery. Collection of detailed history reveals that the carpet in Joe's new apartment was professionally removed last week because the carpet padding was filled with mold. Performance of detailed physical examination finds sinus congestion, swollen cervical lymph nodes, red conjunctivae, and serous fluid behind left tympanic membrane. Abdominal examination reveals no abnormalities associated with inguinal surgical incision, penis, or testicles. Documentation of low medical decision making shows probability of allergic rhinitis due to mold exposure. Recommend OTC Benadryl, and an immunoglobulin blood test is discussed regarding future allergic reactions. Which of the following best reflects the performed E/M service and modifier usage?

   a. Office or other outpatient service, established patient, level 3, with modifier 24

   b. Office or other outpatient service, established patient, level 4, with modifier 24

   c. Office or other outpatient service, established patient, level 3, with modifier 25

   d. No E/M service reportable because the visit occurred during the global period of surgery

8. George is brought into the emergency room after an accident while cutting fruit, which involves a major injury to his left hand. After an expanded problem-focused history and physical examination are documented, the high medical decision making recommends emergent major surgery to repair the damaged radial artery and the radial tendons. Which of the following best reflects the performed E/M service and modifier usage?

   a. Emergency department services, level 5, with modifier 25

   b. Emergency department services, level 3, with modifier 57

   c. Emergency department services, level 5, with modifier 57

   d. No E/M service reportable since this falls within the global period of surgery

9. Stephen is a well-known, 15-year-old patient who presents to Dr. X because of a large painful pimple on his **gluteal crest**. Expanded problem-focused history and problem-focused physical examination reveal this to be a **pilonidal abscess** without sinus tract. Low medical decision making recommends a simple incision and drainage of this pilonidal abscess, which has a 10-day global period of surgery. Stephen is prepped, incision and drainage performed without complication. Wound is packed and does not require suturing. Stephen tolerated the procedure well. Which of the following best reflects the performed E/M service and modifier usage?

   a. Office or other outpatient service, established patient, level 3, modifier 57

   b. Office or other outpatient service, new patient, level 2, modifier 25

   c. Office or other outpatient service, established patient, level 3, modifier 25

   d. No E/M service reportable since only the pilonidal cyst excision should be reported

10. Which of the following is NOT a criterion for reporting modifier 25?

   a. The E/M service has been performed for an identifiably different reason from that of the other performed service or procedure.

   b. The E/M service has been performed by the same physician who performed the other performed service or procedure.

   c. The E/M service occurs on the same day as the other performed service or procedure.

   d. The diagnosis for the separately identifiable E/M service is the same as the diagnosis for the performed service or procedure.

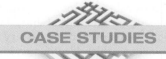

CASE STUDIES

Case Study 17-1

Read the following medical documentation, and then answer the questions that follow.

Stephen returns to Dr. X for a follow-up check 2 days after the excision of the pilonidal abscess on his gluteal crest. No complications noted, and no symptoms of infection or recurrence of pilonidal abscess. During visit, Stephen identifies a different red bump beneath his navel, which has been rubbed raw by the elastic of his underwear. Dr. X documents a problem-focused history, problem-focused physical examination, and medical decision making of low complexity. Dr. X cleans the abraded area with topical solution, applies Neosporin, and then bandages the area. Stephen tolerates the service well.

1. Which of the following best reflects the documented E/M service performed for Stephen?

   a. Office or other outpatient service, established patient, level 2

   b. Office or other outpatient service, new patient, level 1

   c. No E/M service reportable because this occurred during the postoperative period

   d. Preventive medicine service, established patient, level 4

2. Which of the following statements best explains the need for an appended modifier in this case?

   a. A separately identifiable E/M service was performed by the same physician on the same day as the other procedure or service.

b. An unrelated E/M service was performed by the same physician during the postoperative period.

c. An E/M service has been mandated by an outside agency.

d. A decision for surgery has been made by the physician performing the E/M service.

3. Which of the following modifiers should be appended to the E/M service?

a. Modifier 57

b. Modifier 25

c. Modifier 24

d. Modifier 32

Case Study 17-2

Identify the E/M category, subcategory, and criteria for the following case study. Be sure to utilize all prior knowledge. Remember that Appendix D contains the full content of service worksheet.

Patient: David Appleton

Date of admission: December 9, 20XX, 0830 hours

Date of service: December 9, 20XX, 1845 hours

Performing physician: Dr. Frank Gudbuoy

David is an 8-year-old boy admitted 10 hours ago for severe abdominal pain. Mother remembers her son first mentioned the pain on Halloween morning, 5 weeks ago, although there was no trauma or illness precipitating the pain. The patient describes the pain as sharp, rating highest at an 8/10, although the pain is sporadic. Due to the pain, David has missed more than 2 weeks of school at Grand Forks Elementary, where he is a second grader. The pain has not subsided during the past 2 days: mother is very concerned.

History: Aside from the pain, David has been in good health with no recent respiratory or gastrointestinal infections. He usually passes one bowel movement daily without straining, although the BM is described as hard. No pain or burning during urination. David was born with a large gastroschisis, which was repaired with three complex surgeries and a prolonged recovery. He has had no previous issues with postoperative adhesions or abdominal pain before this episode. Overnight, David's pain increased significantly, along with mild temperature increase. David has his legs pulled up tight to his chest. When asked if this helps the pain, he shakes his head briskly.

Physical Exam: Patient pale and sweaty. Eyes clear with no jaundice. Abdomen tense with no rebound. Patient complains of extreme pain during palpation. Exam was discontinued due to David's pain level.

Laboratory: WBC, 14,000. Abdominal MRI performed and reviewed with radiologist, revealing free fluid and significant adhesions between the anterior abdominal wall and the small bowel. The pelvic organs are also involved in the significant adhesions. Discussed case with pediatric surgeon in detail.

Assessment: Adhesive bowel obstruction. Emergent surgical reduction of adhesions scheduled. 80 minutes were spent in counseling family, discussing case with pediatric surgeon, reviewing MRI images and laboratory results.

1. Is content of service documented in this case study? _____

_____

2. Is direct contact with the patient and/or family documented in this E/M service? _____

3. Is time a factor in this E/M service? _____

4. Which E/M service best reflects this documented case study?

_____

5. Should a modifier be appended to the E/M service?

_____

6. If a modifier should be appended to the E/M service, which modifier should be listed?

_____

Coding Challenge

Using your CPT manual, identify the E/M code(s) and modifier that most appropriately reflects each of the following clinical scenarios.

1. Patient is preparing to return to work after suffering a back injury in the workplace. Employer requires the patient to submit comprehensive documentation of a clinical visit with the patient's primary care physician, who is very familiar with the patient. Physician documents a comprehensive history, detailed physical examination, and low medical decision making, and he submits the clinical documentation to the employer along with the appropriate completed forms, which approve the patient for a return to work.

CPT code(s) and E/M modifier: _____

2. Documentation reflects a comprehensive annual evaluation for an established patient, a 58-year-old man with poorly controlled hypertension, frequent headaches, and tingling in his fingers. Annual evaluation is documented by comprehensive history, detailed physical exam, and moderate medical decision making, including counseling regarding appropriate dietary and exercise guidelines. The hypertension, headaches, and tingling are specifically addressed in the medical record with documentation reflecting detailed history and detailed physical examination, along with adjustment of hypertension medication and ordering of labs and oxygen levels.

CPT code(s) and E/M modifier: _____

3. Patient is a 62-year-old woman who is admitted to the hospital with sharp abdominal pain, abdominal distention, dizziness, and rectal bleeding. The initial hospital care documentation reflects a comprehensive history and a detailed physical examination, which identifies an intestinal obstruction due to postoperative intra-abdominal adhesions. Physician recommends emergency exploratory abdominal surgery for reduction of adhesions and identification of obstruction.

CPT code(s) and E/M modifier: _____

4. On 7/12, Dr. G surgically removed a lesion from the left forearm of patient. Three days later, patient returns to Dr. G to examine a nodule found on the right upper arm. Documentation reflects an expanded problem-focused history, problem-focused physical examination, and low medical decision making.

CPT code(s) and E/M modifier: _____

5. On 1/18, established patient is seen by Dr. H regarding a pilonidal abscess. Dr. H documents a detailed history and expanded problem-focused physical examination, and she orders an incision and drainage of the complicated

abscess that afternoon. The global period of surgery for the incision and drainage is 10 days.

CPT code(s) and E/M modifier: _____

6. Patient presents to primary care physician 3 days after being rear-ended by another vehicle. Visit is mandated by patient's automobile insurance company with copies of the documentation requested by the insurance company of the other driver involved in the accident. During the 45-minute visit, physician documents a comprehensive history, comprehensive physical examination, extensive counseling regarding potential therapies for recovery, and a prescription written for 2 days of muscle relaxant and Tylenol 3 for neck pain.

CPT code(s) and E/M modifier: _____

7. A 6-year-old patient admitted with rectal bleeding, fever, and abdominal distention. Ten hours after patient's admission to the hospital, Dr. K documents detailed history, physical examination, and review of radiology images indicating the presence of a foreign body in duodenum with possible perforation. Emergent duodenotomy is scheduled that afternoon.

CPT code(s) and E/M modifier: _____

8. Patient, a 62-year-old woman suffering from sharp abdominal pain, presents to Dr. X, who had previously performed her radical bilateral mastectomy, which has a 90-day global period. During the 35-minute visit, Dr. X identifies that the abdominal pain is not related to the mastectomy, but instead to intra-abdominal postsurgical adhesions related to an emergency appendectomy performed 25 years earlier. Documentation reflects comprehensive history, detailed physical examination, and low medical decision making.

CPT code(s) and E/M modifier: _____

9. During the process of adopting a 2-month-old baby, patient is required to present to a third-party physician for a new patient assessment. Physician documents a comprehensive history, a comprehensive physical examination, and low medical decision making. Physician completes all court-appointed documentation, appends the clinical documentation of the visit, and submits the paperwork directly to the state adoption agency.

CPT code(s) and E/M modifier: _____

10. Dr. F performed an uneventful appendectomy on a 14-year-old patient on June 20. On September 15, the patient presents to Dr. F for abdominal bruising after falling onto the handlebars of a bicycle. Dr. F documents comprehensive history, detailed physical examination, and moderate medical decision making.

CPT code(s) and E/M modifier: _____

11. Patient presents to Fairhaven Urgent Care Clinic to see Dr. Q to address a 1.5 cm laceration on his right palm. Dr. Q documents a detailed history and physical examination, as well as low medical decision making, and performs a simple repair of the laceration.

CPT code(s) and E/M modifier: _____

12. Patient is admitted to the hospital for severe lower right abdominal pain with suspected appendicitis. Ten hours after admission, the attending physician documents a fever of 101.7 with significant guarding and elevated white blood count. Detailed history and physical examination are documented, and an emergency appendectomy is scheduled, with ruptured appendix suspected.

CPT code(s) and E/M modifier: _____

gluteal crest the groove that separates the two rounded buttocks, running from the base of the spine (sacrum) to the perineum (tissue between the anus and either the vaginal opening or the scrotum)

pilonidal abscess the growth of pus and infection within a pilonidal cyst; may require treatment with antibiotics and/or surgical excision

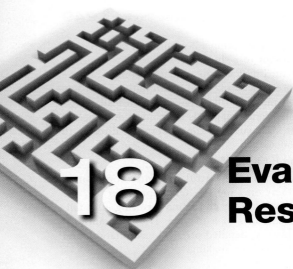

18 Evaluation and Management: Resources and Summary

Learning Objectives

After completing this chapter, you should be able to do the following:

- Spell and define the key terms and abbreviations presented in this chapter
- Define incident-to services
- Identify information and tools outside *Current Procedural Terminology*
- Recognize resources available through the Centers for Medicare and Medicaid Services
- Describe the purpose of the National Correct Coding Initiative (NCCI)
- Summarize the essence of E/M coding

Key Terms and Abbreviations

CMS-1500
Column 1/Column 2
controlled substance
Drug Enforcement Agency
hospital outpatient edits
incident to
medically unlikely edit (MUE)
"Medicare Claims Processing Manual"
midlevel practitioner

Mutually Exclusive Codes
National Correct Coding Initiative (NCCI)
national provider identifier (NPI)
National Uniform Claims Committee (NUCC)
nonphysician practitioner (NPP)
physician NCCI Edits
place of service codes
present on admission
shared/split visit
unit of service

INTRODUCTION

An E/M service code reflects a specific clinical encounter in healthcare: A physician spends time with an individual patient in order to provide healthcare and professional services specifically for that individual. Every E/M service category represents a specific intent for an E/M service, from office or other outpatient

CPT is a registered trademark of the American Medical Association.

to critical care. Category-specific guidelines address the requirements for each category of service and are informed by the intent of the performed service, the nature of the patient's presenting problem, and the context of the visit itself.

Understanding the composition of an E/M service provides a strong foundation for comprehending each category of service. *Current Procedural Terminology,* the "1995 Documentation Guidelines for Evaluation and Management Services," and the "1997 Documentation Guidelines for Evaluation and Management Services" are three essential tools for understanding the actual performance and documentation of E/M services, as well as selecting the correct code to best reflect the performed service.

There are other tools available to medical coders that can deepen their understanding of these healthcare services and even improve their confidence with E/M services. This chapter explores these useful tools and essential information every coder should know when preparing to step into E/M service coding.

A GLIMPSE INTO INCIDENT-TO SERVICES

Physicians function as part of a complex team of varied healthcare professionals. As the field of healthcare has changed, this team of healthcare professionals has grown to include nurse practitioners, physician assistants, and clinical nurse specialists. Even though these important healthcare providers may not have the level of education and experience of physicians, their skill, education, and knowledge provide tremendous assistance in the management of a patient's medical care; they are referred to as **midlevel practitioners** or **nonphysician practitioners (NPPs)**. These NPPs are authorized to practice medicine and are licensed and registered with the state in which they practice medicine. Even as a physician may prescribe medications during a patient's care, an NPP may also be authorized to prescribe medication for the patient during the course of treatment and care.

Because of the complex nature of prescription medication, only qualified healthcare professionals who are properly trained, licensed, registered with, and *authorized by* the state in which they practice may prescribe medications for patients. Prescribed medication is considered a **controlled substance** because its use must be monitored and controlled by the prescribing physician or NPP during the course of treatment. In the third element of medical decision making—risk of complication, comorbidity, or mortality—the table of risk indicates that introduction and continued management of prescription medication increases the level of risk to the patient. However, whether these substances are referred to as medications, prescriptions, or pharmaceuticals, they can provide healing, recovery, and continued health for millions of patients suffering from a myriad of pathologies, conditions, and diseases. Since not all medication is the same, the **Drug Enforcement Agency** has developed an identifying schedule that rates these controlled substances according to the medical usefulness of the chemical compound *and* the risk for potential abuse of the biochemical compound. Schedule 1 substances have no inherently medical purpose and pose a high risk of abuse for the user, whereas Schedule 5 substances are generally used for pain relief, control of diarrhea, and relief or suppression of coughs and pose minimal risk of abuse for the user.

Prescribing controlled substances is only part of the broad field of practice provided by midlevel practitioners. NPPs work in partnership with physicians to provide quality healthcare for patients through a variety of services, which are often integral to the physicians' services. However, since NPPs are, by definition, *not* physicians, the reporting and billing of the clinical, medical, and professional services they provide are different from the reporting and billing of the clinical, medical, and professional services provided by physicians. When the NPP provides incidental services that are integral to the physician's overall services for a patient, these specific services are considered to be **incident to** the physician's services. The term *incident to* is a billing phrase used by CMS to help identify, report, and appropriately bill incidental clinical, medical, or professional services performed by an NPP that are integral to a physician's overall care of a patient. There are a number of incident-to E/M services that may be performed by NPPs; consequently, to help healthcare professionals understand such services, CMS maintains extensive, complex regulations that can be reviewed. In order for the service provided by an NPP to be considered incident to the physician's services, the service must be an important part of the physician's overall care of the patient. This means that the physician has initiated the course of treatment and is continuing to manage the patient's care and that the clinical, medical, or professional service provided by the NPP is only one part of the physician's overall management and care of the patient's condition. In other words, the services provided by the NPP play a minor part in the patient's care in relation to the physician's management and care of the patient. Within the context of E/M services, although the NPP-provided services incident to a physician's services may occur in a wide variety of categories and settings, most of these incident-to services are follow-up visits for established patients with well-known problems.

midlevel practitioner see *nonphysician practitioner*

nonphysician practitioner (NPP) a qualified healthcare professional who is not a physician but who is authorized to practice medicine, is licensed and registered with the state in which he or she practices medicine, and is authorized to prescribe controlled substances during the management and treatment of a patient; also called a midlevel practitioner

controlled substance prescribed medication or drugs that must be monitored and controlled by the prescribing physician or NPP during the course of treatment

Drug Enforcement Agency the federal law enforcement agency responsible for the identification and control of drug use, abuse, and smuggling in the United States

incident to a billing phrase used by CMS to help identify, report, and appropriately bill incidental clinical, medical, or professional services performed by an NPP that are integral to the physician's overall care of the patient

Example: Incident to

Jack presents to Well-Health Physicians for a follow-up visit 12 days after the excision of a severely ingrown toenail. In addition, Jack is concerned because his nasty, barking cough has not subsided. Nurse D, a family nurse practitioner (FNP) who works at Well-Health Physicians, sees Jack because Jack's primary care provider, Dr. G, is currently with another patient in the clinic suite. Nurse D collects an expanded problem-focused history, performs an expanded problem-focused physical examination, and makes medical decisions of low complexity. During the visit, Nurse D identifies that Jack is responding well to the respiratory treatment and recommends that Jack purchase an air humidifier with a HEPA air filter. Nurse D identifies that Jack's left big toe is recovering within normal limits with some minimal swelling. Nurse D changes the dressing and recommends a warm Epsom salt bath twice a day for 2 more days. Return for follow-up is recommended only if toe pain prevents standing or walking, any discharge is noted, or surrounding skin becomes hot, notably red, and swelling increases.

Jack is an established patient with Well-Health Physicians and presents for a follow-up visit regarding his cough and his postoperative toe care. Because this service is integral to Jack's care and Dr. G is readily available in the office suite at the time of Jack's visit, this visit meets the requirements for an E/M service that is incident to Dr. G's care of Jack.

Shared/Split Visits

Reporting incident-to services requires specific personal identifying information in the form of a **national provider identifier (NPI)**. The NPI is a unique number required by Medicare to identify each individual qualified healthcare provider and each individual healthcare organization. This NPI must be used when reporting any performed healthcare service, thereby clearly identifying the qualified healthcare provider who provided the E/M service. If a physician performs the service, it is reported using the physician's NPI. If both a physician and an NPP have participated in the performance of one E/M service, it may be considered a split, or shared, visit, otherwise known as a **shared/split visit**.

Shared/split visits may be reported only if incident-to requirements have been met. When the service is shared or split between a physician and an NPP *and* the incident-to requirements have been met, the E/M service may be reported under the supervising physician's NPI. However, if incident-to requirements have not been met, the split/shared service must be reported under the NPI of the NPP. As with incident-to regulations, CMS maintains and updates extensive regulations for reporting shared/split E/M service visits; however, these regulations are too broad and expansive to review in this chapter. CMS does provide annual updates for the complex professional relationship between physicians and NPPs within the context of E/M services, and these updates can easily be accessed on the CMS website. They may also be specifically identified in the Medicare Claims Processing Manual.

national provider identifier (NPI) a unique number required by Medicare to identify each individual qualified healthcare provider and each individual healthcare organization; must be used when reporting any healthcare service that has been performed by the individual provider and/or healthcare organization

shared/split visit a clinical situation in which both a physician and an NPP have participated in the performance of one E/M service; must meet all incident-to requirements

Example: Shared/Split Visit

Tony is a 45-year-old established patient who presents to Healthy-Street Clinic for significant midchest pain radiating along his jaw and accompanied by heartburn and abdominal pain, as well as a follow-up for his skin rash, tinea versicolor. Dr. M, Tony's primary care physician, collects an expanded problem-focused history, performs a problem-focused physical examination, and makes medical decisions that are low in complexity. Dr. M diagnoses possible GERD and orders an upper GI series to determine acid reflux. When Dr. M is required to address an urgent clinical issue with another patient in the office suite, Nurse B, a family nurse practitioner practicing with Healthy-Street Clinic, enters the visit room to assess the status of Tony's tinea versicolor. Tony has been using Dandruff-B-Gone Extra Strength shampoo topically twice daily for the past 2 weeks, and he states the rash has become less apparent. However, Tony is very frustrated with the treatment. Nurse B identifies a significant decrease in the spread of tinea versicolor and recommends that Tony switch treatment to OTC topical clotrimazole, such as Lotrimin or Lotrimin Ultra to minimize frustration but continue positive results.

Nurse B is an NPP, specifically an FNP, and shares this service with Dr. M. Incident-to requirements have been met with this visit; therefore, it qualifies as a shared/split visit and can be billed under Dr. M's NPI number. If incident-to requirements had not been met, this visit would have been billed under Nurse B's NPI number.

Exercise 18.1   Established Patient: Follow-up for Julian's Sore Face

Read the medical documentation, and then use your CPT manual and prior knowledge to answer the following questions.

Sarah, a 26-year-old established patient, presents to the clinic with complaints of chest congestion, nasal discharge, and fatigue. Dr. H documents an expanded problem-focused history, a physical examination, and medical decision making of moderate complexity. Sarah is diagnosed with Streptococcal pharyngitis and prescribed amoxicillin with NSAIDs for pain relief. Per patient's request, RN provides Sarah with extensive tobacco cessation materials, although Sarah defers any counseling on smoking cessation.

1. Has content of service been reported in this medical documentation? If so, identify the level of each component.
   a. Has content of service been documented? _____
   _____
   b. Category of service: _____
   _____
   c. Subcategory of service: _____
   _____
   d. Specific E/M code: _____
   _____

2. If an E/M service has been identified, please include your rationale supporting the identified category, subcategory, and specific E/M code.
   a. Rationale for category of service: _____
   _____
   b. Rationale for subcategory of service: _____
   _____
   c. Rationale for specific E/M code: _____
   _____

3. Should a modifier be appended to the selected E/M service code? _____
   a. If a modifier should be appended, which of the four modifiers should be appended: 24, 25, 32, or 57?
   b. Explain the reason this modifier should be appended.
   _____
   _____

4. Does this provided service meet incident-to requirements? _____
   Why or why not? _____

HELPFUL INFORMATION AND TOOLS

E/M coding reflects the wide range of professional and clinical services intended to provide care, maintain health, and treat illness for every patient seen by a physician or nonphysician provider. Because the variations of circumstances prompting E/M services can become overwhelming, the CPT manual offers guidelines and requirements for documenting and reporting each category of E/M services. However, other useful educational resources are available that provide practical guidelines and a greater understanding of the appropriate reporting of evaluation and management services. These resources can be found at the Centers for Medicare and Medicaid Services.

Centers for Medicare and Medicaid Services

In 1965, President Lyndon B. Johnson signed two federal programs into law that were intended to protect vulnerable Americans from the devastating costs of illness and disease—Medicare and Medicaid. Medicare is a federal program intended for Americans 65 years of age or older. Medicaid is a partnership between federal and state agencies to provide for low-income children and adults and for individuals with disabilities. These federal programs have been managed and overseen by CMS.

Over the years, CMS has changed and grown in an effort to meet the needs of vulnerable Americans. In its long history of promoting wellness and protecting vulnerable Americans from devastating costs, CMS has been a consolidating force in healthcare. As mentioned previously, CMS collaborated with the AMA to publish the 1995 and 1997 "Documentation Guidelines for Evaluation and Management Services."

Central to CMS is the **CMS-1500** form, the standardized paper claim form utilized by physicians and clinicians to bill for services provided in a noninstitutional healthcare setting. With the advent of electronic health records and the upcoming implementation of the 10th revision of the International Classification of Diseases, otherwise known as ICD-10, the **National Uniform Claims Committee (NUCC)** began a redesign of the CMS-1500 in 2009 to accommodate these changes. At the time this text went to press, the NUCC's revision of the CMS-1500 form had been submitted to the CMS and the Office of Management and Budget for approval. During the approval process, the proposed revision of the CMS-1500 should be available for public comment in order to include the healthcare community in the discussion. However, until the revised CMS-1500 form is implemented, the current CMS-1500 form is the standard paper claims form.

CMS-1500 the official standardized claim form that must be completed and utilized when submitting any Medicare or Medicaid claim

National Uniform Claims Committee (NUCC) a national organization composed of multidisciplinary volunteers dedicated to providing authoritative guidance on the standards for content and data for noninstitutional healthcare claims; maintains and updates the CMS-1500 claim form

"Medicare Claims Processing Manual" a 38-chapter compendium of guidelines for reporting healthcare claims; maintained and updated by CMS

present on admission the diagnosis or diagnoses for which a patient has been admitted to an inpatient facility

place of service codes the numeric codes that identify the specific settings in which the E/M services occurred

National Correct Coding Initiative (NCCI) developed in 1996, a set of guidelines intended to reduce incorrect coding and improper overpayments or underpayments through the identification of codes that may or may not be utilized together or that are medically unlikely

medically unlikely edit (MUE) the NCCI edits table that identifies the maximum number of times a specific code may be reported during a unit of service for one patient

unit of service the specific episode of healthcare service as determined by the category of service

physician NCCI edits the NCCI edits applicable to claims submitted by physicians and nonphysician practitioners

hospital outpatient edits the NCCI edits applicable to claims submitted by hospitals, skilled nursing facilities, and home health agencies

Column 1/Column 2 the NCCI edits table that identifies the codes that may or may not be utilized together, as well as whether a modifier is allowed or required in order for the service to be correctly reported

CMS has been recognized as a leader in the field of healthcare reporting and management but does not dictate policy for private insurance payers, even though many private payers do follow CMS guidelines for reporting and payment. To facilitate communication and the increased education coming from CMS headquarters, which is located in Maryland, 10 different regional offices across the country help with implementation of, support for, and compliance with state Medicaid and federal Medicare guidelines.

"Medicare Claims Processing Manual"   CMS maintains and updates the **"Medicare Claims Processing Manual"**, a 38-chapter compendium of guidelines for reporting healthcare claims. Each chapter is dedicated to a different aspect of reporting healthcare services and is revised and updated as needed, annually or more frequently if changes in policy require updates. Chapter 12, "Physician and Non-Physician Practitioners," includes an extensive section on reporting E/M services, specifically addressing incident-to guidelines, E/M modifiers, and global periods of surgery. As the chapter title suggests, the regulations and requirements included extend to NPPs as well.

Chapter 25 of the manual provides extensive directions for the correct completion and processing of the UB-04 healthcare claim form, whereas Chapter 26 provides equally detailed instructions for the correct completion and processing of the CMS-1500 healthcare claim form. Both of these chapters include directions for correctly identifying the place where the service occurred, which is represented by a series of numbers in both forms. Some of the important instructions include directions regarding **present on admission** diagnosis (or diagnoses), for which a patient has been admitted to an inpatient facility, and **place of service codes**, which identify the specific settings in which E/M services have occurred. The "Medicare Claims Processing Manual" can be reviewed on the CMS website, www.cms.gov, to gain further insight into each aspect of the healthcare process, especially E/M services.

National Correct Coding Initiative (NCCI)   Ultimately, the intent of CMS has been to improve the quality of life for vulnerable Americans and reduce excessive costs through ensuring correct coding. To help achieve this goal, CMS developed the **National Correct Coding Initiative (NCCI)** in 1996 to reduce incorrect coding and improper overpayments and underpayments. Although the NCCI was developed specifically for Medicare and Medicaid benefits, this helpful tool may be used regardless of the specific payer and is utilized daily by countless coders nationwide. Updated quarterly throughout the year, the NCCI proves tremendously useful in identifying whether two codes may be reported together, are mutually exclusive, or are medically unlikely.

A **medically unlikely edit (MUE)** refers to the CMS regulation regarding the maximum number of times a specific code may be reported during a **unit of service** for one patient. A unit of service represents a specific episode of healthcare service, as determined by the category of that service. Determining the unit of service is dependent on the reporting time of the service (e.g., minutes, hours, or days) and the estimated cost or value of the service. For example, a hospital observation service represents a different category of service from that of an emergency department service; however, the concept of a unit of service represents one complete and reported episode of care in either category.

Understanding the intent of each service category reveals the purpose of the MUE. For instance, the newborn care service code that reports the initial hospital or birthing center care of a newborn infant admitted and discharged on the same date may be reported only once per unit of service. There is obvious common sense behind this MUE: A newborn infant can be born only once. Therefore, reporting this specific service more than once is medically unlikely. CMS updates the MUE quarterly.

Along with the many different medical services listed in the NCCI edits, E/M service codes are identified in both the **physician NCCI edits** and the **hospital outpatient edits**. These two NCCI categories of edits list separate guidelines in the form of different tables that can be used to correctly report E/M services: **Column 1/Column 2** and **Mutually Exclusive Codes (MEC)**, which are both updated quarterly.

The Column 1/Column 2 NCCI edits table identifies the codes that may or may not be utilized together, as well as whether a modifier is allowed or required in order for the service to be correctly reported. For example, the level 1 initial observation care code, 99218, may not be reported in conjunction with the level 1 subsequent nursing facility care code, 99307. However, 99218 may be reported with level 1 new patient home service but only if the correct modifier is appended to fully express the context of the performed service.

The Mutually Exclusive Codes table identifies the E/M codes that may never be reported together. For example, the level 4 emergency department service, 99284, may never be reported in conjunction with the initial hospital or birthing center care for a normal, healthy newborn admitted and discharged on the same date.

Example: Using the NCCI Edits

Johnny is an established patient who presents with a barking cough and gastrointestinal upset. Patient has no complaints of nasal drainage. Cough lozenges and cough suppressants have not helped his throat or cough, although he jokes that whiskey helps his discomfort most. Johnny's girlfriend recently moved out after months of arguing about his drinking, but Johnny is dismissive about her departure. Johnny admits that his drinking has increased significantly in the past 6 months but says it has not affected his work. Although the acute illness causing Johnny's cough has resolved, his cough has been exacerbated by the significant increase in alcohol use. A detailed history is collected, expanded problem-focused physical examination is performed, and the medical decision making is low in complexity. More than half of this 35-minute visit was spent in counseling behavior change regarding his alcohol use, including identifying physiologic markers indicative of negative effects on Johnny's health and life.

According to the Column 1/Column 2 table of NCCI physician edits, individual behavior change intervention code 99408 may not be reported in conjunction with office or other outpatient visits. Therefore, only the office or other outpatient E/M service for Johnny's cough should be reported, 99214. This level is determined by the intraservice time, which has been clearly documented.

Mutually Exclusive Codes (MEC) the NCCI edits table that identifies the E/M codes that may never be reported together

---

Exercise 18.2 E/M Modifiers

Read the medical documentation, and then use your CPT manual and prior knowledge to answer the following questions.

Oliver is a 3-year-old new patient presenting with urinary urgency and incontinence. Nurse K, nurse practitioner, sees Oliver and collects a detailed history, performs a detailed physical examination, and makes medical decisions of low complexity. Urinalysis reveals no infection, and KUB reveals healthy ureters, bladder, and urethra, although significant stool is identified in colon. Nurse K identifies that Oliver's urinary incontinence is due to constipation and Oliver's unwillingness to interrupt his play. Nurse K assures Oliver's mother that this is normal and not a cause for concern. Nurse K recommends a timed voiding schedule to allow Oliver the opportunity to interrupt his playtime and empty his bladder. Increased fiber and fluids recommended for constipation, with follow-up in 1 week to re-evaluate constipation.

1. Has content of service been reported in this medical documentation? If so, identify the level of each component.

   a. Has content of service been documented? _____

   b. Category of service: _____

   c. Subcategory of service: _____

   d. Specific E/M code: _____

2. If an E/M service has been identified, please include your rationale supporting the identified category, subcategory, and specific E/M code.

   a. Rationale for category of service: _____

   b. Rationale for subcategory of service: _____

   c. Rationale for specific E/M code: _____

3. Should a modifier be appended to the selected E/M service code? _____

4. If a modifier should be appended, which of the four modifiers should be appended: 24, 25, 32, or 57? _____

   Explain the reason this modifier should be appended.

5. Does this provided service meet incident-to requirements? _____

   Why or why not? _____

EVALUATION AND MANAGEMENT: A SUMMARY

Every E/M service is documented in a patient's record. This medical documentation tells the story of the patient's health and care. The medical documentation also provides the foundation for the continuation of care for the patient and coordination of care for the clinician, as it records pertinent facts, specific findings, observations, assessments, diagnoses, and recommendations for treatment. Ultimately, medical documentation proves to be the connection between clinician, patient, insurance payer, other medical healthcare agencies, and any other party involved in providing healthcare for the patient. However, whereas the medical documentation records the performed service, the service code reports it. The medical documentation and the individual service code are two parts of the whole E/M experience.

In reviewing a documented E/M service, several elements must be identified before the correct service code can be selected. The medical documentation not only records the encounter between the physician and the patient, but also identifies the setting in which it occurred, as well as the patient's previous experience with this specific physician or healthcare agency. In addition, the medical documentation identifies the intent of the service in the chief complaint, the nature of the presenting problem, and/or the physician's diagnosis or diagnoses.

Medical documentation drives healthcare, providing the record of the service and the patient's story of health. However, the specific E/M service code reports the performed service. Each code in the CPT manual represents a specific constellation of components, elements, and factors, each of which distinguishes a different aspect of the service. Each specific code relates to a specific category of service, subcategory, and content of service, intraservice time, and severity of presenting problem. Understanding what is involved in each identified code affords a certain confidence that the specific code does indeed reflect the documented service.

Exercise 18.3 Hospital Inpatient: Cheerleading Injury

Read the medical documentation, and then use your CPT manual and prior knowledge to answer the following questions.

Samantha is a 14-year-old who has been admitted to the hospital this afternoon with chest pain and difficulty breathing after a fall during cheerleading practice. Rib fractures identified, and pneumothorax suspected. As evening has progressed, Samantha's breathing difficulties and pain have steadily increased, and radiology reveals equalizing pressure between pleural space and lungs. Hemothorax identified on radiology image. Samantha prepped for tube thoracotomy (32551), which has a global period of surgery of 0 days.

1. Has content of service been reported in the medical documentation? If so, identify the level of each component.
   a. Has content of service been documented? _____
      _____
   b. Category of service: _____
      _____
   c. Subcategory of service: _____
      _____
   d. Specific E/M code: _____
      _____

2. If an E/M service has been identified, please include your rationale supporting the identified category, subcategory, and specific E/M code.
   a. Rationale for category of service: _____
      _____
   b. Rationale for subcategory of service: _____
      _____
   c. Rationale for specific E/M code:_____
      _____

3. Should a modifier be appended to the selected E/M service code? _____

4. If a modifier should be appended, which of the four modifiers should be appended: 24, 25, 32, or 57? _____
   _____
   Explain the reason this modifier should be appended.
   _____
   _____

5. Does this provided service meet incident-to requirements?_____
   Why or why not? _____
   _____

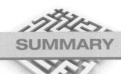

SUMMARY

- The term *incident to* is a billing phrase used by CMS to help identify, report, and appropriately bill incidental clinical, medical, or professional services performed by an NPP when those provided services are integral, although incidental, to the physician's overall care of the patient. In such a case, the physician has initiated the course of treatment for the patient, and the service provided by the NPP plays a minor part in the physician's ongoing management of the patient's care. A shared/split visit identifies an E/M service visit during which an NPP

and a physician have both participated in the performance of the service and the incident-to requirements have been met. CMS maintains and updates extensive guidelines regarding the identification and reporting of incident-to services and shared/split visits.

- CMS manages and provides oversight for Medicare and Medicaid. CMS has been a leader in healthcare guidelines and regulation. In collaboration with the National Uniform Claims Committee, CMS maintains and updates the UB-04 claim form and the CMS-1500, which should be completed and used when submitting any Medicare or Medicaid claim. Ten different regional offices provide oversight and support throughout the country. Even though CMS does not dictate policy for private insurance payers, the CMS coding regulation guidelines provide leadership and direction for clinicians, coders, and many others in various aspects of healthcare.

- The "Medicare Claims Processing Manual," a 38-chapter compendium of guidelines for reporting healthcare claims, is maintained and updated by CMS and may be viewed on the CMS website, www.cms.gov. Chapter 12 includes extensive guidelines and regulations for the correct reporting of E/M services, NPPs, incident-to services, shared/split visits, the correct use of modifiers, and global periods of surgery. Chapter 25 is dedicated to the correct completion and submission of the UB-04 claim form, whereas Chapter 26 details the completion and use of the CMS-1500 claim form. In addition to the many helpful tools maintained by CMS, the National Correct Coding Initiative is intended to increase correct coding through the identification of codes that may or may not be utilized together. Known as the NCCI edits, these tools identify medically unlikely edits, or the maximum number of times a specific code may be reported during one unit of service, or episode of care. The NCCI edits also identify the hospital outpatient edits, which include two different resources useful for correct coding. Column 1/Column 2 edits table identifies the codes that may or may not be utilized together, as well as identifying whether a modifier is allowed in a particular situation. The Mutually Exclusive Code edits table identifies E/M service codes that may never be reported together.

- During the process of selecting an E/M service code, two different components are considered. The medical documentation of the service records the performed service, whereas the service code reports it. The documented service not only records the encounter between the physician and the patient; it also identifies the setting in which the service has occurred, the patient's previous experience with this specific physician or healthcare agency, and the intent of the service in the chief complaint, the nature of the presenting problem and/or the physician's diagnosis or diagnoses. The specific service code is the other component. Each specific code represents a specific category of service, subcategory, and content of service, intra-service time, and severity of the presenting problem. Coders can have confidence in the direction and support provided by the 1995 and 1997 DGs, *Current Procedural Terminology*, and the CMS guidelines.

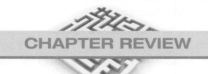

CHAPTER REVIEW

Multiple Choice

Choose the letter that best answers each question or completes each statement.

1. Which of the following is considered a nonphysician practitioner?
   a. A nurse practitioner
   b. A midlevel practitioner
   c. A clinical nurse specialist
   d. All of the above

2. Which of the following best defines an incident-to service?
   a. A billing phrase used by CMS to help identify, report, and appropriately bill incidental clinical, medical, or professional services performed by an NPP when those services are integral to the physician's overall care of the patient
   b. The term used to describe a clinical situation in which both a physician and an NPP have participated in the performance of one E/M service
   c. The term that represents a specific episode of healthcare service as determined by the category of provided service
   d. Prescribed medication or drugs, which must be monitored and controlled by the prescribing physician or NPP during the course of treatment

3. Which of the following best defines the National Correct Coding Initiative?
   a. A unique number that is required by Medicare to identify each individual qualified healthcare provider and each individual healthcare organization and that must be used when reporting any healthcare service performed by the individual qualified healthcare provider and/or individual healthcare organization
   b. A tool intended to reduce incorrect coding and improper overpayments and underpayments through the identification of codes that may or may not be utilized together, that are medically unlikely, or that are mutually exclusive of one another
   c. A billing mechanism defined by CMS to help identify, report, and appropriately bill incidental clinical, medical, or professional services performed by an NPP when those provided services are integral to the physician's overall care of the patient
   d. A federal program intended for Americans 65 years of age or older

4. Which of the following best defines Medicare?
   a. A partnership between federal and state agencies to provide healthcare for low-income children and adults and for individuals with disabilities
   b. A federal program intended for Americans 65 years of age or older
   c. The federal law enforcement agency responsible for the identification and control of drug use, abuse, and smuggling in the United States
   d. An initiative intended to reduce incorrect coding and improper overpayments and underpayments through the identification of codes that may or may not be utilized together, that are medically unlikely, or that are mutually exclusive of one another

5. Which of the following best defines Medicaid?

    a. A unique number that is required by Medicare to identify each individual qualified healthcare provider and each individual healthcare organization and that must be used when reporting any healthcare service performed by the individual qualified healthcare provider and/or individual healthcare organization

    b. An organization involved in managing the finances related to a patient's healthcare services

    c. A partnership between federal and state agencies to provide healthcare for low-income children and adults and for individuals with disabilities

    d. The federal law enforcement agency responsible for the identification and control of drug use, abuse, and smuggling in the United States

6. Which of the following best describes the "Medicare Claims Processing Manual"?

    a. The NCCI edits table that identifies the E/M codes that may never be reported together

    b. A 38-chapter compendium of guidelines for reporting healthcare claims that is maintained and updated by CMS

    c. The tool that identifies the maximum number of times a specific code may be reported during a unit of service for one patient

    d. The official standardized claim form that must be completed and used when submitting any Medicare or Medicaid claim

7. Which of the following best defines a controlled substance?

    a. The official, standardized claim form that must be completed and used when submitting any third-party claim

    b. Prescribed medication or drugs, which must be monitored and controlled by the prescribing physician or NPP during the course of treatment

    c. The official standardized claim form that must be completed and used when submitting any Medicare or Medicaid claim

    d. The diagnosis or diagnoses for which a patient has been admitted to an inpatient facility

8. Which of the following best defines a shared/split visit?

    a. The diagnosis or diagnoses for which a patient has been admitted to an inpatient facility

    b. A specific episode of healthcare service as determined by the category of provided service

    c. A clinical situation in which both a physician and an NPP have participated in the performance of one E/M service

    d. A billing phrase used by CMS to help identify, report, and appropriately bill incidental clinical, medical, or professional services performed by an NPP when those provided services are integral to the physician's overall care of the patient

9. Which of the following best describes a medically unlikely edit?

    a. The NCCI edits table that identifies the maximum number of times a specific code may be reported during a unit of service for one patient

    b. The NCCI edit applicable to claims submitted by physicians and nonphysician practitioners

    c. The NCCI edits table that identifies the codes that may or may not be utilized together, as well as whether a modifier is allowed or required in order for a service to be correctly reported

    d. The NCCI edits table that identifies the E/M codes that may never be reported together

10. Which of the following best describes a mutually exclusive code?

    a. The NCCI edit applicable to claims submitted by physicians and nonphysician practitioners

    b. The NCCI edits table that identifies the maximum number of times a specific code may be reported during a unit of service for one patient

    c. The NCCI edits table that identifies the E/M codes that may never be reported together

    d. The NCCI edits table that identifies the codes that may or may not be utilized together, as well as whether a modifier is allowed or required in order for a service to be correctly reported

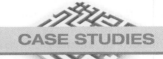

CASE STUDIES

Case Study 18-1

Read the following medical documentation, and then answer the questions that follow.

Stephen is an established patient who returns to Dr. X for a pilonidal abscess on his gluteal crest and another pilonidal cyst beneath his navel. Stephen is 2 months status post excision of pilonidal abscess on his gluteal crest. Dr. X documents an expanded problem-focused history, expanded problem-focused physical examination, and medical decision making of moderate complexity. The pilonidal abscess is not related to the original pilonidal abscess that was excised 2 months ago; however, the associated sinus tract may have developed because of the original

abscess. Dr. X recommends excision of pilonidal abscess of the gluteal crest with possible marsupialization to prevent recurrence; this surgery has a global period of surgery of 90 days. Hot compresses and antibiotic therapy recommended for pilonidal cyst below Stephen's navel. Surgery is scheduled for next week.

1. Has content of service been reported in the medical documentation? If so, identify the level of each component.

    a. Has content of service been documented?_____

    _____

    b. Category of service:_____

    _____

c. Subcategory of service:_____

d. Specific E/M code: _____
_____

2. If an E/M service has been identified, include your rationale supporting the identified category, subcategory, and specific E/M code.
   a. Rationale for category of service: _____
   _____
   b. Rationale for subcategory of service: _____
   _____
   c. Rationale for specific E/M code: _____
   _____

3. Should a modifier be appended to the selected E/M service code?_____

4. If a modifier should be appended, which of the four modifiers should be appended: 24, 25, 32, or 57?_____
   _____
   Explain the reason this modifier should be appended. _____
   _____

5. Does this provided service meet incident-to requirements?
   _____
   Why or why not?_____

Case Study 18-2

Identify the E/M category and subcategory for the following case study, as well as the documented findings and criteria that support the identified category and subcategory. Be sure to utilize all prior knowledge. Remember that Appendix D contains the full content of service worksheet.

Hospital Consultation

Date: 07-16-XX

Chief Complaint: Abdominal pain

History: I was asked by Dr. Goodtummy from the Children's Health Clinic of Metropolis Emergency Department to perform an initial consult on Becca Rawling. She is an otherwise previously healthy 17-year-old woman who has had severe abdominal pain lasting 3+ days, accompanied by constipation, fever, and nausea. On the evening of 07-14-XX, patient felt especially ill with sharp periumbilical pain and nausea. She missed her high school softball game, which her mother states is highly unusual, as her daughter is an avid softball player. On the morning of 07-15-XX, she was awakened by intense lower right abdominal pain and vomited three times that day with no appetite during the course of that day. Her pain increased in severity from a 7/10 to 10/10 when her mother brought her to the hospital for admission. Currently, she is lying in bed, moving her legs in bicycle like motion in an attempt to minimize the pain.

Review of Systems: Becca has been healthy with no history of surgeries or major illnesses. Patient's last menstrual period was 2 weeks ago and was normal. She has experienced no dysuria or foul-smelling urine prior to onset of symptoms. Bowel movements have been daily with no pain or straining, and there has been no change of bowel habits prior to symptoms. No rashes were noted, and there has been no exposure to illness. No cough, chest pain, or joint pain reported in recent weeks; however, patient reports extreme dizziness over past week. As stated previously, patient is very active in her high school softball league and has been doing well in Monterey High School, where she is in the 11th grade. She lives at home with mother, and father is currently serving in Afghanistan as a military chaplain. Mother has history of irritable bowel syndrome.

Exam: T,101.1; weight, 136.25; heart rate, 106. She is very uncomfortable in bed, and her face is significantly flushed due to her fever. Her eyes are glassy but clear and without jaundice. Neck soft without masses. Although patient's moaning has interfered with full auscultation, lungs and heart sounds are clear of rattles, crackles, or murmur with a regular heart rate and rhythm. No swelling of finger knuckles or ankles. Abdomen is guarded and tight with no rebound; patient expresses extreme discomfort when palpation is attempted.

Laboratory: WBC, 36,000: Abdominal X-ray film reviewed: showed pneumoperitoneum throughout lower peritoneum with thick mass in LRQ.

Assessment: Suspected abscessed appendix with likely perforation.

Plan: To operating room for exploratory laparotomy.

1. Is content of service documented in this case study?_____
   _____

2. If content of service is documented, identify the overall levels for each component.
   History: _____
   Physical examination:_____
   Medical decision-making complexity: _____

3. Is direct contact with the patient and/or family documented in this E/M service? _____

4. Is time a factor in this E/M service?_____
   _____

5. Which E/M service code best reflects this documented case study? _____

6. Should a modifier be appended to the E/M service?_____
   _____

7. If a modifier should be appended to the service, which modifier should be listed? _____

APPENDIX A

Instructions for Accessing the "1995 Documentation Guidelines for Evaluation and Management Services"

Written cooperatively by the American Medical Association (AMA) and the Centers for Medicare and Medicaid Services (CMS), the "1995 Documentation Guidelines for Evaluation and Management Services" established definitive regulations and guidelines that physicians could use when documenting the E/M service visits performed. This clarification provided consistency in how these services were documented, by defining each individual content of service element.

The "1995 Documentation Guidelines for Evaluation and Management Services" is considered in the public domain and can be easily downloaded from the Internet and either saved or printed for future reference. Given the importance of this resource, CMS has developed a specific section of the website dedicated to outreach and education for many aspects of provision and reimbursement associated with Medicare and Medicaid services. This outreach and education division of CMS is known as the Medicare Learning Network (MLN). The MLN lists the original "1995 Documentation Guidelines for Evaluation and Management Services" in its section of the website titled "Documentation Guidelines for Evaluation and Management." The document can be accessed by following these steps:

1. Go to the website for the Centers for Medicare and Medicaid Services, www.cms.gov.
2. Click on the "Outreach and Education" link on the CMS website.
3. Find the section entitled Medicare Learning Network (MLN).
4. Click on the MLN Educational Web Guides link.
5. Click on the Documentation Guidelines for Evaluation and Management Services link.
6. Click on the 1995 Documentation Guidelines for Evaluation and Management Services to download the document.

The "1995 Documentation Guidelines for Evaluation and Management Services" is a 15-page, 163 KB, .pdf document that contains these sections:

- Introduction and general principles of medical record documentation
- Documentation of E/M services
- Documentation of history
- Documentation of 1995 body area/organ system physical examination
- Documentation of medical decision making
- Documentation of services dominated by counseling or coordination of care

The introduction of the documentation guidelines inspired consistency in how E/M services were documented but conflict in the documentation of the performed physical examination. Whereas documenting the collected history elements and the medical decision-making elements remained consistent across different physician specialties, documentation of the performed physical examination became problematic because of the ambiguities in the guidelines for the body area and organ system physical examination. As a result, the AMA and CMS cooperatively developed the "1997 Documentation Guidelines for Evaluation and Management Services" and formatted a more exacting set of guidelines for documenting the physical examination—the general multisystem physical examination and the single organ–system physical examination.

Like the "1995 Documentation Guidelines for Evaluation and Management Services," the "1997 Documentation Guidelines for Evaluation and Management Services" is considered in the public domain and can be accessed by following some simple steps:

1. Go to the website for the Centers for Medicare and Medicaid Services, www.cms.gov.
2. Click on the Outreach and Education link.
3. Find the Medicare Learning Network (MLN).
4. Click on the MLN Educational Web Guides link.
5. Click on the Documentation Guidelines for Evaluation and Management Services link.
6. Click on the 1997 Documentation Guidelines for Evaluation and Management Services link to download the document.

The "1997 Documentation Guidelines for Evaluation and Management Services" is a 48-page, 442 KB, .pdf document that can be saved or printed and contains the following sections:

- Introduction and general principles of medical record documentation
- Documentation of E/M services
- Documentation of history
- Documentation of physical examination guidelines
- General multisystem physical examination
- Single organ–system physical examination
    - Cardiovascular single organ system physical examination
    - Ear, nose, throat, and mouth single organ system physical examination
    - Eye single organ system physical examination
    - Genitourinary single organ system physical examination
    - Hematologic/lymphatic/immunologic single organ system physical examination
    - Musculoskeletal single organ system physical examination
    - Neurologic single organ system physical examination
    - Psychiatric single organ system physical examination
    - Respiratory single organ system physical examination
    - Skin single organ system physical examination
- Documentation of medical decision making
- Documentation of services dominated by counseling or coordination of care

APPENDIX C
The Anatomy of the Evaluation and Management Medical Documentation

COLOR KEY FOR IDENTIFIED SECTIONS

Even though every patient is a unique individual, there is an overarching consistency among nearly all documented E/M service visits that corresponds to the content of service elements. Appendix C utilizes a different color to identify each individual content of service element throughout one example of service documentation. The intent of this appendix is to provide an illustration of how the content of service elements stand apart but also function together in reflecting any E/M service.

Patient: Georgia Downsen   DOB: 07/27/89   DOS: 04/26/2012

Healthy Family Care
Family Physicians
Midwest Town, USA
Dr. Marguerite Owen

History of Present Illness
Review of Systems
Past, Family, and Social History
Physical Examination
Medical Decision Making: Number of Diagnoses and/or Management Options
Medical Decision Making: Amount and/or Complexity of Data to Be Reviewed
Medical Decision Making: Risk of Complication, Comorbidity, and/or Mortality
New Patient
Site of Service (Place of Service)

Georgia is a 22-year-old new patient, presenting to the Healthy Family Care Clinic with complaints of chest pain, shortness of breath, difficulty breathing, and a recent, sudden weight gain of 10 pounds. Patient is 7 weeks postpartum, having relocated to the area 1 month ago from Indiana. Patient's pregnancy complicated by gestational diabetes at 26 weeks and preeclampsia at 31 weeks. Bed rest was prescribed at 37 weeks and continued until induction at 39 weeks. Labor was complicated by 2 hours of prolonged labor, and emergency C-section was performed, delivering a 9.92-lb healthy infant female. This was Georgia's first pregnancy. Due to a change in her husband's job, she moved to Midwest Town with husband and baby daughter. Although patient denies postpartum anxiety or depression, she describes moving away from her friends and family as "challenging," especially since she could not lift anything heavier than 10 lbs. Two weeks after relocating to Midwest Town, Georgia began experiencing sharp chest pain, dyspnea, diarrhea, orthopnea, lower leg edema, and a dry cough. These symptoms continued to increase over the next 2 weeks. Then, during the past 2 days, she has been unable to sleep supine secondary to shortness of breath, and instead she has had to sleep seated in a recliner. She has been unable to carry or hold her 7-week-old daughter or perform simple chores around the house secondary to shortness of breath. She reports significant pain in the center of her chest associated with palpitations, which patient describes as a "scary fluttering." Lower leg edema has increased significantly over the past 5 days; she has been unable to wear her socks, and her shoes no longer fit.

ROS

Const: Patient reports excessive sweating over the past 2 days, requiring her to change her shirt two to three times a day. No complaint of fever. Patient's husband reports patient has been very flushed over the past 2 days with signs of dizziness.

Psych: Patient reports feeling very anxious over the past 2 weeks, especially when her shoes didn't fit her feet and none of her pants fit her anymore.

Chest: Reported the presentation of a dry, hacking, unproductive cough 2 weeks ago, which was nonresponsive to any OTC treatment. No report of chest pain until 2 days ago. Negative for nasal congestion.

Extremities: Patient reported she first noticed progressive swelling of her ankles when it was harder to pull her socks onto her feet. Numbness in her toes noted yesterday. Negative for bruising, although patient states she does bruise easily. Negative for joint pain.

GU: Postpartum history has been uneventful until the sudden presentation of symptoms. Negative for vaginal bleeding. Patient is breastfeeding without difficulty, although excessive sweating has caused discomfort and a rash on the underside of her breasts.

GI: Patient reports watery diarrhea for 5 days.

PFSH

This was patient's first pregnancy, complicated by gestational diabetes at 26 weeks and preeclampsia at 31 weeks. Patient was on bed rest from 37 weeks to 39 weeks, when labor was induced. Emergency C-section was performed for failure to progress. No history of tobacco or alcohol use.

Mother: History of obesity, type II diabetes, and atherosclerosis. Maternal history of five pregnancies and three live births. Two pregnancies ended in miscarriage at 9 weeks and 24 weeks gestation, respectively. Of the three live births, two pregnancies complicated by preeclampsia and gestational diabetes, and all three births delivered infants over 8.5 lbs. All live births were vaginal.

Father: Died 3 years ago of esophageal cancer. 25-year history of smokeless tobacco.

Physical Exam

Const: T, 98.1; pulse, 148; BP, 179/120. Patient appears flushed and agitated, but pleasant and cooperative.

Head and Neck: EOMI; PERRLA. Conjunctivae clear. Nasal passages are patent and clear. Tympanic membranes are clear upon otoscopic inspection. Palpation of face reveals no tenderness. Uvula, tonsils, tongue, and buccal mucosa are normal upon inspection. No cervical, clavicular, mandibular, or submental lymphadenopathy. Slight cervical and clavicular soft tissue edema noted.

Chest: Heart irregular rate and rhythm. Grade 2/6 soft holosystolic murmur identified, loudest at the right sterna border with inspiration. Auscultation reveals squeak and friction rub, with diminished lung sounds. Patient's breathing is labored and deep without wheezes, rhonchi, or crackles. No indication of tactile fremitus. Base of lungs dull to percussion. Significant dyspnea noted with minimal exertion on ambulation.

Abdomen: Soft, distended. Bowel sounds present. Diffuse tenderness to palpation but without guarding or rebound. Surgical incision clean, dry, and intact.

Genital: Deferred

Extremities: Muscle strength 4/5 throughout bilateral upper extremities. No numbness or tingling in hands or fingers. Significant generalized edema noted throughout lower extremities, with 4+ pitting edema noted along length ankle and foot. No inguinal lymphadenopathy noted.

Laboratory Tests: Patient is hyponatremic: sodium, 115 mEq/L; hypokalemic: potassium, 3.1 mEq/L. BUN, 45 mg/dl; creatinine, 1.5 mg/dl; WBC, 11,000; RBC, 3.9; BNP, 889 pg/ml; hemoglobin, 10.5 g/dl.

Radiology Results: Chest X-ray without consolidation or infiltrate. Pulmonary congestion noted with mild bilateral pleural effusions. Cardiomegaly.

Impression: Presumptive peripartum cardiomyopathy

Assessment: Georgia's medical records from Indiana have been received and reviewed at length, as well as extensive conversation with Dr. Andres, Georgia's obstetrician, who had ordered extensive monitoring of Georgia's preeclampsia and gestational diabetes. Her prenatal course was uneventful, and there was no indication of eclampsia tendencies or potential HELLP syndrome during pregnancy. According to Dr. Andres, the induction of labor was scheduled in accordance with the patient's move to Midwest Town, and Dr. Andres expressed confidence in Georgia's compliance with postoperative activity restrictions during her family's move.

Plan: I spoke with cardiologist Dr. Verihart at length, discussed Georgia's medical history, physical examination, lab results, and chest X-ray in order to coordinate care for Georgia's complicated case. An echocardiogram, electrocardiogram, and BNP were ordered with results to be sent to Dr. Verihart's office. While waiting for laboratory results and consultation with Dr. Verihart, will start Lasix 40 mg daily and lisinopril 5 mg daily. Further follow-up per Dr. Verihart.

History (chief complaint included)	Problem-Focused	Expanded Problem-Focused	Detailed	Comprehensive
History of Present Illness Location, severity, timing, mod fact, quality, duration, context, assoc s/s	Brief (1 finding)	Brief (2–3 findings)	Ext. (4+ findings, or 3 chronic problems)	Ext. (4+ findings, or 3 chronic problems)
Review of Systems Constitutional, ENT/M, respiratory, GU, skin/breast, endocrine, all/imm, eyes, CV, GI, musculoskeletal, psychiatric, neurologic, hem/lymph	None	Pert. (1 system)	Extended (2–9 systems)	Complete (10+ systems)
Past, Family, and Social History New/initial/consults	Pertinent (1–2 elements)	Pertinent (1–2 elements)	Pertinent (1–2 elements)	Complete (3 elements)
Past, Family, and Social History Established patient/subsequent hospital	Pertinent (1 element)	Pertinent (1 element)	Pertinent (1 element)	Complete (2–3 elements)

Physical Examination	Problem-Focused	Expanded Problem-Focused	Detailed	Comprehensive
1995 PE	A limited examination of affected body area or organ system (1 body area/organ system)	A limited examination of the affected body area or organ system and other symptomatic or related organ systems (2–4 body areas/organ systems)	An extended examination of the affected body area(s) or organ system(s) and other symptomatic or related body areas or organ systems (5–7 body areas/organ systems)	A general multisystem examination or complete examination of a single organ system and other symptomatic or related body areas or organ systems; should include 8 or more of the 12 organ systems (8+ body systems OR organ systems, but they cannot be mixed)
1997 General Multisystem	1–5 elements identified by a bullet	At least 6 elements identified by a bullet	At least 2 elements identified by a bullet from each of 6 areas/systems OR at least 12 elements identified by a bullet in 2 or more areas/systems	Performance of all elements identified by a bullet in at least 9 organ systems or body areas and documentation of at least 2 elements identified by a bullet in each of the examined areas/systems
1997 Single Organ System	1–5 elements identified by a bullet, whether in a shaded or unshaded border	At least 6 elements identified by a bullet, whether in a shaded or unshaded border	At least 12 elements identified by a bullet, whether in a shaded or unshaded border (Eye & psychiatric: at least 9 elements identified by a bullet, whether in a shaded or unshaded border)	All elements identified by a bullet within each shaded border and at least 1 element identified by a bullet within each unshaded border

Complexity of Medical Decision Making	Straightforward	Low	Moderate	High
Number of Diagnoses and/or Management Options	Established presenting problem, stable or improving	Established presenting problem, worsening	New presenting problem, without workup	New presenting problem, with workup
Amount and/or Complexity of Data to Be Reviewed	Ordering or reviewing diagnostic data	Obtaining old records or additional history from someone other than patient	Discussion of diagnostic results with physician who performed diagnostic testing	Independent visualization of image, tracing, or scan by physician performing the E/M service
Risk of Complication, Comorbidity, and/or Mortality	Minimal	Low	Moderate	High

abdomen   the body area extending from the lowest rib to the pelvic bones, encompassing the small and large intestines; liver; spleen; bladder; muscles, tendons, and connective tissue of the abdomen; veins and arteries of the abdomen (including the aorta)

abdominal CT scan   the CT scan used to identify structure, anatomy, and pathologies within the patient's abdominal cavity

abrasion   a minor wound of the skin that is most commonly identified as a scrape; caused by friction

accessory muscles   supplemental muscles that provide support or aid to essential organs, tissues, or structures

activities of daily living (ADLs)   the activities necessary for an independent person to perform in order to live alone, including, but not limited to, grooming oneself, feeding oneself, cooking, and getting dressed

acute myocardial infarction   a heart attack, specifically the period of time when the circulation of blood within the heart is obstructed

add-on service codes   numeric codes representing E/M services that may be reported only in conjunction with a different E/M service and may never be listed independently

adenoids   lymphatic tissue located behind the nose, in the roof of the nasopharynx

admission   the formal acceptance of the patient's care by the hospital, nursing home, domiciliary care provider, boarding or rest home, or other healthcare facility where the patient will remain overnight

admitting physician   physician responsible for completion of documentation specific to the hospital inpatient setting, including documentation intended to facilitate coordination of care with other physicians, nurses, and any other clinical staff who will provide care and treatment for the patient

allergic   the internal, physiologic reaction to substances or factors that cause a heightened sensitivity within the human body; often documented in conjunction with the immunologic system

ambulatory healthcare facility   any healthcare facility that provides same-day care for the patient

American Medical Association (AMA)   the largest, nonprofit professional organization for physicians and medical students in the United States

amount of data   the quantity of data that has been reviewed and interpreted by the physician performing the E/M service

amphoric breath sound   an abnormal hollow, blowing sound heard during auscultation of the lungs; can be indicative of an abnormal opening into the bronchus or pneumothorax or an obstruction of the bronchus

anatomy   the physical structure of the human body

ankle jerk reflex   also known as "Achilles reflex"; reveals the rate of contraction of the calf muscles and tendons when the Achilles tendon is struck; tests the neurologic reflexes that occur when the Achilles tendon is sharply struck by a physician during a physical examination

annual nursing facility assessment   the standardized protocols intended to assess and measure the patient's progress, ability, and function throughout the patient's stay in the nursing facility

anteroposterior   view from the front to the back of the body, as in the direction of an X-ray image

anticoagulant   a category of pharmaceutical medication intended to reduce or prevent the abnormal or pathological clotting of blood

aorta   the large artery leading away from the heart to the lower part of the human body; includes five sections—ascending aorta, arch of the aorta, and descending aorta, which divides into the thoracic aorta and the abdominal aorta

Apgar assessments   five different assessments at the time of birth that determine the patient's blood flow, heart rate, respiratory function, and neurologic function

apical   referring to the tip, as in an apical pneumothorax, which is the accumulation of air or gas in the pleural cavity at the tip of the lung

arterial blood gases   the oxygen and carbon dioxide content of the blood as measured in diagnostic laboratory tests

arterial pH   measurement of the acidity within the blood: levels lower than 7.35 suggesting acidosis and levels higher than 7.45 suggesting alkalosis

arterial puncture   puncturing the walls of an artery with a hypodermic needle for the purpose of drawing blood; like venipuncture, may also be used in the delivery of therapeutic treatment

arteriogram   a radiologic view of the arterial structure achieved by injecting contrast medium into the artery and using X-rays

assessing the risk   identifying the level of risk of complication, comorbidities, or mortality posed to the patient by the presenting problem; refers to the ordered or performed diagnostic tests or the management option selected by the performing physician

assisted living facility   a residential facility with self-contained apartments, or units, that provides assessment of the resident's needs as well as healthcare support 24 hours a day, 7 days a week, in addition to other services

associated signs and symptoms   a report or observation of evidence of pathology or disease in the patient's physiology, such as blood in urine, *and/or* subjective observations of physical experience such as pain or discomfort

atraumatic   without sign or indication of trauma or injury

atrophy   the decrease of mass in a muscle, organ, or other tissue, most often caused by changes in nutrition or disease

auricle   external surface of the ear that can be easily visualized, most commonly referred to as the external ear, earlobe

auscultation   listening to the sounds produced in an organ or body cavity

AVantage A/H5N1 Flu test   a minimally invasive test involving a nasal or throat swab, used to quickly determine whether a person has been infected with the H5N1 avian flu

azithromycin   an antibiotic, commonly known as Zithromax, often used to treat respiratory infections and other bacterial infections

Babinski test   checks the neurologic reaction of the toes and soles of the feet when the bottoms of the feet are stroked;

provides a neurologic indication for the physician, depending on where the soles of the feet are stroked, which causes the toes and feet to curl in different manners

back the body area extending from the lowest part of the neck down to the top of the buttocks, including, but not limited to, the spinal cord and the bones, muscles, tendons, and other connective tissue of the back

behavior change intervention services services intended to promote change in a behavior that could be considered an illness, such as obesity, use of or addiction to tobacco, alcohol use or abuse

beneficiary an individual who receives the benefit of a service or program; most commonly used in reference to private, state, and federal health and/or medical insurance policies

benign prostatic hypertrophy enlargement of the cells within the prostate; also known as benign prostatic hyperplasia

bilaterally on both sides

birthing room one designated room or area specially equipped to deal with the delivery and care of newborns

body area one of seven specific anatomic regions that make up the entire human body

bowel obstruction anything that prevents the normal flow and function of the small or large intestines; may be caused by a foreign body, a pathological process, anatomical defect, or abnormal collection of waste

brief history of present illness documentation of one to three history-of-present-illness standardized descriptions

bronchi the anatomical tube that connects the trachea (windpipe) and the lungs

bronchoscopy the act of inserting a cylindrical fiber optic tube with a video function into the airway; allows direct visualization of the mucosal tissues of the airways for diagnostic purposes

broviac catheter a small, flexible, tubular instrument threaded into a large vein and inserted into one of the large chambers of the heart; used to deliver medication or nutrition to the central venous system

bruit a murmur or other unusual sound identified in the heart, most commonly identified by listening with a stethoscope

cardiac catheterization the insertion of a catheter into a chamber of the heart for the purpose of diagnosis, measurement, and investigation; may be accomplished through an incision in the femoral artery in the groin

cardiac electrophysiological tests invasive and noninvasive diagnostic testing to determine and understand any abnormal heart rhythms; as a treatment, may also be used for therapeutic purposes

cardiac stress test measurement of the heart function and the ability to respond to stress caused by physical activity or pharmacologic stimulation in a controlled clinical environment

cardiopulmonary function the heartbeat that pumps the blood to the lungs during respiration

cardiothoracic surgeon a physician specially trained to investigate and repair the internal structure and function of the organs of the chest, including, but not limited to, the lungs, heart, mediastinum, and pleura

cardiovascular the organ system related to the flow of blood from the heart to the lungs and through the body—including, but not limited to, the function of the heart, dispersal of oxygenated blood through the entire body, and the return of de-oxygenated blood to the lungs for re-oxygenation, veins, arteries, and capillaries

care plan oversight the management and/or coordination of any multifaceted or multidisciplinary treatment plans for a patient's healthcare; requires the participation of the supervising physician

carotid one of two large arteries that carry blood from the chest to the head

cataract a disease of the eye that causes clouding of the ocular lens

category the group of CPT codes that identify evaluation and management services performed in a similar healthcare setting or location

Cefotaxime a broad spectrum antibiotic used for infections of the skin, bones, respiratory tract, and urinary tract; septicemia; and other infections

ceftriaxone an antibiotic

Centers for Medicare and Medicaid Services (CMS) the administrative branch of the U.S. Department of Health and Human Services responsible for the oversight of Medicare and Medicaid services, including guidelines, regulation, payment for services, coverage policies, and many other aspects

central nervous system failure the breakdown of the human central nervous system through pathology, illness, disease, or injury

cerebrovascular accident also known as a stroke; an occlusion or blockage of vessels in the brain caused by an embolus, thrombus, or other pathology that can cause lack of blood flow in the tissues of the brain

cervical referring to lymph nodes located in the neck

chest the body area between the collarbone and the lowest rib; encompasses, but is not limited to, the lungs, heart, ribs, trachea, bronchioles, mediastinal cavity, including the thoracic diaphragm, which is the sheet of muscle that separates the organs within the chest cavity from the organs within the abdominal cavity

chest compressions the manual compression of the chest for the purpose of restoring heart function; most often associated with cardiopulmonary resuscitation

chief complaint the patient's description of the specific health issue, complaint, or disease for which the patient came to the clinician

choanae the funnel-shaped channels that form large openings through which air leaves the nose; also referred to as *posterior nares*

clinical speech reception thresholds determination of a patient's ability to hear, retain, and repeat two-syllable words prompted by the physician

clinician a healthcare professional dedicated to the care and treatment of patients in a healthcare setting; includes a physician, nurse practitioner, registered nurse, or other trained healthcare professional who is most commonly licensed through an overarching professional organization

CMS-1500 the official standardized claim form must be completed and utilized when submitting any Medicare or Medicaid claim

cog wheel a specific form of muscular rigidity caused by tension in the muscles

colitis inflammation of the colon, or large intestine

colostomy an abnormal opening that is surgically created to allow the release of feces from the body via an opening other than the anus

Column 1/Column 2 the NCCI edits table that identifies the codes that may or may not be utilized together, as well as whether a modifier is allowed or required in order for the service to be correctly reported

comorbidity a secondary or additional disease or illness that is separate from the presenting problem but that occurs at the same time as the presenting problem

complete the level of review of systems that includes 10 or more organ systems in the medical documentation

complexity of data identification of how multifaceted, difficult, or intricate the presented data are, as well as the level of difficulty the data present to the physician performing the E/M service

complicating pneumonia opportunistic pneumonia that develops as a result of an illness, often a secondary infection

complication a pathological development that is not an inherent part of the presenting problem but that occurs in a patient during the management of the patient's presenting problem

comprehensive history the fourth level of documented history, requiring an extended HPI, complete ROS, and complete PFSH

computed tomography (CT) scan known as computed tomography, or CT; a specific radiological diagnostic test that creates a three-dimensional image of the inside of the human body or cavity

conjunctivae the inner surface of the eyelids and the surface of the eyeball

constitutional referring to the anatomy and functions of the human body that provide the underlying sense and experience of health—such as body temperature, weight, height, pulse rate, paleness or flushed skin—any of which factors, if disturbed, may indicate ill health or disease

content of service the three elements that are considered the building blocks of evaluation and management services: history, physical examination, and medical decision making

context narration of the circumstance or event that occurred prior to or coincidentally with the onset of the patient's sign, symptom, or disease; may or may not be related to the sign or symptom

contracture an abnormal tightening or shortening of muscles, usually in the extremities, that permanently limits the movement of the body part

contraindications physiologic, diagnostic, or medical reasons that indicate that a specific medication, therapy, treatment, or plan of care would be undesirable, unwise, or impossible to prescribe for a patient's health

contrast medium a substance that is relatively impenetrable by X-rays or other forms of radiation; used in diagnostic radiol-ogy such as arteriograms, X-rays, and magnetic resonance imaging

controlled substance prescribed medication or drugs that must be monitored and controlled by the prescribing physician or NPP during the course of treatment

convalescent care healthcare services provided for a patient who is recovering from an illness; also referred to as recuperative care

coordination of care managed sharing of medical findings, management options, and treatment plans between two or more participants in the patient's healthcare

costovertebral angle the angular space of the back between the lowest rib and the vertebrae, which is most commonly located over the kidneys

counseling the dialogue between the physician and the patient during which the physician provides additional information regarding the disease process, expected prognosis, diagnostic procedures or results, treatment or management options, the necessity for compliance, or any other unanswered questions from the patient and/or family

counseling risk factor reduction (services) E/M services intended to encourage an intentional avoidance of disease or conditions associated with high-risk factors

crackles abnormal, sharp sounds that can be heard during auscultation of the lungs

cranial nerves the 12 nerves that connect the brain to 12 various sensory and motor sections of the head, or cranium

crepitation a crackling or grating sound; in the lungs, associated with lung disease; also occurs when two ends of a broken bone rub together

critical care personalized, continuous care provided for one specific patient whose health has been abruptly damaged by an illness, injury, or disease that simultaneously poses a significant and definite threat to the patient's life

culdocentesis an invasive diagnostic procedure that requires the placement of a needle in the rectouterine pouch, or the space between the uterus and the rectum, for the purpose of extracting fluid

***Current Procedural Terminology* (CPT)** the book of numeric and alphanumeric codes that identify and describe the healthcare service provided to the patient; maintained and published annually by the AMA

cystitis inflammation of the bladder

data information that could help facilitate the diagnosis of the presenting problem; includes the results of diagnostic testing, the patient's old medical records, and additional history from the patient's family or caretaker

day management refers to the inclusion of any services provided to the patient during the entire process of discharging the patient from observation care status

deep tendon reflexes one of many neurologic tests that provide indication of the integrity of the central nervous system and the peripheral nervous system; include Babinski test, ankle jerk reflex, and the knee jerk reflex

deep vein thrombosis a medical emergency involving the formation of a clot in a vein deep within the body, most commonly a lower extremity; causes severe pain, redness, significant warmth and swelling of the affected area, engorgement of superficial veins of the affected limb, and can lead to a pulmonary embolism if the clot dislodges and travels to the lung

delivery room a designated room or area specially equipped to deal with the delivery and care of newborns

detailed history the third level of documented history, requiring an extended HPI, extended ROS, and pertinent PFSH

diabetic ketoacidosis a potentially life-threatening complication due to diabetes mellitus and a lack of insulin in the body

diagnostic data information obtained by the physician that identifies the internal structure, status, physiology, or pathology within the patient's body through tests that facilitate identification and diagnosis of the presenting problem

diagnostic laparoscopy an invasive surgical procedure that involves an incision in the abdominal wall and inflation of the abdominal cavity to allow the insertion of a small scope for examining the abdominal cavity and internal organs

diagnostic results the results of any laboratory, pathology, radiology, medical, or other diagnostic testing to determine a final diagnosis; may be presented in a variety of forms, including, but not limited to, a report, itemized results, images, scans, or compiled records

diagnostic testing a specific test used to determine the internal function, status, structure, and/or pathology occurring within the patient; includes laboratory tests, radiology rests, or even endoscopies

diaphragmatic related to the diaphragm, the sheet of muscle that separates the organs within the chest cavity from the organs within the abdominal cavity

diaphragmatic rupture a tear or created abnormality of the muscle that aids inspiration and separates the thoracic cavity and the abdominal cavity

differential diagnosis the process by which a physician identifies a diagnosis through the elimination of different pathologies

dilated intestinal loops the swelling and bulging of the intestines caused by a buildup of gases or fluid produced by infection and/or obstruction within the intestines

direct contact the presence of the patient (or the patient's family) with the performing physician or in the team conference during the E/M service

dislocation the displacement of a joint, bone, organ, or structure from its normal position

Documentation Guidelines (DGs) standardized requirements for medical documentation as defined by the Centers for Medicare and Medicaid Services in 1995 and 1997

domiciliary referring to the home or other dwelling in which a person lives and which is the person's legal place of residence; may be a multioccupant building or a private home

Drug Enforcement Agency the federal law enforcement agency responsible for the identification and control of drug use, abuse, and smuggling in the United States

drug therapy requiring intensive monitoring for toxicity any prescription drug with a significantly higher risk of potentially harmful side effects that may require regular monitoring for appropriate dosing and identification of the onset of potentially harmful side effects or contraindications

duration the measurement of elapsed time since the patient began to experience the sign, pain, discomfort, or symptom, either by identifying the starting point; the length of time the symptom, pain, or discomfort has impacted the patient's life; or the point of time when a complication arose during the management of a chronic condition

ears the anatomic organ and system within the human body related to hearing, such as the earlobe, ear canal, and eardrum; often documented in conjunction with the nose, throat, and mouth and abbreviated as ENT/M

echocardiography the graphic recording of the electric activity of the heart, utilizing ultrasound to create images of the heart

echoencephalography a diagnostic scan that utilizes ultrasound waves to study the brain

edema an abnormal collection of fluids between the cells of an organ or in intercellular tissues, a body cavity, or an extremity

effective serum osmolality the concentration of chemicals dissolved in the serum of the blood, including sodium, chloride, bicarbonate, proteins, glucose, and others

effusion the abnormal collection of fluid in a body cavity or organ

electrocardiogram a graphic recording of the electric activity of the heart through the placement of electrodes along the surface of the skin

electroencephalogram a graphic record of the electric the electric waves of the brain through the placement of electrodes along the surface of the scalp

embolus clotted blood or other material that breaks free within the circulatory system and could cause an obstruction of the blood flow

emergency medical technician (EMT) a specially trained medical professional capable of performing medical services such as resuscitation, cardiac monitoring, and other services

emergent surgery a surgical procedure that is essential in order to save the life of the patient

endocrine the anatomic system of organs and tissues within the human body that relates to the excretion, or release, of hormones into the blood; influences growth, metabolism, and many other functions and includes the thyroid, pancreas, adrenals, and pituitary gland

endoscopies internal observation of the structure of the human body, organs, vessels, tubes, or cavities, using an instrument known as an endoscope

epiglottis the flap of tissue that covers and protects the larynx during the act of swallowing

established patient a patient who has received professional, medical, or other healthcare services from a specific physician, or from another physician of the exact same specialty and subspecialty who also belongs to the same group practice, during the 3 years prior to the evaluation and management service in question

established patient complete PFSH documentation supporting two or three of the three PFSH elements for an established patient of the clinician or facility

established patient pertinent PFSH documentation supporting one of the three PFSH elements for an established patient of the clinician or facility

established problem any patient's presenting problem that has already been diagnosed by the performing physician

established problem, stable or improving a patient's presenting problem that has already been diagnosed by the performing physician and that has remained stable or shows improvement

established problem, worsening a patient's presenting problem, which has already been diagnosed by the performing physician, and has become worse

eustacian tube a tube or passage linking the middle ear to the throat, which helps to regulate internal air pressure and drain mucus

evaluation a review and/or assessment of a patient to ascertain a clinical judgment of the patient's diagnosis, current health status, and/or condition

evidentiary checklist the specifically identified clinical, pathological, and anatomic findings that are listed in the 1997 Documentation Guidelines for the general multisystem physical examination and single organ system physical examination

exacerbation worsening in severity of a disease, syndrome, or any symptoms thereof

examination of gait a physician's examination of the patient's natural method, form, and process of movement; provides indicators about neuromuscular function, as well as balance, sense of space, and other indicators

examination of station a physician's examination of the patient's natural method, form, and process of standing or sitting still; provides indicators about neuromuscular function, balance, and other indicators

excised surgically removed (e.g., a specific part of the human anatomy)

expanded problem-focused history the second level of documented history, requiring a brief HPI, pertinent ROS, and pertinent PFSH

expectoration spitting up, coughing up, or clearing one's throat by coughing and spitting out collected mucus

explored surgically investigated (e.g., a specific portion of the human anatomy)

extended the level of review of systems that includes between two and nine organ systems in the medical documentation

extended history of present illness documentation of four or more of the history-of-present-illness standardized descriptions

extra-ocular movements an indication of the coordinated function of the seven muscles that control the movement of the eye; typically occur during a physical examination when a patient is instructed to look up, to the side, or down or to track a moving finger; considered "intact" when the movements are within normal limits

extrauterine outside the womb

extremity the body area of the arms and legs, including the joints of the arms and legs; the muscles, tendons, and connective tissue; phalanges (fingers and toes); the circulatory veins, arteries, and vessels; the lymphatic vessels and nodes

exudates the collection of fluid that is secreted from inflamed, infected, or swollen cells or tissues; can include pus

eyes the anatomic organ and tissue system within the human body related to vision, such as the eyeball, conjunctiva (white of the eye and inside of eyelids), the eyelids, eyelashes, tear ducts, and optic nerve

face-to-face time the time the physician spends in the presence of the patient collecting history, performing the physical examination, determining the medical decision making, providing counseling to the patient, and/or coordinating care during the E/M service

false vocal cords the mucus membrane that covers the true vocal cords

family history the medical history of the patient's immediate family, which may or may not be relevant to the health of the patient; any hereditary and/or lifestyle health factors of the patient's immediate family that could provide further insight into the physiology of the patient and any cause of the patient's current condition

fee-for-service program in healthcare, a specific service that establishes a standard of payment, acknowledging the amount of work involved in the provision of that service, care, or treatment

femoral arteries the large arteries found in the upper thigh, or along the femur

femur the large bone located in the thigh that extends from the hip bone to the knee

fetal contraction stress test ultrasound measurement of the fetal heartbeat during uterine contractions prior to birth

fetus the term that identifies an unborn human young from the 8th week of gestation up to birth

finger rub test an auditory test that identifies how well the patient can hear the sound of a finger and thumb being rubbed together beside the patient's ear

flaccid loose, flabby, weak

forward flexion bending forward

fremitus vibrations that can be felt externally when breathing or speaking; if respiratory, indicates excessive secretions that vibrate when air flows through the lungs

gallop abnormal third or fourth beat that makes the heartbeat sound like a galloping horse

gastrointestinal the organ system related to the intake, digestion, and processing of food and the disposal of solid waste products; includes every part of the digestive system from the lips of the mouth to the anus

gastroschisis a congenital defect that is identified at birth, characterized by a defect in the abdominal wall that allows intestinal contents to protrude outside the abdominal cavity; requires surgical intervention to return intestinal contents to the abdominal cavity and repair the abdominal wall

gastrostomy tube a tube that is inserted directly into the stomach through the abdominal wall; introduces nutrients to patients who are unable to take nourishment through the mouth

general multisystem physical examination physical examination that follows the requirements listed in the 1997 Documentation Guidelines for documentation; includes an evidentiary checklist of anatomic, physiologic, and pathologic findings identified by bullets in the guidelines

general surgeon a physician specially trained to investigate and repair the internal structure and function of abdominal organs, as well as treating disease and injury through manual manipulation

genitalia the body area related to the male and female sex organs; includes, but is not limited to, the male penis and testicles and the female vagina, uterus, and fallopian tubes

genitourinary any part of the human body relating to either the production of urine—such as kidneys, ureters, and urethra—or reproduction and the male/female genitalia—such as the uterus, ovaries, and vagina for women and the testicles, penis, and prostate for men

global period of surgery the period of time recognized for a patient's full recovery after surgery; accounts for the materials, services, and procedures that are required for the performance of and recovery from a surgical procedure

gluteal crest the groove that separates the two rounded buttocks, running from the base of the spine (sacrum) to the perineum (tissue between the anus and either the vaginal opening or the scrotum)

gravida a woman's state of pregnancy; often used with a number to indicate how many pregnancies the woman has experienced

groin a triangular area of the body between the pelvic bones, including, but not limited to, the pelvic muscles, tendons, and hip bones

hard palate the hard part of the roof of the mouth

head the body area above the chin; includes, but is not limited to, the head hair, brain, eyes, eyelids, ears, nose, sinuses, oropharynx, nostrils, teeth, gums, tongue, lips

healthcare the promotion and preservation of physical health and well-being through clinical assessment, diagnosis, treatment, and, if necessary, management of disease and illness

heart failure the failure of the heart to pump blood

heart failure with acute pulmonary edema the failure of the heart to pump blood, combined with the collection of fluid within the pulmonary tissues, leading to intense difficulty breathing

HELLP syndrome a life-threatening condition occurring during pregnancy that is often associated with preeclampsia; characterized by destruction of red blood cells, elevated liver enzymes, and low platelet count

hematologic the blood and blood-producing organs, structures, and anatomy of the human body, including, but not limited to, the bone marrow and the spleen; often documented in conjunction with the lymphatic system

hemodynamically regarding the movement of blood through the patient's body

hemorrhages excessive bleeding

hepatosplenomegaly enlargement of the liver and spleen

hereditary referring to an inherited condition, disease, or syndrome that is passed through bloodlines, or from parent to offspring or extended relative to descendant, such as grandparent to grandchild

high medical decision making one of the four levels of medical decision making that reflects a very intricate process of diffi-

cult or extreme decisions, difficult coordination of diagnostic tests or results, complex diagnosis or diagnoses, or convoluted management options, all of which may involve a high risk to the patient

history the first of three components of the E/M content of service; addresses the history of present illness (the patient's personal experience of this illness), the review of the patient's organ systems (status of the patient's health before this illness), and any aspects of the patient's past, family, and social history that may relate to this illness

history of present illness any of eight standardized descriptions with which the patient may provide a visceral, personalized description of the specific health issue, complaint, or disease for which the patient came to the clinician

home care agency the provider of the coordinated care of different healthcare professionals and/or therapists—including nursing care; speech, physical, or occupational therapy; and even home aid workers who can provide assistance with light chores—for a patient who is residing in a private home or domiciliary residence

homeostasis the physical state when vital organ systems not only function within normal limits, but function together to ensure the normal physiology of a patient

hospice care the provision of medical, emotional, psychological, and spiritual support by interdisciplinary healthcare and other skilled professionals, specifically for patients who are terminally ill

hospital outpatient edits the NCCI edits applicable to claims submitted by hospitals, skilled nursing facilities, and home health agencies

human chorionic gonadotropin (hCG) also known as the "pregnancy hormone"; measured to identify the gestation stage of pregnancies

hydrocodone cough suppressant a cough suppressant combined with a narcotic analgesic, or pain reliever

hyperextended bent to an extreme angle farther than the normal range of motion

immunologic pertaining to the physiological reaction of a patient's immunity and any reactions to external or internal factors, pathologies, or substances; often documented in conjunction with the allergic system

incident to a billing phrase used by CMS to help identify, report, and appropriately bill incidental clinical, medical, or professional services performed by an NPP that are integral to the physician's overall care of the patient

incisional biopsy the incision and removal of part of a lesion for the purpose of diagnosis

indomethacin an NSAID used to reduce fever, pain, swelling, and stiffness; used in the treatment of various conditions, including rheumatoid arthritis and patent ductus arteriosus

induration abnormal hardening of tissues

infant a child from birth to approximately 1 year of age, or about the time the infant learns to walk

infraorbital referring to the area below the orbital cavity of the eye

initial comprehensive preventive medicine services the first preventive medicine service performed for a patient by the physician

inpatient hospital a category of E/M services that occur when the patient has been admitted to a hospital setting for the purpose of evaluation and/or treatment

integumentary the organ system that covers the exterior of the human body in protective tissues, including, but not limited to, the epidermis, dermis, sweat glands, body hair, toenails, and fingernails; also known as skin

intensive care the critical care provided by a team of healthcare professionals operating on a unit that is dedicated to the critical care of patients

intercostal muscles the muscles between the ribs that contract during respiration

intermediate care facilities transitional facilities that provide rehabilitative care for patients who require care and services for a short period of time

internationalized normalized ratio (INR) a measure of the coagulation tendency of the blood, used to monitor anticoagulant therapy; may also be called a prothrombin (PT) test

intra-abdominal adhesions fibrous bands that form between organs and/or tissues within the abdominal cavity, most commonly after an injury or during postoperative recovery; often referred to as internal scar tissue

intramuscular within a muscle; for example, describing an injection into the muscle tissue

intraservice time the amount of time the physician spends performing an E/M service

intrauterine within the uterus

intussusception an intestinal condition in which part of the small intestine folds in on itself, thereby creating a telescope-like compression as the walls of the small intestine rub together; requires emergency intervention

jaundice yellowing of skin, mucus membranes, and the whites of the eyes caused by an excess of bile in the tissues

ketones chemicals toxic to the function of the body that are built up as a result of low insulin

kyphoplasty a percutaneous surgical procedure that utilizes fluoroscopic radiologic guidance and is used to repair collapsed or fractured vertebrae; involves the placement of a small balloon into which a specific kind of cement is injected, thereby reducing the deformity caused by the fracture or the collapse (sometimes referred to as "balloon kyphoplasty")

laboratory a facility that provides scientific study of clinical specimens such as blood, fluids, or other tissues for the purpose of identifying information about the health of the patient, specifically in relation to diagnosis

labored breathing mechanical dysfunction of respiration due to disease or injury

lactation the production of milk in the mammary glands in females

laparotomy the major, invasive surgical procedure that creates a large incision along the abdominal cavity to explore, repair, remove, or transplant organs or tissues between the diaphragm and the pelvis

larynx the section of the throat that contains the voice box

laxity the condition of abnormal loosening of tissues, as in a loss of firmness in skin

Legionnaire's disease a potentially life-threatening infection caused by an aerobic bacterium, which often causes a virulent form of pneumonia

location the specific anatomic area in or on the body in which signs and symptoms have occurred

long-term care facilities facilities that provide extended healthcare services for patients who require extensive or ongoing care, therapeutic support, or assistance with activities of daily living

low birth weight weight of a newborn baby that is between 3.3 pounds and 5.5 pounds, or 1500 grams to 2500 grams, at the time of birth

low medical decision making one of the four levels of medical decision making that reflects a more complicated combination of medical decision-making elements but does not warrant a significant or substantial level of medical decision making

lumbar puncture an invasive diagnostic procedure that requires the placement of a needle between two spinal vertebrae for the purpose of extracting cerebrospinal fluid; may also be used for therapeutic purposes

luxation the act of dislocating a bone, organ, or joint out of alignment

lymphatic the organ system responsible for the production, flow, and processing of lymphatic fluid, a clear fluid that contains white blood cells, circulates through the human body in lymphatic vessels, and is filtered by lymph nodes; significantly impacts a patient's immunity, as well as several other elements of health; often documented in conjunction with the hematologic system

malrotation an emergent condition in which the bowels become twisted; can cause ischemia of the bowels and necrotic bowel

management identification of an appropriate clinical treatment to promote the patient's health, recovery, and wellness

management option documentation of any existing or initiated method of treatment, care, or management of the presenting problem; could range from something as simple as getting a little rest, to having an invasive medical procedure

mandated ordered to occur at the request of another organization, agency, or company

Medicaid a healthcare program that works in cooperation with each of the states to provide assistance for low-income children and adults, as well as individuals with disabilities; founded in 1965 and monitored by the Center for Medicare and Medicaid Services

medical decision making clinical identification of the level of risk and complexity posed to the patient by the current health complaint, as well as the risk posed by any proposed diagnostic or treatment options

medical documentation the record of healthcare provided to the patient at the healthcare facility, which may be in the form of handwritten or typed narratives, reported diagnostic results, diagnostic images or scans, or other records

medically unlikely edit (MUE) the NCCI edits table that identifies the maximum number of times a specific code may be reported during a unit of service for one patient

Medicare a federal healthcare insurance program that provides insurance for people of the United States over the age of

65 and for those with disabilities or anyone with end-stage renal disease; founded in 1965 and administered by the Center for Medicare and Medicaid Services

"Medicare Claims Processing Manual" a 38-chapter compendium of guidelines for reporting healthcare claims; maintained and updated by CMS

methotrexate an antineoplastic antimetabolite that acts as a folic acid antagonist as well as an immunosuppressive agent for autoimmune diseases such as rheumatoid arthritis; also used in the medical treatment of ectopic pregnancies

midlevel practitioner see *nonphysician practitioner*

moderate medical decision making one of the four levels of medical decision making that reflects more complicated coordination on the part of the physician performing the E/M service but does not pose an excessive risk to the patient

modifying factor any treatment taken by a patient in an attempt to alleviate or change the sign or symptom; may include over-the-counter or prescription medication, a specific activity or therapy, such as ice packs or massage

morbidity a state of disease, illness, or ill health

mortality actual death of the patient or increased potential for death due to the patient's presenting problem, a drastic worsening of the presenting problem, or associated disease process

mouth the anatomic section of the body that identifies the beginning of digestion, is necessary for production of speech, and includes the tongue, gums, teeth, palate, and taste buds; often documented in conjunction with the ears, nose, and throat and abbreviated as ENT/M

moxifloxan an antibacterial medication used in the treatment of respiratory infections, anthrax, intra-abdominal infections, and other high-risk diseases

multidisciplinary qualified nonphysician healthcare professionals clinicians from different disciplines such as physical therapy, occupational therapy, speech therapy, psychology, other specialties, and nursing

murmur an abnormal heart sound

musculoskeletal the organ system responsible for the structure and movement of the human body, including, but not limited to, the bones, ligaments, tendons, muscles, cartilage, and vertebral discs

Mutually Exclusive Codes the NCCI edits table that identifies the E/M codes that may never be reported together

myocardial infarction a medical emergency during which blood supply to the heart is interrupted, causing the cells of the affected part of the heart to die; more commonly known as a heart attack

nail matrix the structure from which toenails and fingernails grow

nares nostrils

nasal mucosa the layer of moist tissue that covers the inside of the nasal cavity

National Correct Coding Initiative (NCCI) developed in 1996, a set of guidelines intended to reduce incorrect coding and improper overpayments or underpayments through the identification of codes that may or may not be utilized together or that are medically unlikely

national provider identifier (NPI) a unique number required by Medicare to identify each individual qualified healthcare provider and each individual healthcare organization; must be used when reporting any healthcare service that has been performed by the individual provider and/or healthcare organization

National Uniform Claims Committee (NUCC) a national organization composed of multidisciplinary volunteers dedicated to providing authoritative guidance on the standards for content and data for noninstitutional healthcare claims; maintains and updates the CMS-1500 claim form

nature of the presenting problem the physician's clinical identification of the severity of and risk posed by the condition, disease, illness, injury, complaint, or other medical reason for which the patient has presented to the healthcare facility for the E/M service

neck the body area between the chin and the collarbone; includes, but is not limited to, the trachea, larynx (voice box), thyroid, upper esophagus, lymph nodes, neck (cervical) vertebrae, muscles, tendons

negative in the context of a review of systems, refers to the absence of any identifiable symptoms or signs of discomfort; considered to be interchangeable with "none" or "N/A"

neonatal medicine healthcare services provided to a newborn infant from birth up to 28 days of age

neurological the organ system responsible for the electric impulses that control the function and movement of the human body, including, but not limited to, the brain, spinal cord, and complex network of nerves extending throughout the entire body, even into the extremities

new patient a patient who has not received any professional, medical, or other healthcare services from the physician, or from another physician of the same specialty or subspecialty who belongs to the same group practice, during the 3 years prior to the evaluation and management service in question

new patient complete PFSH documentation supporting all three of the PFSH elements for a new patient of the clinician or facility

new patient pertinent PFSH documentation supporting one or two of the three PFSH elements for a new patient of the clinician or facility

new problem patient's presenting problem that is new or unfamiliar to the performing physician

new problem with diagnostic workup an undiagnosed new presenting problem that requires specific laboratory, pathology, or other diagnostic tests to identify the differential diagnosis

newborn an infant from birth to 28 days of life

none (or N/A) the level of review of systems that includes no organ systems in the medical documentation

non–face-to-face physician services services between a physician and an established patient that, unlike any other E/M service, may occur over the phone or via the Internet

noninsulin dependent diabetes commonly referred to as "type II" diabetes; requires no insulin therapy and can be managed through lifestyle and diet

nonphysician practitioner (NPP) a qualified healthcare professional who is not a physician but who is authorized to practice medicine, is licensed and registered with the state in which he or she practices medicine, and is authorized to prescribe controlled substances during the management and treatment of a patient; also called a midlevel practitioner

nonphysician qualified healthcare professional any healthcare professional who is not a physician

normal visual field test an assessment of the scope of the patient's visual field

nose the anatomic organ and structure related to the sense of smell, including the nasal cavity and septum; often documented in conjunction with the ears, throat, and mouth and abbreviated as ENT/M

number of diagnoses the documentation that reflects the physician's familiarity or unfamiliarity with the patient's presenting problem

nursing facility inpatient facility that provides various kinds of healthcare services for patients requiring care on a 24-hour basis

objective referring to any method of impartially measuring patient symptoms or signs; can be repeated with a variety of patients and will provide consistent results—for example, a numeric pain scale of 1–10

observation status the designation given when the patient's clinical presentation requires the physician performing the E/M service to closely monitor the patient's health before a final determination can be made

odorous foul smelling

open procedure an invasive surgical procedure that requires incision through the exterior of the body to access internal organs, structures, or cavities

oral mucosa the layer of moist tissue that covers the inside of the mouth, including the gums, tongue, and roof of the mouth

organ system a specific set of anatomically interconnected tissues, structures, and organs that operate together to perform a specific physiological function within the human body

orientation to person appropriate identification of oneself and the known nearby people; for example, a patient's appropriate identification of him- or herself by name, identifying the physician by name and any family member in the room

orientation to place appropriate identification of the place in which a person finds him- or herself; for example, a patient's appropriate identification of the name of the state, city, town, and clinic in which he or she happens to be sitting for the E/M service visit

orientation to time appropriate identification of the date, month, year

otitis media an infection of the middle ear

otoscope examination instrument with magnifying lens and light that is used to examine the interior of the external surface of the ear as well as the interior tympanic membrane, interior tissues, and structures of the inner ear

outpatient any clinical location that does not require the patient to be admitted for evaluation and management; most commonly identified as a clinical setting to which a patient presents for medical care and then leaves after the service is completed, such as a physician's clinic office

over-the-counter medication any medication that does not require a prescription, such as Tylenol, Advil, or nonprescription allergy medication such as Benadryl

overall history the combined levels of HPI, ROS, and PFSH

oxygenation the normal flow of oxygen to the tissues

palpation determining the status of an organ by pressing, gently pushing, or touching with fingertips, fingers, or palm of hand; for example, palpating the upper left quadrant of the abdomen to determine the size of the spleen

para a woman who has delivered at least one live birth; often used with a number to indicate how many live births the woman has delivered

partial hospital setting a healthcare facility that offers intensive therapeutic treatment or support for a patient whose condition does not warrant admission into an inpatient facility; most commonly provides psychiatric and mental health care

past, family, and social history (PFSH) the third element of history, which is composed of the patient's past medical history, the medical history of the patient's family, and the patient's day-to-day social activities

past history the patient's past medical history that may be pertinent to the chief complaint; includes any childhood illnesses, any surgeries or procedures, injuries, and prescribed medications or treatments

patellar reflex also known as "knee jerk test," which reveals the rate of contraction of the tendons that run along the front of the shinbone when the patellar, or kneecap, tendon is sharply struck

patent ductus arteriosus a congenital abnormality in which the opening between the aorta and the pulmonary artery, which normally closes at birth, remains open

pathology a scientific study of tissues to determine the nature of a disease and its causes, processes, development, and potential consequences

pedal pulse the area in the ankle where the physician can identify the peripheral pulse

pediatric medicine any healthcare services provided to infants older than 29 days but younger than 71 months

per diem measurement by day, per day, or according to the passage of 1 day

percussion tapping to determine resonance in or around an organ or body cavity

percutaneous referring to the introduction of surgical, therapeutic, or diagnostic devices through the skin

perineal pertaining to the skin and tissue at the base of the torso; in males, the tissue space between the scrotum and the anus; in females, the tissue between the vaginal opening and the anus

periodic comprehensive preventive medicine services any preventive medicine services that occur after the first comprehensive preventive medicine service that is performed for a patient by the physician

peritonitis inflammation of the lining of the peritoneum, the membrane lining the inside of the abdominal cavity and all the internal organs within the peritoneal cavity

persistent cyanosis   a symptom of decreased flow of oxygen to the tissues, most often presenting as a bluish coloration of the skin

pertinent   the level of review of systems that includes one organ system in the medical documentation

pertussis   whooping cough

pharyngeal walls   the mucosal tissues covering the surface of the throat, extending from the mouth and nasal cavities down to the tracheoesophageal junction; the sides of the pharynx, through which food passes to the esophagus and air passes to the lungs

pharyngitis   inflammation of the throat

physical examination   the objective clinical assessment of a patient's current health status, performed by a physician during an E/M service visit; identifies the functions, performance, and structure of the patient's physiology and health

physician NCCI Edits   the NCCI edits applicable to claims submitted by physicians and nonphysician practitioners

pilonidal abscess   the growth of pus and infection within a pilonidal cyst; may require treatment with antibiotics and/or surgical excision

pilonidal cyst   literally, "nest of hair"; a collection of hair that has become infected, although it may be asymptomatic; most commonly occurs on the gluteal cleft near the sacrum, or near the base of the back

place of service   the facility or location where the evaluation and management service visit occurs, such as a clinic office or an emergency room

place of service codes   the numeric codes that identify the specific settings in which the E/M services occurred

placental abruption   an abnormal separation of the placenta from the wall of the uterus prior to the birth of a baby; can lead to severe, uncontrollable uterine bleeding

plan of care   the method of treatment, maintenance of health, or plan of therapy prescribed by the physician for the patient's symptoms, condition, diagnosis, or disease

plantar flexion   the motion of pointing toes downward while the patient is standing upright

plantar reflexes   another phrase for the Babinski test, when irritation of the sole of the foot causes contraction of toes and feet

pleuritic   related to pleurisy

pneumatosis intestinalis   the presence of air within the intestines, usually indicative of a life-threatening infection, necrosis, or abscess within the intestines

pneumonitis   inflammation of the lung tissue

pneumo-otoscopy   the use of an otoscope to identify and diagnose otitis media (an infection of the middle ear); utilizes a puff of air to determine how much pressure is behind the eardrum and to assess the mobility of the eardrum

pneumothorax   an abnormal presence of air or gas within the pleural cavity, which can cause pain, difficult breathing, or lung collapse; may be the result of an injury or illness or could be surgically induced as a form of treatment

positive bone scan   a specific kind of diagnostic test that utilizes X-rays to measure the calcium content in the bone, often in the lumbar region of the back

positive pressure ventilation   process of forcing oxygenated air into the lungs through mechanical means

possible diagnosis   considered to be an uncertain likelihood, but one that could be the final diagnosis

posterior   any area of the body located toward the back, or opposite of the front

postpartum   after birth

prescription drugs   any medication prescribed by a physician and dispensed by a pharmacist

present on admission   the diagnosis or diagnoses for which a patient has been admitted to an inpatient facility

probable diagnosis   a diagnosis that is considered to be very plausible by the physician because of the findings, data, and information gathered about the presenting problem and the patient

problem-focused history   the lowest level of documented history, requiring a brief HPI, no ROS, and a pertinent PFSH

progressive severe rheumatoid arthritis   the most severe, debilitating form of rheumatoid arthritis; a chronic, painful, inflammatory disorder that affects the synovial joints of the human body and encompasses a variety of symptoms throughout the body, including the skin, heart, liver, lungs, and kidneys; requires long-term treatment and managed care

prolonged services   services requiring a longer amount of time to perform than the intraservice time typically allows; may occur in an outpatient or an inpatient setting

prone   lying face down

proprioception   subconscious awareness (with eyes closed) of one's body and extremities, including posture and position of arms, legs, hands, and feet; identified in a patient's verbal responses to a physician's queries

psychiatric   the organ system responsible for the emotional and mental health of the human body and the human experience

pulmonary embolism   a medical emergency that involves a blockage of the main artery of the lung or one of the arterial branches within the lungs; caused by a substance or material called an embolus, which obstructs blood flow and increases pressure on the right ventricle of the heart; can cause difficulty breathing, painful and/or rapid breathing, and heart palpitations

pulmonary embolus   obstruction of the pulmonary artery or part of the branches of the pulmonary artery; caused by the presence of an embolus

pulmonary function tests   a thorough evaluation and assessment of the respiratory function through the collection of patient history, physical examination data, chest X-ray, laboratory blood analysis, and intensive respiratory testing, including spirometry and oxygen desaturation during a 6-mile walk on a treadmill

pulmonologist   a physician specializing in the health of the pulmonary, or respiratory, system, as well as the prevention and treatment of diseases related to the respiratory system

pupils equal, round, reactive to light (and accommodation) (PERRLA)   an ocular and neurologic test to identify the dilation of the pupils, and ocular response when a bright light is shined into the patient's eyes

pyelonephritis   inflammation of the kidney and/or renal pelvis, otherwise known as the junction of the kidney and the ureter, or tube that carries urine from the kidney into the bladder; most commonly caused by an infection

pyriform sinuses   a pear-shaped recess near the larynx, which is a common location where food may be caught

quadriceps tendon   the tendon that runs along the back of the thigh, from the hip to the knee

qualified healthcare professionals   healthcare professionals who have education, experience, and expertise to legally practice medicine; includes a wide range of professionals, such as physicians; nurses; physical, occupational, or speech therapists; nutritionists; and more

quality   a subjective description of the pain or discomfort that illustrates the patient's personal experience of the sign or symptom

radiology   a scientific study obtaining images of the body with the use of imaging technologies such as X-ray, ultrasound, computed tomography

rales   an abnormal sound in the lungs, identified by auscultation; characterized by crackles and caused by accumulation of fluid within the trachea, bronchi, or lungs

rapid antigen test   a quick laboratory test to determine whether the patient has strep throat

rebound   a sudden tightening of muscles caused by an autonomic reflex, such as tightening of abdominal muscles because of disease, illness, or injury

regular rate and rhythm (RRR)   refers to a heartbeat with regular rate and rhythm and without any abnormal findings

rehabilitative care   healthcare services—such as therapy, education, and counseling—intended to enable a patient's return to good health in mind and body

repaired   surgically restored or reconstructed (e.g., a specific part of the human anatomy)

respiration   the act of breathing air, which is made up of inspiration and exhalation; requires the function of the lungs, diaphragm, intercostal muscles, and other parts of the anatomy

respiratory   the organ system related to the inspiration of air into the lungs, the oxygenation of blood in the lungs, and the exhalation of de-oxygenated air, including, but not limited to, the lobes of the lungs, the trachea (windpipe), lungs, bronchioles, and alveoli

respiratory failure   failure of the lungs to function

resuscitation   manual establishment of the functions of heart and lungs after a sudden cessation of normal cardiac or respiratory function

review of systems (ROS)   a patient's verbal or written responses to questions posed by the clinician or representative of the clinic; relates to the patient's status of health and the presence or absence of any signs and/or symptoms prior to the clinical visit

Reye's syndrome   a disease of unknown cause that prompts a variety of serious pathological effects on several organs, particularly the brain and liver; strongly correlated with aspirin use in children with fevers, although it also has occurred with no associated aspirin use

rhinitis   inflammation of the mucosal lining of the nasal cavity

rhonchi   the plural form of *rhonchus*; an abnormal sound, similar to loud snoring or whistling, that is heard during lung auscultation and is caused by air rushing through mucosal secretions or swollen tissues of the bronchioles

rub   the abnormal sound of friction caused by inflamed tissues rubbing together; can be caused by respiratory tissues rubbing together or cardiac tissues rubbing together

rule-out diagnosis   a diagnosis intended to do one of two things: either prove that a specific diagnosis is the definitive diagnosis through diagnostic testing, data, and findings, or dismiss it from any future consideration as the final diagnosis of the presenting problem

salivary glands   glands located in the mouth and beneath the tongue that secrete saliva

same physician   the individual physician who has performed the service or procedure in question, or another physician of the same specialty within the practice who has also performed the E/M service

seizure   sudden convulsion, contraction, or uncontrolled movements caused by interruptions of the electric impulses of the brain; may also manifest in sensory disturbances or periods of altered consciousness

selecting overall history   the process by which the levels for each of the individual history elements—HPI, ROS, and PFSH—are reviewed to determine the level of total history

semi-elective surgery   an important surgical procedure that may be postponed for a limited number of days but must be performed to prevent further deterioration of the patient's condition

septum   the natural barrier that divides one body cavity into different sections, as, for example, the nasal septum divides the nasal cavity into separate sections

serous fluid   bodily fluids that may include lymphatic fluid, or fluid that may include white blood cells, plasma proteins, platelets, or red blood cells, or other fluids

serum bicarbonate   also known as HCO_3, a component of blood that is tested to measure the metabolic function of the human body; metabolic acidosis indicated by a low level

severe respiratory distress   extremely difficult breathing that could cause very serious pathological damage unless treated immediately

severity   an objective measurement of the patient's experience of the sign or symptom

shaded border   a dark border outlining a specific system/body area in the 1997 Documentation Guidelines that bears considerable importance to the examination of a single organ system

shared/split visit   a clinical situation in which both a physician and an NPP have participated in the performance of one E/M service; must meet all incident-to requirements

shock   one of several life-threatening conditions that lead to the inadequate flow of blood to the body and a decrease of oxygen in the tissues; can lead to a buildup of toxins in tissues and quickly to brain damage and death; includes distributive shock, hypovolemic shock, and carcinogenic shock

side-to-side flexion   bending from side to side

sign objective evidence of an illness, condition, or pathology that can be scientifically observed and quantified

single organ–system physical examination a physical examination that narrows its focus to the elements supporting one single organ system, according to the requirements listed in the 1997 Documentation Guidelines

site of service the location in which an E/M service visit occurs

skilled nursing facilities facilities that provide housing for chronically ill patients who require a variety of healthcare services, including nursing care; physical, speech, or occupational therapy; rehabilitation; and other services of care

social history the patient's social activities, including employment or school attendance; use of cigarettes, cigars, or other tobacco; the amount of physical activity in which the patient regularly engages; alcohol consumption; sports activities; sexual activity; use of any illicit drugs or substances; and the patient's living situation

soft palate the soft section of the roof of the mouth

solid white exudates secretions covering the back of the throat that might suggest an infection

spastic referring to abnormal spasms of muscles

sputum gram stain a commonly used laboratory test that uses stains to determine specific bacterial infection

status post a term indicating that a person has recently had a significant procedure or experienced a medical event; often preceded by a time designation and followed by a medical procedure, as in "4 days status post appendectomy" to indicate that this individual had an appendectomy 4 days prior

straightforward medical decision making the lowest of the four levels of medical decision making, which reflects a relatively uncomplicated process of medical decision making

Streptococcus pneumonia a bacterial infection that causes pneumonia, sinusitis, ear infections, and many other pathologies

stroke a medical emergency caused by an interruption or disturbance of the blood flow to and through a part of the brain; impairs or prevents the affected part of the brain from functioning; can be one of many types, each of which impacts and impairs the neurological function in different ways

subcategory the ancillary, or secondary, group of CPT codes that identify the type of evaluation and management service performed in the specific place of service

subjective a patient's personalized description or individualized measurement of a specific symptom, which is unique to a specific patient and may not be able to be accurately repeated with any other patient

subluxation a partial dislocation or misalignment of a joint, an organ, or tissues

subsequent provided after the initial E/M service

supervising physician specific physician who may not be the only clinician involved in the observation of this patient, but who is responsible for the observation service provided for the patient

supine lying on the back; often refers to blood pressure that is taken when the patient is lying down

suppurative pus-producing or puslike

symptom a patient's subjective report of the discomfort, pain, illness, or disease currently experienced

systems/body areas the phrase used to identify the 14 different recognized body areas and organ systems that are included in the general multisystem physical examination in the 1997 Documentation Guidelines

table of risk an objective tool to determine the level of risk of complication, comorbidity, and/or mortality in an easy-to-read format

testicular referring to the testicles

thoracentesis an invasive diagnostic procedure that requires the placement of a needle or tube into the space between the two layers of the pleural lining of the chest for the purpose of extracting collected pleural fluid for diagnostic or therapeutic purposes

thoracoabdominal related to the thorax and the abdomen

thoracotomy the major, invasive surgical procedure that creates an incision in the chest wall, retracts the ribs, and dissects the pleural cavity to gain access to the heart, lungs, mediastinum, esophagus, trachea, or other organs, tissues, or structures within the chest cavity

throat the anatomic junction between the nasal cavity, mouth, and upper part of the throat visible in the back of the mouth, which is called the nasopharynx; often documented in conjunction with the ears, nose, and mouth and abbreviated as ENT/M

thyroid the endocrine organ located in the neck

thyromegaly enlargement of the thyroid gland

tibia the larger of the two lower leg bones between the knee and the ankle

tibial tuberosity the rounded protuberance at either end of the tibia

timing a measurable, objective indication of how the pain, discomfort, sign, or symptom has affected or currently affects the patient's day-to-day life

tinea corporis fungal infection of the skin, also known as ringworm

tonsils lymphatic tissue located at the back of the throat

transfer of care the process that occurs when a patient's primary care physician relinquishes the responsibility of some or all of the patient's care to a different physician who has not previously provided any consultation services for the patient

transient ischemic attack commonly referred to as a ministroke; caused by a disruption of blood flow to the brain

transplanted surgically transferred (e.g., a portion of the human anatomy) from one section of the body to another section of the body or from one body to a different but compatible body

true vocal cords the vocal folds responsible for the production of sounds

turbinates three bony projections within each side of the nasal cavity; covered in mucosa; assist in filtering, warming, and humidifying the air inhaled through the nose

tympanic membrane the eardrum

type of service identification of the clinical experience provided for the patient by the clinician or facility

typical time the standardized amount of intraservice time usually spent by a physician performing this specific E/M service

unit of service the specific episode of healthcare service as determined by the category of service

unit/floor time the time the physician spends on the patient's hospital unit or floor, as well as the time the physician spends at the patient's bedside, collecting history, performing the physical examination, making medical decisions, providing counseling to the patient and/or family, and/or coordinating care during the E/M service

unlisted E/M service the E/M service code that can be used to report a performed service that no other service reflects, reports, or identifies

unshaded border a light line outlining a system/body area in the 1997 Documentation Guidelines that bears a lower significance to the examination of a single organ system

urgent surgery a surgical procedure that is very important for the patient's health

urinary meatus the external opening of the urinary system, which allows urine to leave the body

urinary tract infection (UTI) infectious process involving the urethra, bladder, ureters, or any other part of the urinary tract

uvula the tear-drop-shaped fleshy tissue that can be seen dangling in the back of the throat

varicosities enlarged or swollen veins that are commonly identified in the extremities but may be identified in any other part of the human body

venipuncture puncturing the walls of a vein with a hypodermic needle for the purpose of drawing blood; can also be used in the delivery of therapeutic treatment

verbal apraxia a neurological condition that causes an inability of the muscles of the face and mouth to form words

very low birth weight weight of a newborn baby that is less than 3.3 pounds, or 1500 grams, at birth

vital organ system failure the interruption or cessation of normal physiological function of one of the important organ systems that is vital to the normal function of the human body

well-controlled hypertension high blood pressure that is responding well to treatment

wheeze whistling sound that can be heard during auscultation of the lungs

workup documentation of any ordered or requested diagnostic testing to identify the final diagnosis